BEFORE WE ARE
BORN

ESSENTIALS *of* EMBRYOLOGY *and* BIRTH DEFECTS

9th Edition

Keith L. Moore,

BA, MSc, PhD, DSc, FIAC, FRSM, FAAA

Professor Emeritus, Division of Anatomy, Department of Surgery
Former Professor and Chair, Department of Anatomy and
Associate Dean for Basic Medical Sciences
Faculty of Medicine, University of Toronto, Toronto, Ontario, Canada
Former Professor and Head of Anatomy, Faculty of Medicine, University of Manitoba,
Winnipeg, Manitoba, Canada

T.V.N. (Vid) Persaud,

MD, PhD, DSc, FRCPath (Lond.), FAAA

Professor Emeritus and Former Head, Department of Human Anatomy and Cell Science
Professor of Pediatrics and Child Health
Associate Professor of Obstetrics, Gynecology, and Reproductive Sciences, Faculty of
Medicine, University of Manitoba, Winnipeg, Manitoba, Canada
Professor of Anatomy, St. George's University, Grenada, West Indies

Mark G. Torchia,

MSc, PhD

Associate Professor and Director of Development, Department of Surgery
Associate Professor, Department of Human Anatomy and Cell Sciences
Director, Centre for the Advancement of Teaching and Learning, University of Manitoba,
Winnipeg, Manitoba, Canada

ELSEVIER

ELSEVIER

1600 John F. Kennedy Blvd.
Ste 1800
Philadelphia, PA 19103-2899

BEFORE WE ARE BORN, NINTH EDITION

ISBN: 978-0-323-31337-7

Copyright © 2016 by Saunders, an imprint of Elsevier Inc. All rights reserved.
Previous editions copyrighted: 2013, 2008, 2003, 1998, 1993, 1989, 1983, 1974

All rights reserved. No part of this publication may be reproduced or transmitted in any form or by any means, electronic or mechanical, including photocopying, recording, or any information storage and retrieval system, without permission in writing from the publisher. Details on how to seek permission, further information about the Publisher's permissions policies and our arrangements with organizations such as the Copyright Clearance Center and the Copyright Licensing Agency, can be found at our website: www.elsevier.com/permissions.

This book and the individual contributions contained in it are protected under copyright by the Publisher (other than as may be noted herein).

Notices

Knowledge and best practice in this field are constantly changing. As new research and experience broaden our understanding, changes in research methods, professional practices, or medical treatment may become necessary.

Practitioners and researchers must always rely on their own experience and knowledge in evaluating and using any information, methods, compounds, or experiments described herein. In using such information or methods they should be mindful of their own safety and the safety of others, including parties for whom they have a professional responsibility.

With respect to any drug or pharmaceutical products identified, readers are advised to check the most current information provided (i) on procedures featured or (ii) by the manufacturer of each product to be administered, to verify the recommended dose or formula, the method and duration of administration, and contraindications. It is the responsibility of practitioners, relying on their own experience and knowledge of their patients, to make diagnoses, to determine dosages and the best treatment for each individual patient, and to take all appropriate safety precautions.

To the fullest extent of the law, neither the Publisher nor the authors, contributors, or editors, assume any liability for any injury and/or damage to persons or property as a matter of products liability, negligence or otherwise, or from any use or operation of any methods, products, instructions, or ideas contained in the material herein.

Library of Congress Cataloging-in-Publication Data

Moore, Keith L., author.
  Before we are born : essentials of embryology and birth defects / Keith L. Moore, T.V.N. Persaud, Mark G. Torchia.—9th edition.
       p. ; cm.
  Includes bibliographical references and index.
  ISBN 978-0-323-31337-7 (pbk. : alk. paper)
  I. Persaud, T. V. N., author. II. Torchia, Mark G., author. III. Title.
  [DNLM: 1. Embryonic Development. 2. Congenital Abnormalities. 3. Embryology–methods.
4. Fetal Development.   QS 604]
  QM601
  612.6′4–dc23

2014042520

Content Strategist: Meghan Ziegler
Senior Content Development Specialist: Jennifer Ehlers
Publishing Services Manager: Patricia Tannian
Senior Project Manager: Kristine Feeherty
Design Direction: Maggie Reid

MRI cover image from Brugger PC, Mittermayer C, Prayer D: A new look at the fetus: thick-slab T2-weighted sequences in fetal MRI. Eur J Radiol 57:182, 2006, Figure 2. Normal first-trimester fetus cover image from Vandermeer FQ, Wong-You-Cheong J: Ultrasound of the normal and failed first-trimester pregnancy. In Fielding JR, Brown DL, Thurmond AS (eds): Gynecologic Imaging. Philadelphia, Saunders, 2011.

Working together
to grow libraries in
developing countries

www.elsevier.com • www.bookaid.org

Printed in the United States of America

Last digit is the print number: 9 8 7 6 5 4 3 2 1

Shrewsbury Health Library
LSH... ...Hospital
Staffs

BEFORE WE ARE
BORN

ESSENTIALS *of* EMBRYOLOGY *and* BIRTH DEFECTS

Book No.   **05609639**

30121 0 05609639

KEITH L. MOORE

Recipient of the inaugural **Henry Gray/Elsevier Distinguished Educator Award** in 2007—the American Association of Anatomists' highest award for excellence in human anatomy education at the medical/dental, graduate, and undergraduate levels of teaching; the **Honored Member Award of the American Association of Clinical Anatomists (1994)** for significant contributions to the field of clinically relevant anatomy; and the **J.C.B. Grant Award of the Canadian Association of Anatomists (1984)** "in recognition of meritorious service and outstanding scholarly accomplishments in the field of anatomical sciences." In 2008 Professor Moore was inducted as a **Fellow of the American Association of Anatomists**. The rank of Fellow honors distinguished AAA members who have demonstrated excellence in science and in their overall contributions to the medical sciences. In 2012 Dr. Moore received an **Honorary Doctor of Science** degree from The Ohio State University; The **Queen Elizabeth II Diamond Jubilee Medal** honoring significant contributions and achievements by Canadians; and the **Benton Adkins Jr. Distinguished Service Award** for an outstanding record of service to the American Association of Clinical Anatomists.

T.V.N. (VID) PERSAUD

Recipient of the **Henry Gray/Elsevier Distinguished Educator Award** in 2010—the American Association of Anatomists' highest award for excellence in human anatomy education at the medical/dental, graduate, and undergraduate levels of teaching; the **Honored Member Award of the American Association of Clinical Anatomists (2008)** for significant contributions to the field of clinically relevant anatomy; and the **J.C.B. Grant Award of the Canadian Association of Anatomists (1991)** "in recognition of meritorious service and outstanding scholarly accomplishments in the field of anatomical sciences." In 2010 Professor Persaud was inducted as a **Fellow of the American Association of Anatomists**. The rank of Fellow honors distinguished AAA members who have demonstrated excellence in science and in their overall contributions to the medical sciences. In 2003 Dr. Persaud was a recipient of the **Queen Elizabeth II Golden Jubilee Medal**, presented by the Government of Canada for "significant contribution to the nation, the community, and fellow Canadians."

MARK G. TORCHIA

Recipient of the **Norman and Marion Bright Memorial Medal and Award** and the **Silver Medal** of the Chemical Institute of Canada in 1990 for outstanding contributions. In 1993 he was awarded the **TIMEC Medical Device Champion Award**. In 2008 and in 2014 Dr. Torchia was a nominee for the **Manning Innovation Awards**, for innovation talent. Dr. Torchia's most cherished award has been the **Award for Teaching Excellence** in 2011 from the Faculty of Medicine, University of Manitoba, and being asked to address the graduating class of 2014.

In Loving Memory of Marion

My best friend, wife, colleague, mother of our five children, and grandmother of our nine grandchildren, for her love, unconditional support, and understanding. Wonderful memories keep you ever near our hearts.

−KLM and family

For Pam and Ron

I should like to thank my eldest daughter, Pam, who assumed the office duties previously carried out by her mother, Marion. She has also been helpful in so many other ways (e.g., reviewing the text). I am also grateful to my son-in-law, Ron Crowe, whose technical skills have helped me utilize the new technology when I was improving this book.

−KLM

For Gisela

My lovely wife and best friend, for her endless support and patience; our three children— Indrani, Sunita, and Rainer (Ren)—and grandchildren (Brian, Amy, and Lucas).

−TVNP

For Barbara, Muriel, and Erik

Nothing could ever mean more to me than each of you. Thank you for your support and your love.

−MGT

For Students and Their Teachers

To our students: We hope you will enjoy reading this book, increase your understanding of human embryology, pass all of your exams, and be excited and well prepared for your careers in patient care, research, and teaching. You will remember some of what you hear, much of what you read, more of what you see, and almost all of what you experience and understand fully. To their teachers: May this book be a helpful resource to you and your students. We appreciate the numerous constructive comments we have received over the years from both students and teachers. Your remarks have been invaluable to us in improving this book.

Contributors

CONTRIBUTORS

David D. Eisenstat, MD, MA, FRCPC
Professor, Departments of Pediatrics, Medical Genetics and Oncology, Faculty of Medicine and Dentistry, University of Alberta; Director, Division of Pediatric Immunology, Hematology, Oncology, Palliative Care, and Environmental Health, Department of Pediatrics, Stollery Children's Hospital and the University of Alberta; Inaugural Chair, Muriel and Ada Hole Kids with Cancer Society Chair in Pediatric Oncology, Edmonton, Alberta, Canada

Jeffrey T. Wigle, PhD
Principal Investigator, Institute of Cardiovascular Sciences, St. Boniface Hospital Research Centre; Associate Professor, Department of Biochemistry and Medical Genetics, University of Manitoba, Winnipeg, Manitoba, Canada

CRITICAL REVIEWERS

Albert E. Chudley, MD, FRCPC, FCCMG
Professor of Pediatrics and Child Health, University of Manitoba, Winnipeg, Manitoba, Canada; Medical Director, Program in Genetics and Metabolism, Health Sciences Centre and Winnipeg Regional Health Authority, Winnipeg, Manitoba, Canada

Michael Narvey, MD, FRCPC, FAAP
Section Head, Neonatal Medicine, Health Sciences Centre and St. Boniface Hospital; Associate Professor of Pediatrics and Child Health, University of Manitoba, Winnipeg, Manitoba, Canada

FIGURES AND IMAGES (SOURCES)

We are grateful to the following colleagues for the clinical images they have given us for this book and also for granting us permission to use figures from their published works:

Steve Ahing, DDS
Division of Oral Diagnosis and Radiology, Faculty of Dentistry, Department of Pathology, University of Manitoba, Winnipeg, Manitoba, Canada
Figure 18-10BCD

Franco Antoniazzi, MD, and Vassilios Fanos, MD
Department of Pediatrics, University of Verona, Verona, Italy
Figure 19-3

Volker Becker, MD[†]
Pathologisches Institut der Universität, Erlangen, Germany
Figures 8-12 and 8-14

J. Been, MD, M. Shuurman, MD, and S. Robben, MD
Maastricht University Medical Centre, Maastricht, The Netherlands
Figure 11-6B

David Bolender, MD
Department of Cell Biology, Neurobiology, and Anatomy, Medical College of Wisconsin, Milwaukee, Wisconsin, USA
Figure 15-13A

[†]Deceased.

Peter C. Brugger, MD, PhD
Associate Professor/Privat Dozent, Center for Anatomy and Cell Biology, Medical University of Vienna, Vienna, Austria
Cover image (MRI of breech fetus)

Jack C.Y. Cheng, MD
Department of Orthopaedics and Traumatology, The Chinese University of Hong Kong, Hong Kong, China
Figure 15-18

Albert E. Chudley, MD, FRCPC, FCCMG
Department of Pediatrics and Child Health, Section of Genetics and Metabolism, Children's Hospital, University of Manitoba, Winnipeg, Manitoba, Canada
Figures 5-12, 10-30, 12-17AB, 12-24, 13-13, 13-26, 15-24, 15-25, 15-26, 16-10, 16-11, 16-23, 17-14, 19-4, 19-5, 19-6, 19-9, 19-10, 19-12, and 19-14A

Blaine M. Cleghorn, DMD, MSc
Faculty of Dentistry, Dalhousie University, Halifax, Nova Scotia, Canada
Figure 18-10A

Heather Dean, MD, FRCPC
Department of Pediatrics and Child Health, University of Manitoba, Winnipeg, Manitoba, Canada
Figures 13-17, 13-25, and 19-13

Marc Del Bigio, MD, PhD, FRCPC
Department of Pathology (Neuropathology), University of Manitoba, Winnipeg, Manitoba, Canada
Figures 15-10, 16-22, and 16-26

João Carlos Fernandes Rodrigues, MD
Servico de Dermatologia, Hospital de Desterro, Lisbon, Portugal
Figure 18-3

Frank Gaillard, MB, BS, MMed
Department of Radiology, Royal Melbourne Hospital, Melbourne, Victoria, Australia; Radiopaedia.org
Figures 9-8C and 10-17

Gary Geddes, MD
Lake Oswego, Oregon, USA
Figure 15-13B

Barry H. Grayson, MD, and Bruno L. Vendittelli, MD
New York University Medical Center, Institute of Reconstructive Plastic Surgery, New York, New York, USA
Figure 10-31

Christopher R. Harman, MD, FRCSC, FACOG
Department of Obstetrics, Gynecology, and Reproductive Sciences, Women's Hospital and University of Maryland, Baltimore, Maryland, USA
Figure 12-16

Jean Hay, MSc[†]
University of Manitoba, Winnipeg, Manitoba, Canada
Figures 7-2 and 7-4

Health Sciences Centre
Children's Hospital and University of Manitoba, Winnipeg, Manitoba, Canada
Figures 10-13 and 19-7

Lyndon M. Hill, MD
Magee-Women's Hospital, Pittsburgh, Pennsylvania, USA
Figure 12-5

Klaus V. Hinrichsen, MD[†]
Medizinische Fakultät, Institut für Anatomie, Ruhr-Universität Bochum, Bochum, Germany
Figures 10-2 and 10-25

Evelyn Jain, MD, FCFP
Breastfeeding Clinic, Calgary, Alberta, Canada
Figure 10-22

John A. Jane, Sr., MD
Department of Neurological Surgery, University of Virginia Health System, Charlottesville, Virginia, USA
Figure 15-11AB

Dagmar K. Kalousek, MD
Department of Pathology, University of British Columbia; Children's Hospital, Vancouver, British Columbia, Canada
Figures 12-12A and 13-10

James Koenig, MD, FRCPC
Department of Radiology, Health Sciences Centre, Winnipeg, Manitoba, Canada
Figure 14-28D

Wesley Lee, MD
Department of Obstetrics and Gynecology, Division of Fetal Imaging, William Beaumont Hospital, Royal Oak, Michigan, USA
Figure 16-12A

[†]Deceased.

Deborah Levine, MD, FACR
Department of Radiology, Obstetric and Gynecologic
Ultrasound, Beth Israel Deaconess Medical Center,
Boston, Massachusetts, USA
*Figures 7-5B, 16-12B, and cover image (MRI of 27-week
fetus)*

Mina Leyder, MD
Universitair Ziekenhaus Brussels, Brussels, Belgium
Figure 14-19

E. A. (Ted) Lyons, OC, MD, FRCPC, FACR
Departments of Radiology, Obstetrics & Gynecology,
and Human Anatomy & Cell Science, Division of
Ultrasound, Health Sciences Centre, University of
Manitoba, Winnipeg, Manitoba, Canada
*Figures 4-6B, 5-1, 5-10, 6-6, 7-1, 7-9, 8-4, 12-17CD,
and cover image (ultrasound of 9-week fetus)*

Maulik S. Patel, MD
Consultant Pathologist, Surat, India; Radiopaedia.org
Figure 5-13

Martin H. Reed, MD, FRCPC
Department of Radiology, University of Manitoba and
Children's Hospital, Winnipeg, Manitoba, Canada
Figure 12-23

Gregory J. Reid, MD, FRCSC
Department of Obstetrics, Gynecology, and
Reproductive Sciences, University of Manitoba,
Women's Hospital, Winnipeg, Manitoba, Canada
Figure 14-9

Michael and Michele Rice
Figure 7-6

Prem S. Sahni, MD
Formerly of the Department of Radiology, Children's
Hospital, Winnipeg, Manitoba, Canada
Figure 15-14

Gerald S. Smyser, MD
Formerly of the Altru Health System, Grand Forks,
North Dakota, USA
Figures 10-17, 15-11C, and 17-13

Pierre Soucy, MD, FRCSC
Division of Pediatric Surgery, Children's Hospital of
Eastern Ontario, Ottawa, Ontario, Canada
Figures 10-10 and 10-11

Alexandra Stanislavsky, MD
Department of Radiology, Mercy Hospital for Women,
Royal Melbourne Hospital, Melbourne, Victoria,
Australia; Radiopaedia.com
Figure 12-12B

R. Shane Tubbs, PhD, and W. Jerry Oakes, MD
Department of Pediatric Neurosurgery, Children's
Hospital, Birmingham, Alabama, USA
Figure 16-24

Edward O. Uthman, MD
Consultant Pathologist, Houston/Richmond, Texas,
USA
Figure 5-3C

Elspeth H. Whitby, BSc, MB, ChB (Hons), FFDRCSI
Academic Unit of Reproductive and Developmental
Medicine, Department of Academic Pathology,
University of Sheffield, Sheffield, England,
United Kingdom
Figure 16-25

Nathan E. Wiseman, MD, FRCSC
Department of Surgery, Section of Pediatric and
Cardiothoracic Surgery, Children's Hospital, University
of Manitoba, Winnipeg, Manitoba, Canada
Figures 9-8B and 12-15

Preface

efore We Are Born has been in print for more than 43 years. This concise work is based on our larger book, *The Developing Human: Clinically Oriented Embryology, Tenth Edition.*

The ninth edition of *Before We Are Born* has been completely updated to reflect current understanding of clinical human embryology. It provides the essentials of normal and abnormal development. As in earlier editions, *clinically oriented materials* are highlighted in blue color (often called **blue boxes**). Every chapter has been revised thoroughly to reflect new research findings and their clinical significance, as well as new understanding of the developmental biology.

This edition follows the official *international list of embryological terms (Terminologia Embryonica*, 2013). It is important that physicians, nurses, physician assistants, dentists, physical and occupational therapists, other health professionals, scientists, and students in the health professions throughout the world use the same name for each structure.

We have included numerous **new color photographs** of embryos, fetuses (normal and abnormal), neonates (newborns), and children. There are also many new *diagnostic images*: US (ultrasound), CT (computed tomography) scans, and MRI (magnetic resonance imaging) studies of embryos and fetuses.

An important feature of this book is the **Clinically Oriented Questions**, which appear at the end of each chapter. In addition, available through Elsevier's *studentconsult.com* website, there are many helpful **clinical case studies** and questions with answers and explanations. These will benefit students preparing for USMLE Step 1 and similar examinations.

Accompanying this ninth edition of *Before We Are Born* is an innovative set of **17 full-color animations** that will assist students in learning the complexities of embryologic development. These animations are available at **studentconsult.com.** High-resolution animations are available to teachers for their lectures if they have adopted this book or *The Developing Human* (consult your Elsevier representative). When one of the animations is especially relevant to the book's text, an **icon** has been added in the margin.

The **teratology** (studies concerned with birth defects) section has been updated because the study of abnormal development is required for understanding the causes of birth defects and how these may be prevented. *Molecular aspects of developmental biology* have been highlighted throughout the book, especially in areas that appear promising for clinical medicine and future research. Moreover, Chapter 20 is devoted exclusively to more detailed information related to the cellular and molecular basis of embryonic development.

Keith L. Moore
T.V.N. (Vid) Persaud
Mark G. Torchia

Acknowledgments

Many colleagues and students have made invaluable contributions to this ninth edition of *Before We Are Born*. We are indebted to the following colleagues (listed alphabetically) for either critical reviewing of chapters, making suggestions for improvement of this book, or providing some of the new figures: Dr. Steve Ahing, Faculty of Dentistry, University of Manitoba, Winnipeg, Manitoba; Dr. David Bolender, Department of Cell Biology, Neurobiology, and Anatomy, Medical College of Wisconsin, Milwaukee, Wisconsin; Professor Margaret Buckingham, Department of Developmental Biology, Pasteur Institute, Paris, France; Dr. Albert Chudley, Departments of Pediatrics & Child Health and Biochemistry & Medical Genetics, University of Manitoba, Winnipeg, Manitoba; Dr. Blaine M. Cleghorn, Faculty of Dentistry, Dalhousie University, Halifax, Nova Scotia; Dr. Frank Gaillard, Radiopaedia.org, Royal Melbourne Hospital, Melbourne, Victoria; Dr. David F. Gomez-Gil, Chicago, Illinois; Dr. Boris Kablar, Department of Anatomy and Neurobiology, Dalhousie University, Halifax, Nova Scotia; Dr. Sylvia Kogan, Winnipeg, Manitoba; Dr. Deborah Levine, Beth Israel Deaconess Medical Center, Boston, Massachusetts; Dr. Marios Loukas, St. George's University, True Blue, Grenada; Dr. Stuart Morrison, Department of Radiology, Cleveland Clinic, Cleveland, Ohio; Professor Bernard J. Moxham, Cardiff School of Biosciences, Cardiff University, Cardiff, Wales; Dr. Michael Narvey, Department of Pediatrics and Child Health, University of Manitoba, Winnipeg, Manitoba; Dr. Drew Noden, Department of Biomedical Sciences, Cornell University, College of Veterinary Medicine, Ithaca, New York; Dr. Shannon E. Perry, San Francisco State University, San Francisco, California; Dr. Gregory J. Reid, Department of Obstetrics, Gynecology, and Reproductive Sciences, University of Manitoba, Winnipeg, Manitoba; Professor Sir Peter W.J. Rigby, The Babraham Institute, Cambridge, England; Dr. L. Ross, Department of Neurobiology and Anatomy, University of Texas Medical School at Houston, Houston, Texas; Dr. Michael A. Rudnicki, Regenerative Medicine Program, Ottawa Hospital Research Institute, Ottawa, Ontario; Dr. J. Elliott Scott, Departments of Oral Biology and Human Anatomy & Cell Science, University of Manitoba, Winnipeg, Manitoba; Dr. Gerald S. Smyser, formerly of the Altru Health System, Grand Forks, North Dakota; Dr. Alexandra Stanislavsky, Department of Radiology, Mercy Hospital for Women, Royal Melbourne Hospital, Melbourne, Victoria; Dr. Richard Shane Tubbs, Children's Hospital, Birmingham, Alabama; Dr. Edward O. Uthman, Consultant Pathologist, Richmond, Texas; and Dr. Michael Wiley, Department of Surgery, Division of Anatomy, Faculty of Medicine, University of Toronto, Toronto, Ontario.

The illustrations were prepared by Hans Neuhart, president of the Electronic Illustrators Group in Fountain Hills, Arizona. At Elsevier, we are indebted to Ms. Meghan K. Ziegler, Content Strategist, for her continued interest and encouragement. We are especially thankful to Ms. Kel McGowan, Content Development Specialist, for her invaluable insights and many helpful suggestions. Their unstinting support during the preparation of this new edition was greatly appreciated. Finally, we should also like to thank Ms. Kristine Feeherty, Senior Project Manager; Ms. Maggie Reid, Designer; Ms. Amy Naylor, Art Buyer; and Ms. Thapasya Ramkumar, Multimedia Producer, at Elsevier for nurturing this book to completion. This new edition of *Before We Are Born* is the result of their dedication and technical expertise.

Keith L. Moore
T.V.N. (Vid) Persaud
Mark G. Torchia

Contents

Introduction to Human Development

Human development begins at fertilization when an **oocyte** (ovum) from a female is fertilized by a **sperm** (spermatozoon) from a male. Development involves many changes that transform a single cell, the **zygote**, into a multicellular human being. Embryology is concerned with the origin and development of a human being from a zygote to birth. The stages of development before birth are shown in Figure 1-1.

IMPORTANCE OF AND ADVANCES IN EMBRYOLOGY

The study of prenatal stages and mechanisms of human development helps us understand the normal relationships of adult body structures and the causes of **birth defects** (congenital anomalies). Much of the modern practice of obstetrics involves applied or **clinical embryology**. Because some children have birth defects, such as spina bifida or congenital heart disease, the significance of embryology is readily apparent to pediatricians. Advances in surgery, especially in procedures involving the prenatal and pediatric age groups, have made knowledge of human development more clinically significant. In addition, as we discover new information about the development processes, we in turn have a better understanding of many diseases and their process as well as their treatment.

Rapid advances in molecular biology have led to the use of sophisticated techniques (e.g., **recombinant DNA technology**, **chimeric models**, **transgenics**, and **stem cell manipulation**) in research laboratories to explore such diverse issues as the genetic regulation of morphogenesis, the temporal and regional expression of specific genes, and the mechanisms by which cells are committed to form the various parts of the embryo. Researchers continue to learn how, when, and where selected genes are activated and expressed in the embryo during normal and abnormal development.

Development begins at fertilization, approximately 14 days after the onset of the last normal menstrual period. The continuous process begins when a sperm penetrates an oocyte (ovum) and forms a zygote (see Fig. 1-1, first week). The **embryonic period** covers the first 8 weeks of development of an embryo. The **fetal period** begins in the ninth week. Examination of the timetable shows that the most visible advances occur during the third to eighth week.

The critical role of genes, **signaling molecules**, receptors, and other molecular factors in regulating early embryonic development is rapidly being delineated. In 1995, Edward B. Lewis, Christiane Nüsslein-Volhard, and Eric F. Wieschaus were awarded the **Nobel Prize** in Physiology or Medicine for their discovery of genes that control embryonic development. Such discoveries are contributing to a better understanding of the causes of spontaneous abortion and birth defects.

In 1997, Ian Wilmut and colleagues were the first to produce a mammal (a sheep dubbed **Dolly**) by cloning using the technique of somatic cell nuclear transfer. Since then, other animals have been cloned successfully from cultured differentiated adult cells. Interest in human cloning has generated considerable debate because of social, ethical, and legal implications. Moreover, there is concern that cloning may result in an increase in the number of neonates (newborns) with birth defects and serious diseases.

Human embryonic stem cells are pluripotential and capable of developing into diverse cell types. The isolation and culture of human embryonic and other stem cells may hold great promise for the development of molecular therapies.

DESCRIPTIVE TERMS

In anatomy and embryology, special terms of position, direction, and various planes of the body are used. Descriptions of the adult are based on the *anatomical position*; the body is erect, the upper limbs are at the sides, and the palms are directed anteriorly (Fig. 1-2A). The descriptive terms of position, direction, and planes used for embryos are shown in Figure 1-2B to E.

Figure 1–1 Early stages of human development. An ovarian follicle containing an oocyte, ovulation, and phases of the menstrual cycle are shown.

AGE (weeks)

Figure 1–1, cont'd

Figure 1–2 Illustrations of descriptive terms of position, direction, and planes of the body. **A,** Lateral view of an adult in the anatomical position. **B,** Lateral view of a 5-week embryo. **C** and **D,** Ventral views of a 6-week embryo. The median plane is an imaginary vertical plane of section that passes longitudinally through the body, dividing it into right and left halves. A sagittal plane refers to any plane parallel to the median plane. A transverse plane refers to any plane that is at right angles to both the median and frontal planes. **E,** Lateral view of a 7-week embryo. A frontal (coronal) plane is any vertical plane that intersects the median plane at a right angle and divides the body into front (anterior or ventral) and back (posterior, or dorsal) parts. In describing development, it is necessary to use words denoting the position of one part relative to another or to the body as a whole. For example, the vertebral column develops in the dorsal part of the embryo and the sternum is in the ventral part of the embryo.

CLINICALLY ORIENTED QUESTIONS

1. Why do we study human embryology? Does it have any practical value in medicine and other health sciences?

2. Physicians date a pregnancy from the first day of the last normal menstrual period, but the embryo does not start to develop until approximately 2 weeks later (Fig. 1-1). Why do physicians use this method?

The answers to these questions are at the back of this book.

2

Human Reproduction

P uberty begins when secondary sex characteristics appear, usually between the ages of 10 to 13 years in females and 12 to 14 years in males. **Menarche** (first menstrual period) may occur as early as 8 years. *Puberty in females* is largely completed by age 16. *Puberty in males* is also largely completed by age 16; it ends when the first mature sperms are formed.

▶ REPRODUCTIVE ORGANS

1 Reproductive organs produce and transport germ cells (gametes) from the gonads (testes or ovaries) to the site of fertilization in the uterine tube (Fig. 2-1).

Female Reproductive Organs

Vagina
The vagina serves as the excretory passage for menstrual fluid, receives the penis during sexual intercourse, and forms the inferior part of the **birth canal**—the cavity of the uterus and vagina through which the fetus passes (see Fig. 2-1*A* and *B*).

Uterus
The uterus (womb) is a thick-walled, pear-shaped organ (Fig. 2-2*A* and *B*) that consists of two main parts:

- The **body**, the expanded superior two thirds
- The **cervix**, the cylindrical inferior third

7

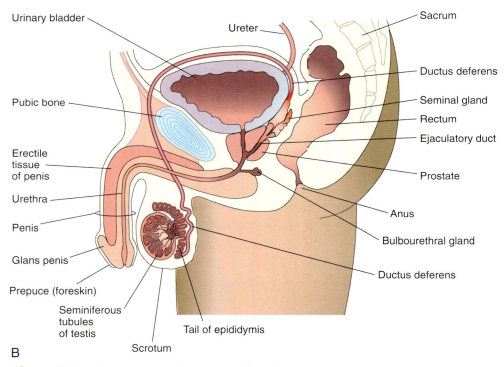

Figure 2–1   Schematic sagittal sections of the pelvic regions of a woman (**A**) and a man (**B**).

The **fundus of the uterus** is the rounded part of the uterine body that lies superior to the orifices of the uterine tubes. The **body of the uterus** narrows from the fundus to the **isthmus**, the constricted region between the body and the **cervix** (see Fig. 2-2*A*). The lumen of the cervix, the **cervical canal**, has a constricted opening, the *os (ostium)*, at each end. The **internal os** communicates with the cavity of the body of the uterus, whereas the **external os** communicates with the vagina. The walls of the body consist of three layers:

- **Perimetrium,** a thin external peritoneal layer
- **Myometrium,** a thick smooth muscle layer
- **Endometrium,** a thin internal layer

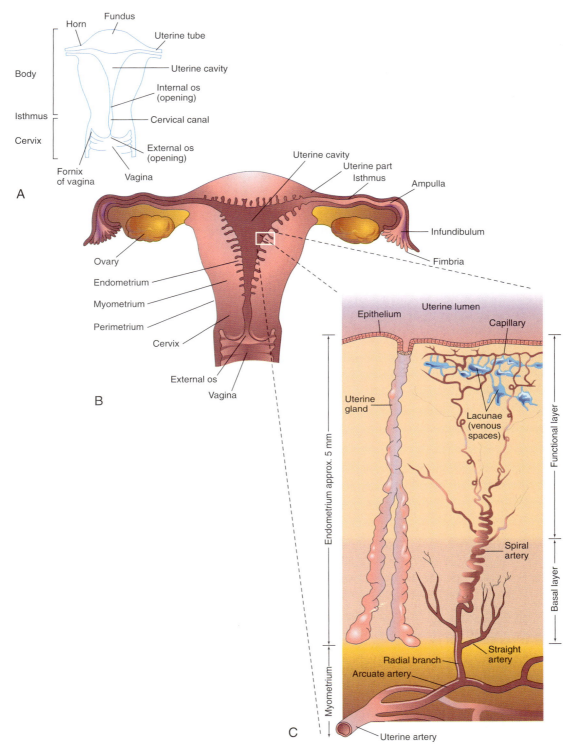

Figure 2–2 Female reproductive organs. **A,** Parts of the uterus. **B,** Diagrammatic frontal (coronal) section of the uterus, uterine tubes, and vagina. The ovaries are also shown. **C,** Enlargement of the area outlined in **B.** The functional layer of the endometrium is sloughed off during menstruation.

At the peak of its development, the endometrium is 4 to 5 mm thick. During the luteal (secretory) phase of the menstrual cycle (see Fig. 2-8), three layers of the endometrium can be distinguished microscopically (see Fig. 2-2C) into the following:

- A compact layer, consisting of densely packed connective tissue around the neck of the uterine glands
- A spongy layer, composed of edematous connective tissue containing the dilated, tortuous bodies of the uterine glands

● A basal layer, containing the blind ends of the uterine glands

The compact and spongy layers—the *functional layer*—disintegrate and are shed at menstruation and after *parturition* (childbirth). The basal layer has its own blood supply and is not cast off during menstruation.

Uterine Tubes

The **uterine tubes**, measuring 10 cm long and 1 cm in diameter, extend laterally from the **horns of the uterus** (see Fig. 2-2*A*). Each tube opens into a horn at its proximal end and into the peritoneal cavity at its distal end. *The uterine tube is divided into the following parts: infundibulum, ampulla, isthmus, and uterine part.* The tubes carry oocytes from the ovaries and sperms to the fertilization site in the ampulla (see Fig. 2-2*B*). The uterine tube also conveys the dividing zygote to the uterine cavity.

Ovaries

The **ovaries** are almond-shaped **reproductive glands** that are located close to the lateral wall of the pelvis on each side of the uterus. The ovaries produce **oocytes** (see Fig. 2-5). When released from the ovary at *ovulation*, the secondary oocyte passes into one of the *uterine tubes*. These tubes open into the *uterus*, which protects and nourishes the embryo and fetus until birth. The ovaries also produce estrogen and progesterone, the hormones responsible for the development of secondary sex characteristics and regulation of pregnancy.

Female External Sex Organs

The female external sex organs are known collectively as the **vulva** (Fig. 2-3). The **labia majora**, fatty external folds of skin, conceal the **vaginal orifice**, the opening of the vagina. Inside these labia are two smaller folds of mucous membrane, the **labia minora**. The **clitoris**, a small erectile organ, is situated at the superior junction of these folds. The vagina and urethra open into a cavity, the **vestibule** (cleft between the labia minora). The vaginal orifice varies with the condition of the **hymen**, a fold of mucous membrane that surrounds the orifice (see Fig. 2-3).

Male Reproductive Organs

The male reproductive organs (see Fig. 2-1*B*) include the penis, testes, epididymis, ductus deferens (vas deferens), prostate, seminal glands, bulbourethral glands, ejaculatory ducts, and urethra. The oval **testes** (testicles) are located in the cavity of the **scrotum**. Each **testis** consists of many highly coiled **seminiferous tubules** that produce sperms. **Immature sperms** pass from the testis into a single, complexly coiled tube, the **epididymis**, where they are stored. From the epididymis, the **ductus deferens** carries the sperms to the ejaculatory duct. This duct descends into the pelvis, where it fuses with the ducts of the seminal glands to form the **ejaculatory duct**, which enters the urethra.

The **urethra** is a tube that leads from the urinary bladder through the penis to the outside of the body. Within the **penis**, *erectile tissue* surrounds the urethra. During sexual excitement, this tissue fills with blood, causing the penis to erect. **Semen** (penile ejaculate) consists of sperms mixed with seminal fluid produced by the *seminal glands*, *bulbourethral glands*, and *prostate*.

GAMETOGENESIS

The sperms and oocytes are highly specialized gametes— **germ cells** (Fig. 2-4). Each of the cells contains half the number of required chromosomes (i.e., 23 instead of 46). The number of chromosomes is reduced during a special type of cell division—**meiosis**. This type of cell division occurs only during **gametogenesis** (formation of germ cells). In males, this process is termed **spermatogenesis**; in females, it is **oogenesis** (Fig. 2-5).

Meiosis

Meiosis consists of two meiotic cell divisions (Fig. 2-6), during which the chromosome number of the germ cells is reduced to half (23, the *haploid* number) of the number in other cells in the body (46, the *diploid* number).

During the **first meiotic division**, the chromosome number is reduced from diploid to haploid. **Homologous chromosomes** (one from each parent) pair during prophase and then separate during **anaphase**, with one representative of each pair randomly going to each pole of the **meiotic spindle**. The spindle connects to the chromosome at the **centromere** (see Fig. 2-6*B*). At this stage, they are **double chromatid chromosomes**. The X and Y chromosomes are not homologs; however, they have homologous segments at the tips of their short arms. They pair in these regions only. By the end of the first meiotic division, each new cell formed (**secondary spermatocyte** or **secondary oocyte**) has the haploid chromosome number of double chromatid chromosomes; therefore, each cell contains half the number of chromosomes of the

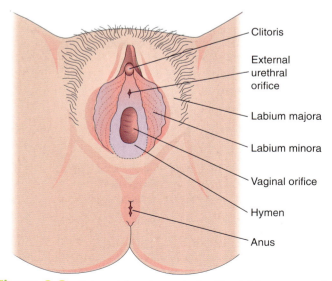

Clitoris

External urethral orifice

Labium majora

Labium minora

Vaginal orifice

Hymen

Anus

Figure 2–3   External female genitalia. The labia are spread apart to show the external urethral and vaginal orifices.

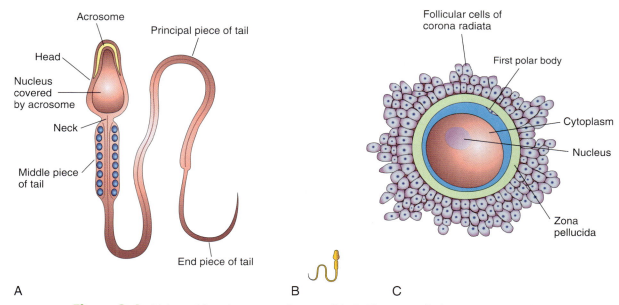

Figure 2–4 Male and female gametes (germ cells). **A,** The parts of a human sperm (×1250). The head, composed mostly of the nucleus, is partly covered by the acrosome, an organelle containing enzymes. **B,** A sperm drawn to approximately the same scale as the oocyte. **C,** The human secondary oocyte (×200) is surrounded by the zona pellucida and corona radiata.

preceding cell (primary spermatocyte or primary oocyte). This separation, or disjunction, of paired homologous chromosomes is the physical basis of segregation, or separation, of allelic genes during meiosis.

The **second meiotic division** follows the first division, without a normal interphase (i.e., without an intervening step of DNA replication). Each double chromatid chromosome divides, and each half, or **chromatid**, is randomly drawn to a different pole of the meiotic spindle; thus, the haploid number of chromosomes (23) is retained. Each daughter cell formed by meiosis has the reduced haploid number of chromosomes, with one representative of each chromosome pair (now a single chromatid chromosome).

Meiosis:

- Provides for *constancy of the chromosome number* from generation to generation by reducing the chromosome number from diploid to haploid, thereby producing haploid gametes.
- Allows *random assortment of maternal and paternal chromosomes* between the gametes.
- Relocates segments of maternal and paternal chromosomes by *crossing over of chromosome segments*, which "shuffles" the genes and produces a recombination of genetic material.

Spermatogenesis

Before puberty, primordial sperms (spermatogonia) remain dormant in the seminiferous tubules of the testes from the late fetal period. At puberty (after 12 years), they begin to increase in number. After several mitotic

cell divisions, the sperms grow and undergo gradual changes that transform them into **primary spermatocytes**—the largest germ cells in the seminiferous tubules (see Fig. 2-5). Each primary spermatocyte subsequently undergoes a reduction division—the *first meiotic division*—to form two haploid **secondary spermatocytes**, which are approximately half the size of primary spermatocytes (see Fig. 2-5). Subsequently, the secondary spermatocytes undergo a *second meiotic division* to form four haploid **spermatids**, which are approximately half the size of secondary spermatocytes. The spermatids are gradually transformed into four **mature sperms** during a process known as **spermiogenesis** (see Fig. 2-5).

During this **metamorphosis** (change in form), the nucleus condenses and the **acrosome** forms (see Fig. 2-4A). The acrosome contains enzymes that probably facilitate the sperm's penetration of the zona pellucida (see Chapter 3, Fig. 3-1). When spermiogenesis is complete, sperms enter the lumina (cavities) of the **seminiferous tubules** (see Fig. 2-1B). The sperms then move to the **epididymis**, where they are stored and become functionally mature. Spermatogenesis requires approximately 2 months for completion. Maturation of sperms—**spermatogenesis**—normally continues throughout the reproductive life of a male.

When ejaculated, the **mature sperms** are free-swimming, actively motile cells *consisting of a head and a tail* (see Fig. 2-4A). The neck of the sperm is the junction between the head and tail. The head of the sperm, forming most of the bulk of the sperm, contains the nucleus. The anterior two thirds of the head are covered by the **acrosome**, a cap-like organelle containing enzymes that facilitate sperm penetration during fertilization. The

NORMAL GAMETOGENESIS

Figure 2–5   Normal gametogenesis: conversion of germ cells into gametes. The illustrations compare spermatogenesis and oogenesis. Oogonia are not shown in this figure because they differentiate into primary oocytes before birth. The chromosome complement of the germ cells is shown at each stage. The number designates the total number of chromosomes, including sex chromosome(s) (shown after the comma). Note: (1) After the two meiotic divisions, the diploid number of chromosomes, 46, is reduced to the haploid number, 23; (2) four sperms form from one primary spermatocyte, whereas only one secondary oocyte results from maturation of a primary oocyte; (3) the cytoplasm is conserved during oogenesis to form one large cell, the oocyte.

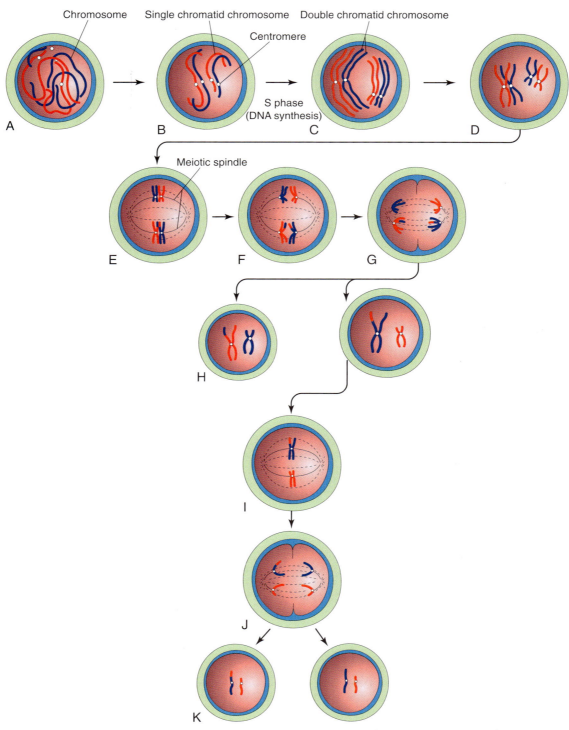

Chromosome   Single chromatid chromosome   Double chromatid chromosome

Centromere

S phase
(DNA synthesis)

A   B   C   D

Meiotic spindle

E   F   G

H

I

J

K

Figure 2–6 Diagrammatic representation of meiosis. Two chromosome pairs are shown. **A** to **D,** Stages of prophase of the first meiotic division. The homologous chromosomes approach each other and pair; each member of the pair consists of two chromatids. Observe the single crossover in one pair of chromosomes, resulting in the interchange of chromatid segments. **E,** Metaphase. The two members of each pair become oriented on the meiotic spindle. **F,** Anaphase. **G,** Telophase. The chromosomes migrate to opposite poles. **H,** Distribution of parental chromosome pairs at the end of the first meiotic division. **I** to **K,** Second meiotic division, which is similar to mitosis, except that the cells are haploid.

tail provides the motility of the sperm, assisting with its transport to the site of fertilization in the ampulla of the uterine tube. *The **tail of the sperm** consists of three parts*: middle piece, principal piece, and end piece. The middle piece contains the energy-producing **mitochondria**, which fuel the lashing movements of the tail. Hox *genes influence microtube dynamics at the molecular level in shaping the head of the sperm and in the formation of the tail.*

Oogenesis

Oogenesis refers to the sequence of events by which oogonia (primordial oocytes) are transformed into primary **oocytes**. The maturation process begins during the fetal period; however, is not completed until after puberty—16 years. During early fetal life, oogonia proliferate by mitosis and enlarge to form **primary oocytes** (see Fig. 2-5). At birth, all primary oocytes have completed prophase (first stage of mitosis) of the *first meiotic division* (see Fig. 2-6). The oocytes remain in prophase until puberty. Shortly before ovulation, a primary oocyte completes the **first meiotic division**. Unlike the corresponding stage of spermatogenesis, the division of cytoplasm is unequal (see Fig. 2-5). The **secondary oocyte** receives almost all the cytoplasm, whereas the **first polar body** receives very little, causing it to degenerate after a short time. At **ovulation** (release of oocyte), the nucleus of the secondary oocyte begins the *second meiotic division*, but progresses only to metaphase.

If the secondary oocyte is fertilized by a sperm, the second meiotic division is completed and a **second polar body** is formed (see Fig. 2-5). The secondary oocyte released at ovulation is surrounded by a covering of amorphous material—the **zona pellucida**—and a layer of follicular cells—the **corona radiata**—(see Fig. 2-4C). The **secondary oocyte** is large, being just visible to the unaided eye.

Up to 2 million primary oocytes are usually present in the ovaries of a neonate. Most of these oocytes regress during childhood so that, by puberty, no more than 40,000 remain. Of these, only approximately 400 oocytes mature into secondary oocytes and are expelled at ovulation (see Fig. 2-5).

Comparison of Male and Female Gametes

Compared with sperms, the oocytes are massive, are immotile, and have an abundance of cytoplasm (see Fig 2-4B and C). In terms of sex chromosome constitution, **there are two kinds of sperms** (see Fig. 2-5): 22 autosomes plus either an X sex chromosome (i.e., 23,X) or a Y sex chromosome (i.e., 23,Y). **There is only one kind of secondary oocyte**: 22 autosomes plus an X sex chromosome (i.e., 23,X). *The difference in sex chromosome complement forms the basis of primary sex determination.*

FEMALE REPRODUCTIVE CYCLES

At menarche (first menstrual period), females undergo monthly reproductive cycles regulated by the **hypothalamus, pituitary gland**, and **ovaries** (Fig. 2-8). These cycles

ABNORMAL GAMETOGENESIS

During gametogenesis, homologous chromosomes sometimes fail to separate—**nondisjunction**—and as a result, some gametes have 24 chromosomes and others only 22 (Fig. 2-7). If a gamete with 24 chromosomes unites with a normal one with 23 chromosomes, a zygote with 47 chromosomes results, as occurs in neonates with **Down syndrome** (see Chapter 19, Fig. 19-4). This condition is called **trisomy 21** because of the presence of three representatives of a particular chromosome instead of the usual two. If a gamete with only 22 chromosomes unites with a normal gamete, a zygote with 45 chromosomes results. This condition—**monosomy**—occurs because only one representative of the particular chromosomal pair is present. Many embryos and fetuses with monosomy die.

prepare the reproductive system for pregnancy. *Gonadotropin-releasing hormone* is synthesized by neurosecretory cells in the hypothalamus. It stimulates the release of two hormones (gonadotropins), which are produced by the anterior pituitary and act on the ovaries:

- *Follicle-stimulating hormone (FSH)* stimulates the development of ovarian follicles and the production of **estrogen** by the follicular cells.
- *Luteinizing hormone (LH)* serves as the "trigger" for ovulation and stimulates the follicular cells and corpus luteum to produce **progesterone**.

These ovarian hormones also produce growth of the endometrium.

Ovarian Cycle

FSH and LH produce cyclic changes in the ovaries (development of ovarian follicles, ovulation, and formation of the corpus luteum), collectively known as the **ovarian cycle**. During each cycle, FSH promotes growth of several primary follicles (Fig. 2-9; also see Fig. 2-8); however, only one of them usually develops into a mature follicle and ruptures, expelling its oocyte (Fig. 2-10).

Follicular Development

Development of an ovarian follicle (see Fig. 2-8 and Fig. 2-9) is characterized by:

- Growth and differentiation of a primary oocyte
- Proliferation of follicular cells
- Formation of the zona pellucida
- Development of a connective tissue capsule surrounding the follicle—*theca folliculi*. Thecal cells are believed to produce an *angiogenic factor* that promotes growth of blood vessels that provide nutritive support for follicular development.

ABNORMAL GAMETOGENESIS

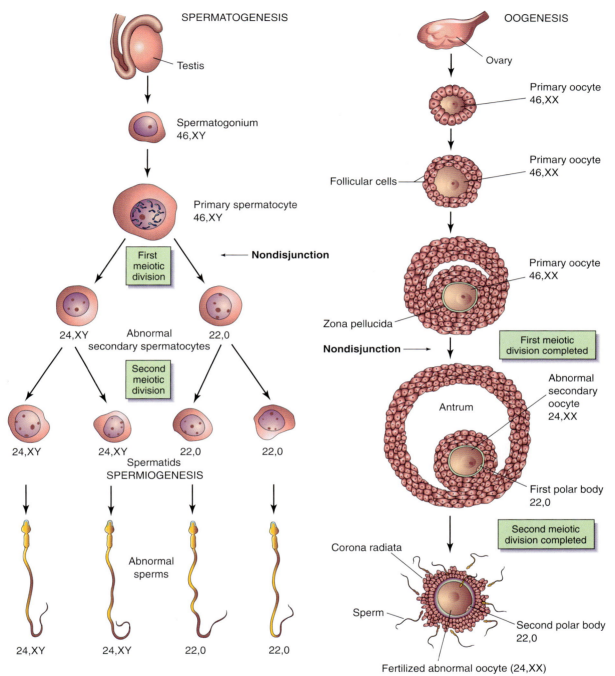

Figure 2–7 Abnormal gametogenesis. The illustrations show how nondisjunction, an error in cell division, results in an abnormal chromosome distribution in gametes. Although nondisjunction of sex chromosomes is illustrated, a similar defect may occur during the division of autosomes (any chromosomes other than sex chromosomes). When nondisjunction occurs during the first meiotic division of spermatogenesis, one secondary spermatocyte contains 22 autosomes plus an X and a Y chromosome, whereas the other one contains 22 autosomes and no sex chromosome. Similarly, nondisjunction during oogenesis may give rise to an oocyte with 22 autosomes and two X chromosomes (as shown) or one with 22 autosomes and no sex chromosome.

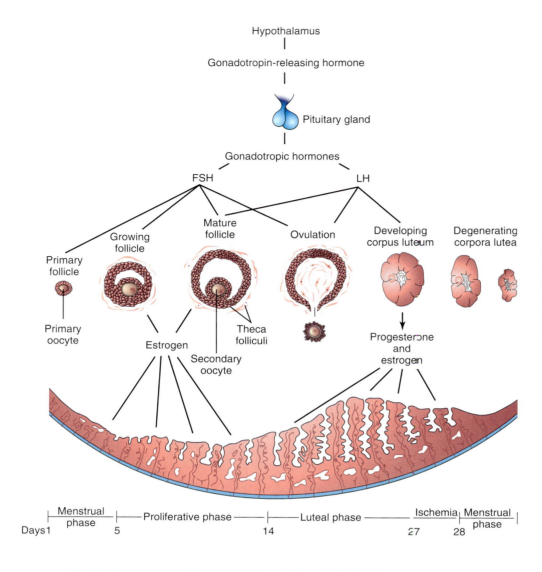

Figure 2–8 Illustrations of the interrelationships among the hypothalamus, pituitary gland, ovaries, and endometrium. One complete menstrual cycle and the beginning of another are shown. *FSH,* Follicle-stimulating hormone; *LH,* luteinizing hormone.

Figure 2–9 Photomicrographs of sections from adult human ovaries. **A,** Light micrograph of the ovarian cortex demonstrating primordial follicles *(P),* which are primary oocytes surrounded by follicular cells (×270). **B,** Light micrograph of a secondary follicle. Observe the primary oocyte and antrum containing the follicular fluid (×132). *(From Gartner LP, Hiatt JL: Color Textbook of Histology, 2nd ed. Philadelphia, Saunders, 2001.)*

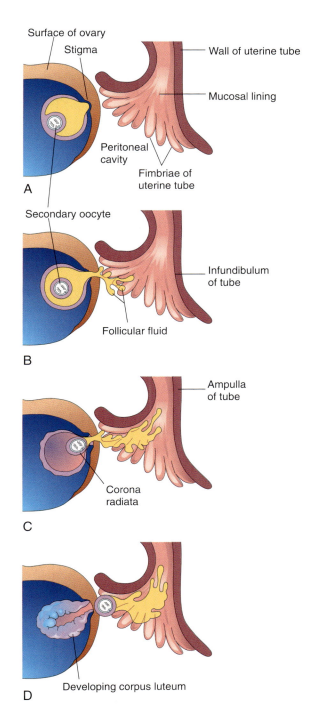

A

Surface of ovary
Stigma
Wall of uterine tube
Mucosal lining
Peritoneal cavity
Fimbriae of uterine tube
Secondary oocyte

B

Infundibulum of tube
Follicular fluid

C

Ampulla of tube
Corona radiata

D

Developing corpus luteum

Figure 2–10 Diagrams **(A–D)** illustrating ovulation. When the stigma ruptures, the secondary oocyte is expelled from the ovarian follicle with the follicular fluid. After ovulation, the wall of the follicle collapses.

▶ Ovulation

The **follicular cells** divide actively, producing a stratified layer around the oocyte (see Fig. 2-9A and B). Subsequently, fluid-filled spaces appear around the follicular cells, which coalesce to form a single cavity, the **antrum**, containing **follicular fluid** (see Fig. 2-9B). When the antrum forms, the ovarian follicle is called a **secondary**

follicle. The primary oocyte is surrounded by follicular cells—the **cumulus oophorus**—that project into the enlarged antrum. The follicle continues to enlarge and soon forms a bulge on the surface of the ovary. A small oval, avascular spot, the **stigma**, soon appears on this bulge (see Fig. 2-10A). Before ovulation, the secondary oocyte and some cells of the cumulus oophorus detach from the interior of the distended follicle (see Fig. 2-10B).

Ovulation follows within 24 hours of a surge of LH production, which appears to be the result of signaling molecules from the granulosa cells. This surge, elicited by a high estrogen level in blood (Fig. 2-11), appears to cause the stigma to rupture, expelling the secondary oocyte along with the follicular fluid (see Fig. 2-10D). Plasmins and matrix metalloproteinases also appear to have some control over stigma rupture.

The expelled secondary oocyte is surrounded by the **zona pellucida**, an acellular glycoprotein coat, and one or more layers of follicular cells, which are radially arranged to form the **corona radiata** and cumulus oophorus (see Fig. 2-4C).

MITTELSCHMERZ AND OVULATION

A variable amount of abdominal pain—*mittelschmerz*—accompanies ovulation in some women. Mittelschmerz may be used as a secondary **sign of ovulation**; however, there are better primary indicators, including slight elevation of basal body temperature, fertile cervical mucus, and change in the cervical position.

ANOVULATION AND HORMONES

Some women do not ovulate because of an inadequate release of gonadotropins. In some women, ovulation can be induced by the administration of **gonadotropins** or an ovulatory agent, resulting in maturation of several ovarian follicles and multiple ovulations. The incidence of multiple pregnancy may increase when ovulation is induced.

ANOVULATORY MENSTRUAL CYCLES

In anovulatory cycles, the endometrial changes are minimal; the proliferative endometrium develops as usual, but ovulation does not occur and no **corpus luteum** forms (see Fig. 2-8). Consequently, the endometrium does not progress to the **luteal phase**; it remains in the proliferative phase until menstruation begins. The estrogen in **oral contraceptives**, with or without **progesterone** (pregnancy hormone), suppresses ovulation by acting on the hypothalamus and pituitary gland; this inhibits secretion of gonadotropin-releasing hormone, follicle-stimulating hormone, and luteinizing hormone.

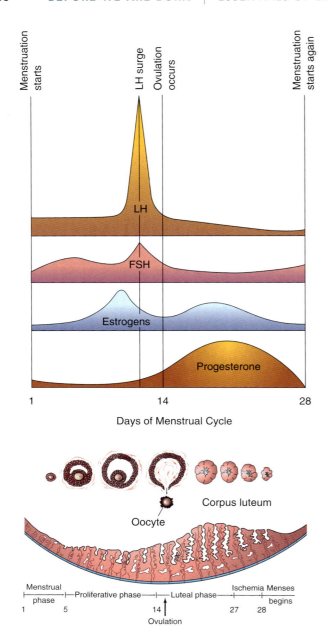

Figure 2–11 Blood levels of various hormones during the menstrual cycle. Follicle-stimulating hormone *(FSH)* stimulates the ovarian follicles to develop and produce estrogens. The level of estrogens rises to a peak just before the luteinizing hormone *(LH)* surge induces ovulation. Ovulation normally occurs within 24 hours after the LH surge. If fertilization does not occur, the blood levels of circulating estrogens and progesterone fall. This hormone withdrawal causes the endometrium to regress and menstruation to start again.

Corpus Luteum

Shortly after ovulation, the ovarian follicle collapses (see Fig. 2-10*D*). Under the influence of LH, the walls of the follicle develop into a glandular structure, the **corpus luteum**, which secretes primarily progesterone and some estrogen. If the oocyte is fertilized, the corpus luteum

enlarges to form a *corpus luteum of pregnancy* and increases its hormone production. Degeneration of the corpus luteum is prevented by *human chorionic gonadotropin* (hCG) (see Chapter 4).

If the oocyte is not fertilized, the corpus luteum degenerates 10 to 12 days after ovulation (see Fig. 2-8). It is then called a *corpus luteum of menstruation*. The degenerated corpus luteum is subsequently transformed into white scar tissue in the ovary, forming the *corpus albicans*.

Menstrual Cycle

The cycle is the period during which the oocyte matures, is ovulated, and enters the uterine tube (see Fig. 2-10*D* and Fig. 2-11). Estrogen and progesterone produced by the ovarian follicles and corpus luteum cause **cyclic changes in the endometrium** of the uterus. These monthly changes in the uterine lining constitute the **menstrual cycle**. The average cycle is 28 days (ranging from 23 to 35 days). Day 1 of the cycle corresponds to the day on which menstruation begins.

Phases of Menstrual Cycle

The cycle is divided into three main phases for descriptive purposes only (see Fig. 2-11). In actuality, *the menstrual cycle is a continuous process*; each phase gradually passes into the next one. The cycles normally continue until the permanent cessation of the **menses** (periodic physiologic hemorrhage). **Menopause** (permanent cessation of menses) usually occurs between the ages of 48 and 55 years.

Menstrual Phase

The first day of menstruation is the beginning of the menstrual phase. The functional layer of the uterine wall is sloughed off and discarded with the menstrual flow, which usually lasts for 4 to 5 days. The menstrual flow (menses), discharged through the vagina, consists of varying amounts of blood combined with small pieces of endometrial tissue. After menstruation, the eroded endometrium is thin (see Fig. 2-8 and Fig. 2-11).

Proliferative Phase

This phase, lasting approximately 9 days, coincides with growth of the ovarian follicles and is controlled by estrogen secreted by the follicles. There is a two- to threefold increase in the thickness of the endometrium during this time (see Fig. 2-8). Early during this phase, the surface epithelium of the endometrium regenerates. The glands increase in number and length, and the spiral arteries elongate (see Fig. 2-2*B* and *C*).

Luteal Phase

The luteal (secretory) phase, lasting approximately 13 days, coincides with the formation, function, and growth of the **corpus luteum** (see Fig. 2-8). The progesterone produced by the corpus luteum stimulates the glandular epithelium to secrete a glycogen-rich, mucoid material. The **uterine glands** become wide, tortuous, and saccular (see Fig. 2-2*C*). The endometrium thickens because of the influence of progesterone and estrogen from the corpus luteum and the increase in fluid in the connective tissue (see Fig. 2-8).

If fertilization does not occur:

- The corpus luteum degenerates.
- Estrogen and progesterone levels decrease and the endometrium undergoes ischemia.
- Menstruation occurs.

Ischemia (reduced blood supply) of the **spiral arteries** occurs by constriction resulting from the decrease in the secretion of progesterone (see Fig. 2-2C). Hormone withdrawal also results in the stoppage of glandular secretions, a loss of interstitial fluid, and a marked shrinking of the endometrium. As the spiral arteries constrict for longer periods, **stasis** (stagnation of blood and other fluids) and patchy ischemic **necrosis** (death) in the superficial tissues occur. Eventually, rupture of vessel walls follows, and blood seeps into the surrounding connective tissue. Small pools of blood form and break through the endometrial surface, resulting in bleeding into the uterus and vagina.

As small pieces of the endometrium detach and pass into the uterine cavity, the torn ends of the spiral arteries bleed into the uterine cavity, resulting in an accumulated loss of 20 to 80 ml of blood. Over 3 to 5 days, the entire compact layer and most of the spongy layer of the endometrium are discarded.

If fertilization occurs:

- Cleavage of the zygote and formation of the blastocyst occur.
- The blastocyst begins to implant on approximately the sixth day of the luteal phase (see Chapter 4, Fig. 4-1A).
- hCG maintains secretion of estrogens and progesterone by the corpus luteum.
- The luteal phase continues and menstruation does not occur.

The menstrual cycles cease during pregnancy, and the endometrium passes into a **pregnancy phase**. With the termination of pregnancy, the ovarian and menstrual cycles resume after a variable amount of time.

▶ TRANSPORTATION OF GAMETES

Oocyte Transport

During ovulation, the fimbriated (fringed) end of the uterine tube comes in close proximity to the ovary (see Fig. 2-10A). The finger-like processes of the tube—*fimbriae*—move back and forth over the ovary. The sweeping action of the fimbriae and the fluid currents produced by them "sweep" the secondary oocyte into the funnel-shaped **infundibulum** of the uterine tube (see Fig. 2-2B and Fig 2-10B). The oocyte passes into the **ampulla** of the tube (see Fig. 2-10B and D), primarily as a result of waves of peristalsis—movements of the wall of the tube characterized by alternate contraction and relaxation.

Sperm Transport

During ejaculation, sperms are rapidly transported from their storage in the **epididymis** to the urethra by peristaltic contractions of the **ductus deferens** (see Fig. 2-1B). Sperms and secretions from the *seminal glands, prostate,* and *bulbourethral glands* form the **semen** (ejaculate). The number of sperms ejaculated ranges from 200 to 600 million. The sperms pass slowly through the cervical canal by movements of their tails (see Fig. 2-4A). Vesiculase, an enzyme produced by the seminal glands, coagulates some of the *semen* and forms a **cervical plug** in the *external os* that may prevent backflow of semen into the vagina. At the time of ovulation, the amount of cervical mucus increases and becomes less viscid (sticky), making it more favorable for sperm transport. Prostaglandins in the semen stimulate uterine motility and help to move the sperms through the uterus to the site of fertilization in the **ampulla** of the uterine tube (see Fig. 2-2B and Fig. 2-10C).

The sperms move 2 to 3 mm per minute. They move slowly in the acidic environment of the vagina, but more rapidly in the alkaline environment of the uterus. Approximately 200 sperms reach the ampulla for fertilization.

SPERM COUNTS

Semen analysis is an important part of evaluating patients for infertility. Sperms account for less than 5% of the volume of semen. The remainder of the ejaculate consists of secretions of the seminal glands (60%), prostate (30%), and bulbourethral glands (5%). The ejaculate of normal males usually contains more than 100 million sperms per milliliter of semen. Although there is much variation in individual cases, men whose semen contains a minimum of 20 million sperms per milliliter, or 50 million in the total specimen, are probably fertile. A man with less than 10 million sperms per milliliter is likely to be sterile, especially when the specimen contains immotile and abnormal sperms. For potential fertility, at least 40% of the sperms should be motile after 2 hours, and some should be motile after 24 hours. Male infertility may result from endocrine disorders, abnormal spermatogenesis, reduced levels of seminal plasma proteins, or obstruction of a genital duct (e.g., the ductus deferens). Male infertility is found in 30% to 50% of involuntarily childless couples.

VASECTOMY

An effective method of contraception in males is **vasectomy**—excision of a segment of the ductus deferens (see Fig. 2-1B). Two to 3 weeks after vasectomy, there are no sperms in the ejaculate, but the amount of seminal fluid is the same as before the procedure.

MATURATION OF SPERMS

Freshly ejaculated sperms are unable to fertilize oocytes. They must undergo a period of conditioning—**capacitation**—lasting approximately 7 hours. During this period, a glycoprotein coat and seminal proteins are removed from the **acrosome**, which partly covers the nucleus of the sperm (see Fig. 2-4A). *Capacitation and acrosome reaction are regulated by src kinase, a tyrosine kinase.* Capacitated sperms show no morphologic changes, but they exhibit increased activity. Sperms are usually capacitated in the uterus or the uterine tubes by substances (including interleukin-6) secreted by these organs.

VIABILITY OF OOCYTES AND SPERMS

Oocytes in the uterine tube are usually fertilized within 12 hours of ovulation. In vitro observations have shown that oocytes cannot be fertilized after 24 hours, and they degenerate shortly thereafter. Most sperms do not survive for more than 24 hours in the female genital tract. Some sperms are captured in folds of the mucosa of the cervix and are gradually released into the cervical canal and pass through the body of the uterus into the uterine tubes. Semen and oocytes can be frozen and stored for many years to be used in assisted reproduction.

CLINICALLY ORIENTED QUESTIONS

1. There have been reports of a woman who claimed that she menstruated throughout her pregnancy. How could this happen?

2. If a woman forgets to take an oral contraceptive and then takes two doses, is she likely to become pregnant?

3. What is *coitus interruptus*? Is it an effective method of birth control?

4. What is the difference between spermatogenesis and spermiogenesis?

5. Is an intrauterine device (IUD) a contraceptive? Explain.

The answers to these questions are at the back of this book.

First Week of Human Development

Development begins at fertilization when a sperm penetrates an oocyte to form a zygote. A **zygote** is a highly specialized, *totipotent cell*, which has the ability to differentiate into any type of cell. It contains chromosomes and genes derived from the mother and father. The zygote divides many times and is progressively transformed into a multicellular human being through cell division, migration, growth, and differentiation (see Chapter 1, Fig. 1-1, first week).

▶ FERTILIZATION

The usual site of fertilization is in the **ampulla**, a saccular dilation of the **uterine tube** (see Chapter 2, Fig. 2-2*B*). If the oocyte is not fertilized, it slowly passes along the tube into the cavity of the uterus, where it degenerates and is resorbed. Fertilization is a complex sequence of coordinated molecular events that begins with the contact between a sperm and an oocyte (Fig. 3-1). Fertilization ends with the intermingling of maternal and paternal chromosomes at **metaphase** (a stage of mitosis) of the first mitotic division of the **zygote** (see Chapter 2, Fig. 2-6). Carbohydrate- and protein-binding molecules on the surface of the **gametes** (oocyte or sperm) are involved in sperm **chemotaxis** (movement of cells) and gamete recognition, as well as in the process of fertilization.

Phases of Fertilization

The phases of fertilization follow (Fig. 3-2; also see Fig. 3-1):

● *Passage of a sperm through the corona radiata of the oocyte.* Dispersal of the follicular cells of the corona radiata results mainly from the action of the enzyme *hyaluronidase*,

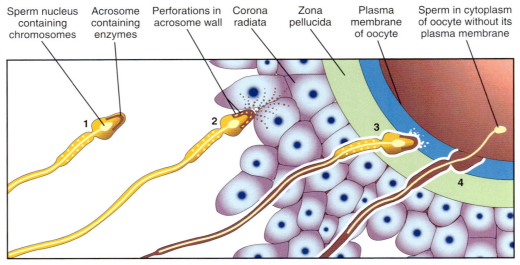

Figure 3–1   Acrosome reaction and sperm penetration of an oocyte. *1*, Sperm during capacitation. *2*, Sperm undergoing the acrosome reaction. *3*, Sperm forming a path through the zona pellucida. *4*, Sperm entering the cytoplasm of the oocyte.

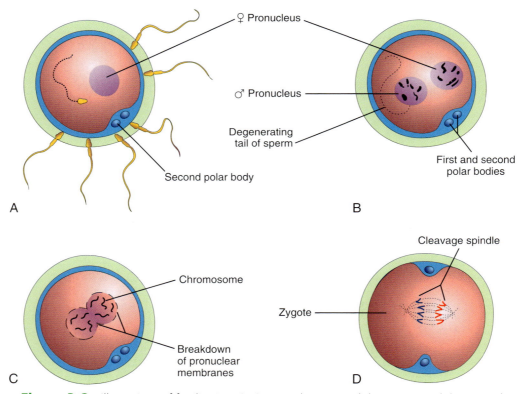

Figure 3–2   Illustrations of fertilization. **A**, A sperm has entered the oocyte and the second meiotic division has occurred, resulting in the formation of a mature oocyte. The nucleus of the oocyte is now the female pronucleus. **B**, The sperm head has enlarged to form the male pronucleus. **C**, The pronuclei are fusing. **D**, The zygote has formed; it contains 46 chromosomes.

which is released from the acrosome of the sperm. *Tubal mucosal enzymes* also appear to assist hyaluronidase. Additionally, movements of the tail of the sperm are important during penetration of the **corona radiata.**

- *Penetration of the zona pellucida.* The formation of a pathway through the **zona pellucida** for the sperm results from the action of enzymes released from the acrosome. The proteolytic enzyme *acrosin*, as well as *esterases* and *neuraminidase*, appears to cause lysis of the zona pellucida, thereby forming a path for the sperm to follow to the oocyte.

- *Fusion of the plasma cell membranes of the oocyte and sperm.* Once the fusion occurs, the contents of cortical granules from the oocyte are released into the perivitelline space, between the oocyte and zona pellucida, resulting in changes in the zona pellucida. These changes prevent other sperms from entering. The cell membranes break down at the area of fusion. The head and tail of the sperm then enter the cytoplasm of the oocyte, but the plasma membrane and mitochondria of the sperm remain behind (see Fig. 3-1 and Fig. 3-2A).
- *Completion of the second meiotic division of the oocyte.* The oocyte completes the second meiotic division and forms a **mature oocyte** and a second polar body (see Fig. 3-2A). The nucleus of the mature oocyte becomes the female pronucleus.
- *Formation of the male pronucleus.* Within the cytoplasm of the oocyte, the nucleus of the sperm enlarges to form the male pronucleus. The tail of the sperm degenerates (see Fig. 3-2B). During growth, the male and female pronuclei replicate their DNA (see Fig. 3-2C).
- *Breakdown of the pronuclear membranes.* Condensation of the chromosomes, arrangement of the chromosomes for mitotic cell division, and the first cleavage division of the zygote occur (see Fig. 3-2D and Fig. 3-3A). The combination of 23 chromosomes in each pronucleus results in a zygote with 46 chromosomes.

Results of Fertilization

Fertilization:

- Stimulates the secondary oocyte to complete the second meiotic division, producing the second polar body (see Fig. 3-2A)
- Restores the normal diploid number of chromosomes (46) in the zygote
- Results in variation of the human species through mingling of maternal and paternal chromosomes
- Determines the chromosomal sex of the embryo; an X-bearing sperm produces a female embryo and a Y-bearing sperm produces a male embryo
- Causes metabolic activation of the oocyte, which initiates cleavage of the zygote

The zygote is genetically unique because half of its chromosomes come from the mother and half are derived from the father. This mechanism forms the basis for *biparental inheritance* and variation of the human species. Meiosis allows independent assortment of maternal and paternal chromosomes among the germ cells. Crossing over of chromosomes, by relocating segments of the maternal and paternal chromosomes, "shuffles" the genes, thereby producing a recombination of genetic material (see Chapter 2, Fig. 2-6). The term **conceptus** refers to the entire products of conception, which include the embryo from fertilization onward and its membranes (e.g., placenta).

CLEAVAGE OF ZYGOTE

Cleavage consists of repeated mitotic divisions of the zygote, resulting in a rapid increase in the number of cells—**blastomeres**. Division of the zygote begins approximately 30 hours after fertilization (see Chapter 1, Fig. 1-1). These blastomeres become smaller with each cleavage division (see Fig. 3-3A to D). During cleavage, the zygote is still surrounded by the zona pellucida.

After the eight-cell stage, the blastomeres change their shape and tightly align themselves against each other—**compaction**. This phenomenon may be mediated by cell surface adhesion glycoproteins. Compaction permits greater cell-to-cell interaction and is a prerequisite for segregation of the internal cells that form the inner cell mass (see Fig. 3-3E). When there are 12 to 32 blastomeres, the conceptus is called a **morula**.

The inner cells of the morula—the **embryoblast** or **inner cell mass**—are surrounded by a layer of flattened blastomeres that form the trophoblast. *Hippo signaling is an essential factor in segregating the inner cell mass from the trophoblast.* An immunosuppressant protein— the **early pregnancy factor**—is secreted by the trophoblastic cells and appears in the maternal serum within 24 to 48 hours after implantation. The early pregnancy factor forms the basis for a pregnancy test applicable during the first 10 days of development.

FORMATION OF BLASTOCYST

Shortly after the morula enters the uterus (about 4 days after fertilization), uterine fluid passes through the zona pellucida to form a fluid-filled space—the **blastocystic cavity**—inside the morula (see Fig. 3-3E). As fluid increases in the cavity, the blastomeres are separated into two parts:

- The **trophoblast**, the thin outer cells that give rise to the embryonic part of the placenta
- The **embryoblast**, a discrete group of blastomeres that is the primordium of the embryo

During this stage of development—*blastogenesis*—the conceptus is called a **blastocyst**. The embryoblast now projects into the **blastocystic cavity** and the trophoblast forms the wall of the blastocyst (see Fig. 3-3E and F). After the blastocyst has floated in the uterine fluid for approximately 2 days, the zona pellucida degenerates and disappears. Shedding of the zona pellucida has been observed in vitro. The shedding permits the blastocyst to increase rapidly in size. While floating freely in the uterine cavity, the blastocyst derives nourishment from secretions of the uterine glands.

Approximately 6 days after fertilization, the blastocyst attaches to the endometrial epithelium (Fig. 3-4A). As soon as it attaches to the epithelium, the trophoblast starts to proliferate rapidly and differentiate into two layers (see Fig. 3-4B):

- The **cytotrophoblast**, the inner layer of cells
- The **syncytiotrophoblast**, the outer layer consisting of a multinucleate protoplasmic mass formed by the fusion of cells

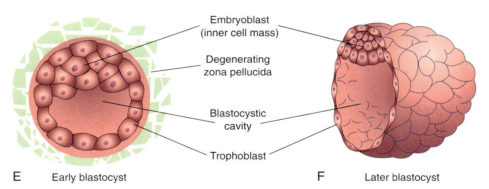

Figure 3–3   Illustrations showing cleavage of the zygote and formation of the blastocyst. **A** to **D** show various stages of cleavage. The period of the morula begins at the 12- to 32-cell stage and ends when the blastocyst forms. **E** and **F** show sections of blastocysts. The zona pellucida disappears by the late blastocyst stage (5 days). Although cleavage increases the number of blastomeres, note that each of the daughter cells is smaller than the parent cells. As a result, there is no increase in the size of the developing embryo until the zona pellucida degenerates. The blastocyst then enlarges considerably **(D)**.

The finger-like processes of the syncytiotrophoblast extend through the endometrial epithelium and invade the endometrial connective tissue. By the end of the first week, the blastocyst is superficially implanted in the compact layer of the endometrium and is deriving its nourishment from the eroded maternal tissues. The highly invasive syncytiotrophoblast rapidly expands adjacent to the embryoblast—the **embryonic pole** (see Fig. 3-4A).

The syncytiotrophoblast produces proteolytic enzymes that erode the maternal tissues, enabling the blastocyst to "burrow" into the endometrium. At the end of the first week, a cuboidal layer of cells, called the **hypoblast**, appears on the surface of the embryoblast, facing the blastocystic cavity (see Fig. 3-4B). Decidual cells also help to control the depth of penetration of the syncytiotrophoblast.

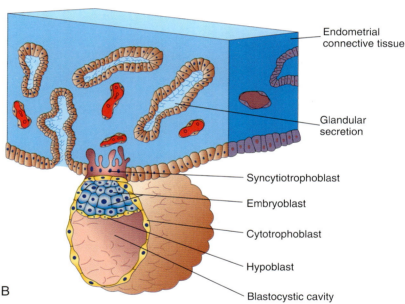

Figure 3–4 Attachment of the blastocyst to the endometrial epithelium during the early stages of its implantation. **A,** At 6 days, the trophoblast is attached to the endometrial epithelium at the embryonic pole of the blastocyst. **B,** At 7 days, the syncytiotrophoblast has penetrated the epithelium and has started to invade the endometrial connective tissue.

IN VITRO FERTILIZATION AND EMBRYO TRANSFER

The process of in vitro fertilization (IVF) of oocytes and transfer of either the dividing zygotes or a blastocyst into the uterus has provided an opportunity for many couples who are infertile. The first of these IVF babies was born in 1978. The steps involved in IVF and embryo transfer are summarized in Figure 3-5. The incidence of multiple pregnancies is higher with IVF than when pregnancy results from normal ovulation. The incidence of spontaneous abortion of transferred embryos is also higher with IVF.

The technique of **intracytoplasmic sperm injection** involves injecting a sperm directly into the cytoplasm of the mature oocyte. This procedure is invaluable in cases of infertility resulting from blocked uterine tubes or *oligospermia* (reduced number of sperms).

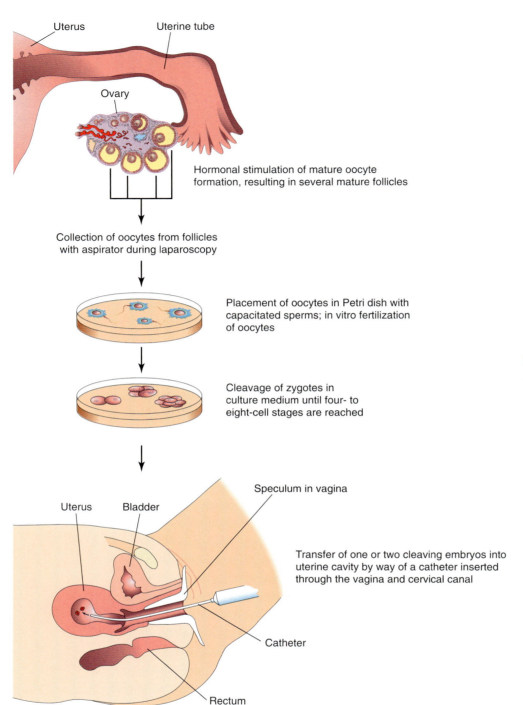

Uterus

Uterine tube

Ovary

Hormonal stimulation of mature oocyte formation, resulting in several mature follicles

Collection of oocytes from follicles with aspirator during laparoscopy

Placement of oocytes in Petri dish with capacitated sperms; in vitro fertilization of oocytes

Cleavage of zygotes in culture medium until four- to eight-cell stages are reached

Speculum in vagina

Uterus   Bladder

Transfer of one or two cleaving embryos into uterine cavity by way of a catheter inserted through the vagina and cervical canal

Catheter

Rectum

Figure 3–5 In vitro fertilization and embryo transfer procedures.

PREIMPLANTATION DIAGNOSIS OF GENETIC DISORDERS

Using currently available techniques, a cleaving zygote known to be at risk for a specific genetic disorder may be diagnosed before implantation during IVF. The sex of the embryo can be determined from a blastomere taken from a six- to eight-cell zygote and analyzed by DNA amplification of sequences from the Y chromosome. This procedure has been used to determine chromosomal sex in cases in which a male embryo would be at risk for a serious X-linked disorder. The polar body may also be tested for disorders when the mother is the carrier.

ABNORMAL EMBRYOS AND SPONTANEOUS ABORTIONS

Many early embryos abort spontaneously. The early implantation stages of the blastocyst are critical periods of development that may fail to occur because of inadequate production of progesterone and estrogen by the corpus luteum (see Chapter 2, Fig. 2-8). Clinicians occasionally see a patient whose last menstrual period was delayed by several days and whose last menstrual flow was unusually profuse. Very likely, such patients have had an early spontaneous abortion. *The overall early spontaneous abortion rate is believed to be approximately 45%.* Early spontaneous abortions occur for a variety of reasons, an important one being the presence of **chromosomal abnormalities**.

CLINICALLY ORIENTED QUESTIONS

1. Although women do not commonly become pregnant after they are 48 years old, very elderly men may still be fertile. Why is this? Is there an increased risk of Down syndrome or other congenital anomalies in the child when the father is older than 50 years of age?

2. Are there oral contraceptives for men? If not, what is the reason?

3. Is a polar body ever fertilized? If so, does the fertilized polar body give rise to a viable embryo?

4. What is the most common cause of spontaneous abortion during the first week of development?

5. Could a woman have dissimilar twins as a result of one oocyte being fertilized by a sperm from one man and another one being fertilized by a sperm from another man?

6. When referring to a zygote, do the terms *cleavage* and *mitosis* mean the same thing?

7. How is the cleaving zygote nourished during the first week?

8. Is it possible to determine the sex of a cleaving zygote developing in vitro? If so, what medical reasons would there be for doing so?

The answers to these questions are at the back of this book.

C H A P T E R

4

Second Week of Human Development

I mplantation of the blastocyst is completed during the second week of development. As this process takes place, changes occur, producing a **bilaminar embryonic disc** composed of two layers, the epiblast and hypoblast (Fig. 4-1*A*). The **embryonic disc** gives rise to germ layers that form all the tissues and organs of the embryo. Extraembryonic structures forming during the second week include the amniotic cavity, amnion, **umbilical vesicle** (yolk sac), connecting stalk, and chorionic sac.

Implantation of the blastocyst is completed during the second week and normally occurs in the endometrium, usually superiorly in the body of the uterus and slightly more often on the posterior than on the anterior wall. The actively erosive **syncytiotrophoblast** invades the endometrial connective tissue that supports the uterine capillaries and glands. As this occurs, the blastocyst slowly embeds itself in the endometrium. Syncytiotrophoblastic cells from this region displace endometrial cells in the central part of the implantation site. The endometrial cells undergo *apoptosis* (programmed cell death), which facilitates implantation. Proteolytic enzymes produced by the syncytiotrophoblast are involved in this process. The uterine connective tissue cells around the implantation site become loaded with glycogen and lipids. Some of these cells—**decidual cells**—degenerate adjacent to the penetrating syncytiotrophoblast. The syncytiotrophoblast engulfs these degenerating cells, providing a rich source of *embryonic nutrition*. As the blastocyst implants, more trophoblast contacts the endometrium and continues to differentiate into two layers (see Fig. 4-1*A*):

- The *cytotrophoblast*, a layer of mononucleated cells that is mitotically active. It forms new trophoblastic cells that migrate into the increasing mass of *syncytiotrophoblast*, where they fuse and lose their cell membranes.
- The syncytiotrophoblast, a rapidly expanding, multinucleated mass in which no cell boundaries are discernible.

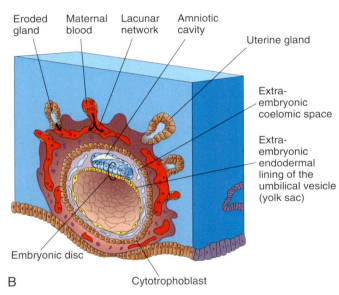

Figure 4–1   Implantation of blastocyst. The actual size of the conceptus is approximately 0.1 mm. **A,** Illustration of a section of a partially implanted blastocyst (approximately 8 days after fertilization). Note the slit-like amniotic cavity. **B,** Illustration of a section through a blastocyst at approximately 9 days.

Figure 4–2   Illustration of sections of two implanted blastocysts at 10 days **(A)** and 12 days **(B)**.

The **syncytiotrophoblast** produces a hormone, **human chorionic gonadotropin** (hCG), that enters the maternal blood in the lacunae in the syncytiotrophoblast (Fig. 4-1B). **hCG** maintains the development of spiral arteries in the myometrium and formation of the syncytiotrophoblast. It also forms the basis for pregnancy tests. Highly sensitive assays are available for detecting hCG at the end of the second week even though the woman is probably unaware that she is pregnant.

FORMATION OF AMNIOTIC CAVITY, EMBRYONIC DISC, AND UMBILICAL VESICLE

As implantation of the blastocyst progresses, changes occurring in the embryoblast result in the formation of a

flattened, almost circular, bilaminar plate of cells—the **embryonic disc**—consisting of two layers (see Fig. 4-1B and Fig. 4-2B):

- The **epiblast**, the thicker layer, consisting of high, columnar cells related to the amniotic cavity
- The **hypoblast**, the thinner layer, consisting of small, cuboidal cells adjacent to the exocoelomic cavity

Concurrently, a small cavity appears in the embryoblast, which is the primordium of the **amniotic cavity** (Fig. 4-1A). Soon, amniogenic (amnion-forming) cells—*amnioblasts*—separate from the epiblast and organize to form a thin membrane, the **amnion**, which encloses the amniotic cavity.

The **epiblast** forms the floor of the amniotic cavity and is continuous peripherally with the amnion. The **hypoblast** forms the roof of the **exocoelomic cavity** and is continuous with the cells that migrated from the hypoblast to form the **exocoelomic membrane**. This membrane surrounds the blastocystic cavity and lines the internal surface of the cytotrophoblast.

The **exocoelomic membrane and cavity** soon become modified to form the **primary umbilical vesicle**. The *embryonic disc* then lies between the amniotic cavity and primary umbilical vesicle (see Fig. 4-1*B*). The outer layer of cells from the umbilical vesicle endoderm forms a layer of loosely arranged connective tissue, the **extraembryonic mesoderm** (see Fig. 4-1*B*).

As the amnion, embryonic disc, and primary umbilical vesicle form, **lacunae** (small spaces) appear in the syncytiotrophoblast (see Figs. 4-1*B* and Fig. 4-2). The lacunae are soon filled with a mixture of maternal blood from ruptured endometrial capillaries and cellular debris from eroded uterine glands. The fluid in the lacunae—*embryotroph*—passes to the embryonic disc by diffusion. The communication of the eroded uterine vessels with the lacunae represents the beginning of the **primordial *uteroplacental circulation*.** When maternal blood flows into the lacunae, oxygen and nutritive substances become available to the extraembryonic tissues over the large surface of the syncytiotrophoblast. Oxygenated blood passes into the lacunae from the *spiral endometrial arteries* in the endometrium (see Chapter 2, Fig. 2-2*C*); deoxygenated blood is removed from the lacunae through endometrial veins.

The **10-day conceptus** (embryo and extraembryonic membrane) is completely embedded in the endometrium (see Fig. 4-2*A*). For approximately 2 more days, there is a defect in the endometrial epithelium that is filled by a **closing plug**, a fibrinous coagulum of blood. By day 12, an almost completely regenerated uterine epithelium covers the closing plug (see Fig. 4-2*B*). As the conceptus implants, the endometrial connective tissue cells undergo a transformation—the **decidual reaction**—resulting from cyclic adenosine monophosphate and progesterone signaling. The cells swell because of the accumulation of glycogen and lipid in their cytoplasm, and they are then called *secretory decidual cells*. The primary function of the decidual reaction is to provide an immunologically privileged site for the conceptus.

In the **12-day embryo**, adjacent syncytiotrophoblastic lacunae have fused to form **lacunar networks** (see Fig. 4-2*B*), the *primordia of the intervillous space of the placenta* (see Chapter 8). The endometrial capillaries around the implanted embryo become congested and dilated to form sinusoids, which are thin-walled terminal vessels that are larger than ordinary capillaries. The syncytiotrophoblast then erodes the **sinusoids** and maternal blood flows into the lacunar networks. The degenerated endometrial stromal cells and glands, together with the maternal blood, provide a rich source of material for *embryonic nutrition*. Growth of the bilaminar embryonic disc is slow compared with the growth of the trophoblast.

As changes occur in the trophoblast and endometrium, the extraembryonic mesoderm increases and isolated **extraembryonic coelomic spaces** appear within it (see

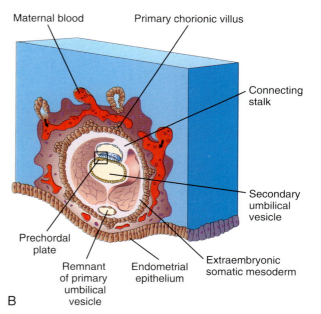

Figure 4–3 Sections of implanted embryos. **A,** At 13 days. Note the decrease in the relative size of the primary umbilical vesicle and the appearance of primary chorionic villi. **B,** At 14 days. Note the newly formed secondary umbilical vesicle.

Fig. 4-2*B*). These spaces rapidly fuse to form a large, isolated cavity, the **extraembryonic coelom** (Fig. 4-3*A*). This fluid-filled cavity surrounds the amnion and umbilical vesicle, except where they are attached to the **chorion** by the **connecting stalk**. As the extraembryonic coelom forms, the primary umbilical vesicle decreases in size and a smaller, **secondary umbilical vesicle** forms (Fig. 4-3*B*). During formation of the secondary umbilical vesical, a large part of the **primary umbilical vesicle** is pinched off. The umbilical vesicle contains no yolk; however, it may have a role in the selective transfer of nutritive materials to the embryonic disc.

DEVELOPMENT OF CHORIONIC SAC

2 The end of the second week is characterized by the appearance of primary chorionic villi (see Fig. 4-3*A* and Fig. 4-4*A* and *C*). Proliferation of the cytotrophoblastic cells produces cellular extensions that grow into the overlying syncytiotrophoblast. The cellular projections form primary chorionic villi, the first stage in the development of the chorionic villi of the placenta. The extraembryonic coelom splits the extraembryonic mesoderm into two layers (see Fig. 4-3*A*):

● The *extraembryonic somatic mesoderm*, which lines the trophoblast and covers the amnion

● The *extraembryonic splanchnic mesoderm*, which surrounds the umbilical vesicle

The growth of these cytotrophoblastic extensions is believed to be induced by the underlying **extraembryonic somatic mesoderm**. The extraembryonic somatic mesoderm and the two layers of trophoblast form the **chorion**. The chorion forms the wall of the chorionic sac (see Fig. 4-3*A*). The embryo, amniotic sac, and umbilical vesicle are suspended in the **chorionic cavity** by the connecting stalk (see Fig. 4-3*B* and Fig. 4-4*B*). Transvaginal ultrasonography (endovaginal sonography) is used to measure the diameter of the chorionic sac. This measurement is valuable for evaluating early embryonic development and pregnancy outcome.

EXTRAUTERINE IMPLANTATION SITES

Blastocysts sometimes implant outside the uterus. These implantations result in **ectopic pregnancies**; 95% to 98% of ectopic implantations occur in the uterine tubes, most often in the ampulla and isthmus (see Chapter 2, Fig. 2-2*B*, and Fig. 4-6*A* and *B*). **Ectopic tubal pregnancy** occurs in approximately 1 in 200 pregnancies in North America. A woman with a tubal pregnancy has the usual signs and symptoms of pregnancy; however, she may also experience abdominal pain (from distention of the uterine tube), abnormal bleeding, and irritation of the pelvic peritoneum.

The *causes of tubal pregnancy* are often related to factors that delay or prevent transport of the cleaving zygote to the uterus (e.g., blockage of uterine tube). Ectopic tubal pregnancies usually result in rupture of the uterine tube and hemorrhage into the peritoneal cavity during the first 8 weeks, followed by death of the embryo.

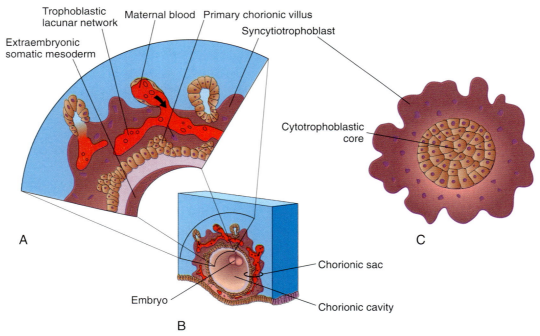

Figure 4–4   **A,** Illustration of a section of the wall of the chorionic sac. **B,** Illustration of a 14-day conceptus showing the chorionic sac and the chorionic cavity. **C,** Transverse section through a primary chorionic villus.

INHIBITION OF IMPLANTATION

The administration of relatively *large doses of estrogen* ("morning-after pills") for several days, beginning shortly after unprotected sexual intercourse, usually does not prevent fertilization; however, it often prevents implantation of the blastocyst. Normally, the endometrium progresses to the luteal phase of the menstrual cycle as the zygote forms, undergoes cleavage, and enters the uterus. A large amount of estrogen, however, disturbs the normal balance between estrogen and progesterone that is necessary to prepare the endometrium for implantation.

An **intrauterine device** (IUD) inserted into the uterus through the vagina and cervix usually interferes with implantation by causing a local inflammatory reaction. Some IUDs contain slow-release progesterone, which interferes with the development of the endometrium so that implantation does not usually occur. Copper-based IUDs appear to inhibit migration of sperm in the tube, while levonorgestrel-based IUDs alter the quality of cervical mucus and endometrial development.

▶ IMPLANTATION SITES OF BLASTOCYSTS

3 Blastocysts usually implant in the uterine endometrium in the superior part of the body of the uterus, slightly more often on the posterior than on the anterior wall of the uterus (Fig. 4-5). Implantation of a blastocyst can be detected by ultrasonography at the end of the second week (Fig. 4-6).

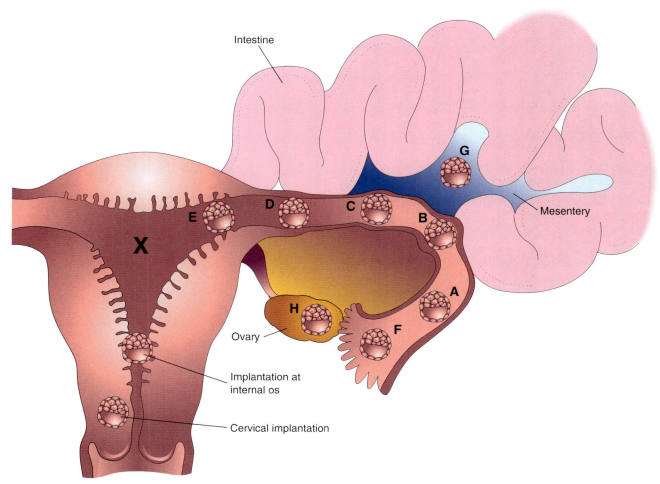

Figure 4–5   Implantation sites of blastocysts. The usual site in the posterior wall of the body of the uterus is indicated by an *X*. The approximate order of frequency of ectopic implantations is indicated alphabetically (**A,** most common, **H,** least common). **A** to **F,** tubal pregnancies; **G,** abdominal pregnancy; **H,** ovarian pregnancy. Tubal pregnancies are the most common type of ectopic pregnancy. Although appropriately included with uterine pregnancy sites, a cervical pregnancy is often considered to be an ectopic pregnancy.

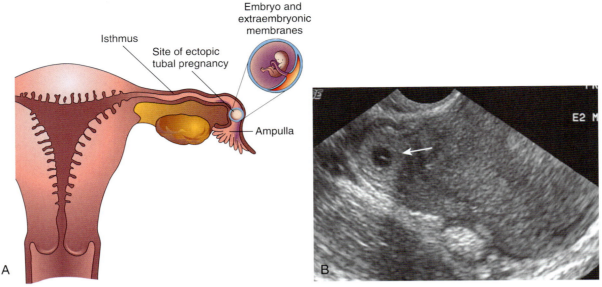

Figure 4–6   **A,** Coronal section of the uterus and uterine tube illustrating an ectopic pregnancy in the ampulla of the uterine tube. **B,** Endovaginal axial scan of the uterine fundus and isthmic portion of the right uterine tube. The ring-like mass is a 4-week ectopic chorionic (gestational) sac in the tube *(arrow)*.

CLINICALLY ORIENTED QUESTIONS

1. What is meant by the term *implantation bleeding*? Is this the same as *menses* (menstrual fluid)?

2. Can a drug taken during the first 2 weeks of pregnancy cause abortion of the embryo?

3. Can an ectopic pregnancy occur in a woman who has an intrauterine device?

4. Can a blastocyst that implants in the abdomen develop into a full-term fetus?

The answers to these questions are at the back of this book.

Third Week of Human Development

R apid development of the embryo from the trilaminar embryonic disc during the third week is characterized by:

- Appearance of the primitive streak
- Development of the notochord
- Differentiation of three germ layers

The third week of development occurs during the week of the first missed menstrual period, that is, 5 weeks after the first day of the last normal menstrual period. *Cessation of menstruation is often the first indication that a woman may be pregnant.* Approximately 5 weeks after the last normal menstrual period (Fig. 5-1), a normal pregnancy can be detected with ultrasonography.

GASTRULATION: FORMATION OF GERM LAYERS

Gastrulation is the process by which the bilaminar embryonic disc is converted into a **trilaminar embryonic disc** (Fig. 5-2A to H). Each of the three germ layers (ectoderm, endoderm, and mesoderm) of the embryonic disc gives rise to specific tissues and organs (see Chapter 6, Fig. 6-4).

Figure 5–1 Endovaginal ultrasonogram of a conceptus 3 weeks after conception implanted in the posterior endometrium, showing the umbilical vesicle. The endometrium completely surrounds the conceptus. *A*, Amnion; *UV*, umbilical sac; *E*, endometrium.

Gastrulation is the beginning of **morphogenesis**—development of body form and structure of various organs and parts of the body. It begins with the formation of the **primitive streak** (see Fig. 5-2*B* and *C*).

Primitive Streak

4   At the beginning of the third week, the **primitive streak** appears on the dorsal aspect of the embryonic disc (see Fig. 5-2*B*). This thickened linear band results from proliferation and migration of cells of the epiblast to the median plane of the embryonic disc (see Fig. 5-2*D*). As soon as the primitive streak appears, it is possible to identify the embryo's craniocaudal axis (cranial and caudal ends), dorsal and ventral surfaces, and right and left sides. As the primitive streak elongates by the addition of cells to its caudal end, its cranial end proliferates to form the **primitive node** (see Fig. 5-2*E* and *F*). Concurrently, a narrow **primitive groove** develops in the primitive streak that ends in a small depression in the primitive node, the **primitive pit** (see Fig. 5-2*F*). Shortly after the primitive streak appears, cells leave its deep surface and form **mesoderm**, a loose network of embryonic connective tissue known as mesenchyme (see Figs. 5-2*H* and Fig. 5-3*B* and *C*) that forms the supporting tissues of the embryo.

Under the influence of various embryonic growth factors, including bone morphogenetic protein signaling, epiblast cells migrate through the **primitive groove** to become endoderm and mesoderm (see Fig. 5-3*B*). Mesenchymal cells have the potential to proliferate and differentiate into diverse types of cells, such as fibroblasts, chondroblasts, and osteoblasts. *Recent studies indicate that signaling molecules (nodal factors) of the transforming growth factor-β superfamily induce the formation of mesoderm.*

The *primitive streak* actively forms **mesoderm** until the early part of the fourth week; thereafter, its production slows down. The streak diminishes in relative size and becomes an insignificant structure in the sacrococcygeal region of the embryo (Fig. 5-4*A* to *D*).

Notochordal Process and Notochord

Some mesenchymal cells migrate cranially from the primitive node and pit, forming a median cellular cord, the **notochordal process** (see Fig. 5-2*G*, Fig. 5-4*B* to *D*, and Fig. 5-5*A* to *C*). This process soon acquires a lumen, the **notochordal canal** (see Fig. 5-5*C* and *D*). The notochordal process grows cranially between the ectoderm and endoderm until it reaches the **prechordal plate**, a small, circular area of cells that is an important organizer of the head region (see Fig. 5-2*C*). The rod-like notochordal process can extend no farther because the prechordal plate is firmly attached to the overlying ectoderm. Fused layers of ectoderm and endoderm form the **oropharyngeal membrane** (Fig. 5-6*C*) located at the future site of the oral cavity (mouth).

Mesenchymal cells from the primitive streak and the notochordal process migrate laterally and cranially between the ectoderm and endoderm until they reach the margins of the embryonic disc. These mesenchymal cells are continuous with the extraembryonic mesoderm that covers the amnion and the umbilical vesicle (see Fig. 5-2*D* and *F*). Some cells from the primitive streak migrate cranially on each side of the notochordal process and around the prechordal plate. They meet cranially to form the cardiogenic mesoderm in the **cardiogenic area**, where the **heart primordium** begins to develop at the end of the third week (see Fig. 5-9*B*). Caudal to the primitive streak, there is a circular area—the **cloacal membrane**—that indicates the future site of the anus (see Fig. 5-5*A* and *D*).

The **notochord** is a cellular rod that:

- Defines the axis of the embryo and gives it some rigidity
- Serves as the basis for the development of the axial skeleton (such as the bones of the head and vertebral column)
- Indicates the future site of the vertebral bodies

The **vertebral column** forms around the notochord, which extends from the oropharyngeal membrane to the primitive node. The notochord degenerates and disappears as the bodies of the vertebrae form, but parts of it persist as the *nucleus pulposus* of each intervertebral disc. The notochord functions as the primary inductor in the early embryo. It induces the overlying embryonic ectoderm to thicken and form the **neural plate** (see Fig. 5-4*B* and *C* and Fig. 5-6*A* to *C*), the primordium of the central nervous system.

Allantois

The **allantois** appears on approximately day 16 as a small, sausage-shaped *diverticulum* (outpouching) from the caudal wall of the umbilical vesicle into the *connecting stalk* (Fig. 5-5*B*, *C*, and *D* and Fig. 5-6*B*). The allantois is involved with early blood formation and is associated

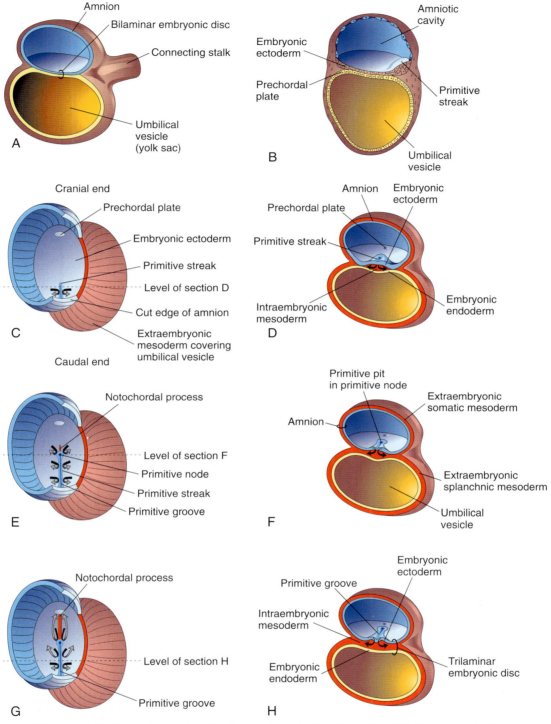

Figure 5–2 Formation of the trilaminar embryonic disc (days 15 to 16). The *arrows* indicate invagination and migration of the mesenchymal cells between the ectoderm and the endoderm. **C, E,** and **G,** Dorsal views of the embryonic disc early in the third week, exposed by removal of the amnion. **A, B, D, F,** and **H,** Transverse sections through the embryonic disc at the levels indicated.

Figure 5–3 **A,** Dorsal view of a 16-day embryo. The amnion has been removed to expose the embryonic disc. **B,** Illustration of the cranial half of the embryonic disc during the third week. The disc has been cut transversely to show the migration of mesenchymal cells from the primitive streak to form the mesoblast that soon organizes to form the intraembryonic mesoderm. **C,** Sagittal section of a trilaminar embryo showing ectoderm *(Ec)*, mesoderm *(M)*, and endoderm *(En)*. Also visible are the amniotic sac *(A)*, the umbilical vesicle *(U)*, and chorionic villi *(CV)*.

with the urinary bladder as well. The blood vessels of the allantois become the umbilical arteries and veins.

NEURULATION: FORMATION OF THE NEURAL TUBE

Neurulation includes the formation of the neural plate and neural folds and closure of these folds to form the neural tube. These processes are completed by the end of the fourth week, when closure of the **caudal neuropore** occurs (see Chapter 6, Fig. 6-11*A* and *B*).

Neural Plate and Neural Tube

As the notochord develops, it induces the overlying embryonic ectoderm over it to thicken and form an elongated **neural plate** of thickened neuroepithelial cells (see Fig. 5-5C). The ectoderm of the neural plate

(neuroectoderm) gives rise to the **central nervous system (CNS)—the brain and spinal cord** and other structures such as the retina. At first, the neural plate corresponds in length to the underlying **notochord**. It appears cranial to the primitive node and dorsal to the notochord and the mesoderm adjacent to it (see Fig. 5-4*B*). As the notochord elongates, the neural plate broadens and eventually extends cranially as far as the **oropharyngeal membrane** (see Fig. 5-4*C*). Eventually the neural plate extends beyond the notochord.

On approximately day 18, the neural plate invaginates along its central axis to form a median longitudinal **neural groove** that has **neural folds** on each side (see Fig. 5-6*F* and *G*). The neural folds are particularly prominent at the cranial end of the embryo and are the first signs of brain development (Fig. 5-7*C*). By the end of the third week, the neural folds have begun to move together and fuse, converting the neural plate into the **neural tube, the primordium of the brain vesicles and spinal cord** (see

Prechordal plate

Cranial end

Embryonic
ectoderm

Primitive
node

Primitive
streak

Caudal end

A 15 days

Oropharyngeal
membrane

Neural
plate

Notochordal
process

Newly
added
cells

Cloacal membrane

B 17 days

Neural
groove

C 18 days

Neural fold

Notochord deep
to neural groove

D 21 days

Figure 5–4 **A** to **D,** Dorsal views of the embryonic disc, showing how it lengthens and changes shape during the third week. The primitive streak lengthens by the addition of cells at its caudal end; the notochordal process lengthens by the migration of cells from the primitive node. At the end of the third week, the notochordal process is transformed into the notochord.

Fig. 5-7F and Fig. 5-8). Neural tube formation is a complex cellular and multifactorial process involving genes and extrinsic and mechanical factors (see Chapter 16). The neural tube soon separates from the surface ectoderm as the neural folds meet (see Fig. 5-8E). The free edges of the ectoderm fuse so that this layer becomes continuous over the neural tube and the back of the embryo. Subsequently, the surface ectoderm differentiates into the epidermis of the skin. Neurulation is completed during the fourth week (see Chapter 6).

Neural Crest Formation

As the neural folds fuse to form the neural tube, some *neuroectodermal cells* lying along the crest of each neural fold lose their epithelial affinities and attachments to neighboring cells (see Fig. 5-8A to C). As the neural tube separates from the surface ectoderm, these **neural crest cells** migrate dorsolaterally on each side of the neural tube. They form a flattened irregular mass, the **neural crest,** between the neural tube and the overlying surface ectoderm (see Fig. 5-8D and E). The neural crest soon separates into right and left parts that migrate in a wave to the dorsolateral aspects of the neural tube (see Fig. 5-8F). Neural crest cells also migrate widely within the mesenchyme. Neural crest cells differentiate into various cell types (see Chapter 6, Fig. 6-4), including the spinal ganglia and the ganglia of the **autonomic nervous system.** The ganglia of cranial nerves V, VII, IX, and X are partially derived from neural crest cells. Neural crest cells also form the sheaths of the peripheral nerves and the pia mater and arachnoid mater (see Chapter 16).

DEVELOPMENT OF SOMITES

16

As the notochord and neural tube form, the intraembryonic mesoderm on each side proliferates to form a thick, longitudinal column of **paraxial mesoderm** (see Fig. 5-6G and Fig. 5-7B). Each column is continuous laterally with the **intermediate mesoderm,** which gradually thins into a layer of **lateral mesoderm.** The lateral mesoderm is continuous with the extraembryonic mesoderm that covers the umbilical vesicle and amnion (see Chapter 4, Fig. 4-3B). Toward the end of the third week, the **paraxial mesoderm** differentiates and begins to divide into paired cuboidal bodies, or **somites,** on each side of the developing neural tube (see Fig. 5-7C and E). The somites form distinct surface elevations on the embryo and appear somewhat triangular on transverse section (see Fig. 5-7D and F). Because the somites are so prominent during the fourth and fifth weeks, they are used as one of several criteria for determining an embryo's age (see Chapter 6, Table 6-1).

The first pair of somites appears at the end of the third week (see Fig. 5-7C) near the cranial end of the notochord. Subsequent pairs form in a craniocaudal sequence. Somites give rise to most of the *axial skeleton* and the associated musculature, as well as to the adjacent dermis of the skin.

Somite formation from the paraxial mesoderm is preceded by expression of the forkhead transcription factors Fox C1 and C2. The craniocaudal segmental pattern of the somites is regulated by the Delta-Notch (Delta 1 and Notch 1) signaling pathway. A molecular oscillator, or clock, has been proposed as the mechanism responsible

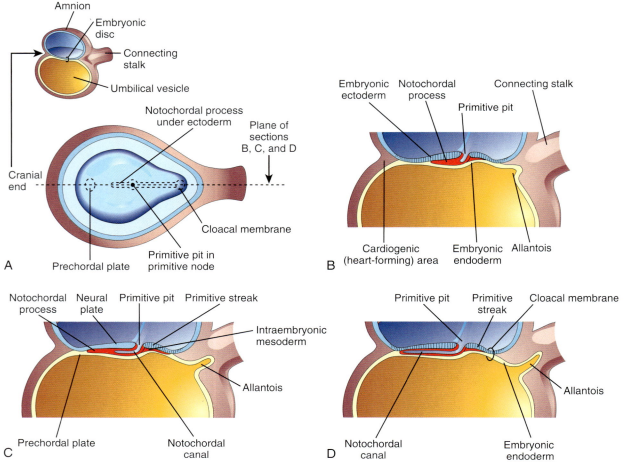

Figure 5–5 Illustrations of the development of the notochordal process. The small sketch at the upper left is for orientation. **A,** Dorsal view of the embryonic disc (at approximately 16 days), exposed by removal of the amnion. The notochordal process is shown as if it were visible through the embryonic ectoderm. **B, C,** and **D,** Median sections, at the same plane as shown in **A,** illustrating successive stages in the development of the notochordal process and canal. The stages shown in **C** and **D** occur at approximately 18 days.

for the orderly sequencing of the somites. The size and shape of somites are determined by cell-cell interactions.

DEVELOPMENT OF INTRAEMBRYONIC COELOM

The intraembryonic coelom (body cavity) first appears as small, isolated, **coelomic spaces** in the lateral intraembryonic mesoderm and cardiogenic (heart-forming) mesoderm (see Fig. 5-7A to D). These spaces coalesce to form a single, horseshoe-shaped cavity—the **intraembryonic coelom** (see Fig. 5-7E and F). The coelom divides the lateral mesoderm into two layers (see Fig. 5-7F):

- A somatic, or *parietal (**somatopleure**),* layer that is continuous with the extraembryonic mesoderm covering the amnion

- A splanchnic, or *visceral (**splanchnopleure**),* layer that is continuous with the extraembryonic mesoderm covering the umbilical vesicle

The somatic mesoderm and overlying embryonic ectoderm form the embryonic body wall (see Fig. 5-7F), whereas the splanchnic mesoderm and the underlying embryonic endoderm form the wall of the gut. During the second month, the intraembryonic coelom is divided into three body cavities: *pericardial cavity, pleural cavities,* and *peritoneal cavity* (see Chapter 9).

EARLY DEVELOPMENT OF CARDIOVASCULAR SYSTEM

At the end of the second week, embryonic nutrition is obtained from the maternal blood by diffusion through the extraembryonic coelom and umbilical vesicle. The

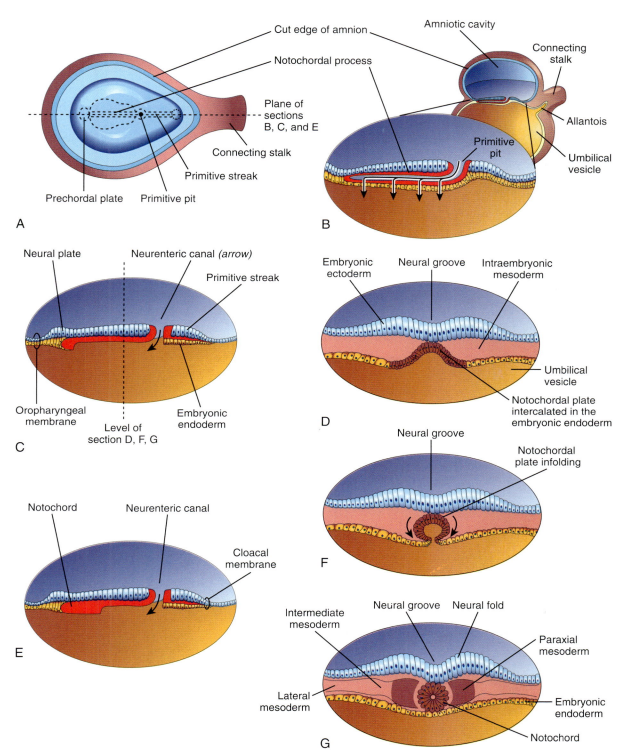

Figure 5–6 Development of the notochord by transformation of the notochordal process. **A**, Dorsal view of the embryonic disc (at approximately 18 days), exposed by removing the amnion. **B**, Three-dimensional median section of the embryo. **C** and **E**, Similar sections of slightly older embryos. **D, F,** and **G**, Transverse sections of the trilaminar embryonic disc shown in **C** and **E**.

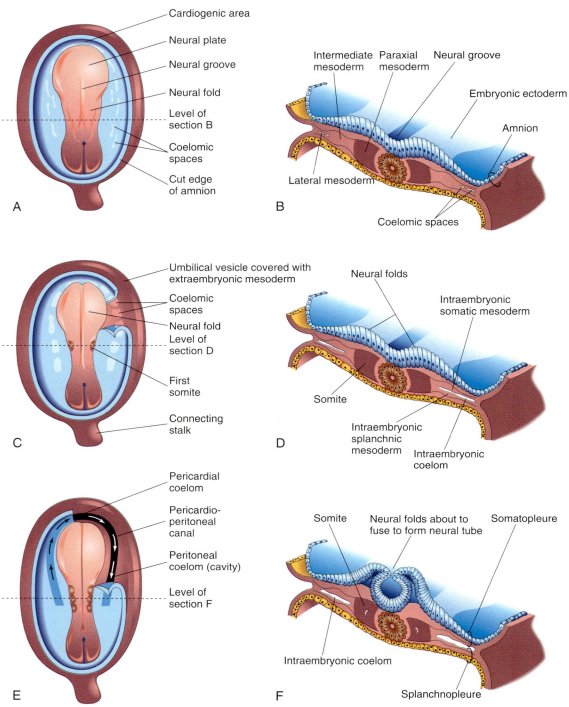

Figure 5–7   Illustrations of embryos 19 to 21 days old, illustrating the development of the somites and the intraembryonic coelom. **A, C,** and **E,** Dorsal view of the embryo, exposed by removal of the amnion. **B, D,** and **F,** Transverse sections through the embryonic disc at the levels shown. **A,** A presomite embryo of approximately 18 days. **C,** An embryo of approximately 20 days, showing the first pair of somites. A portion of the somatopleure on the right has been removed to show the isolated coelomic spaces in the lateral mesoderm. **E,** A three-somite embryo (approximately 21 days old), showing the horseshoe-shaped intraembryonic coelom, exposed on the right by removal of part of the somatopleure.

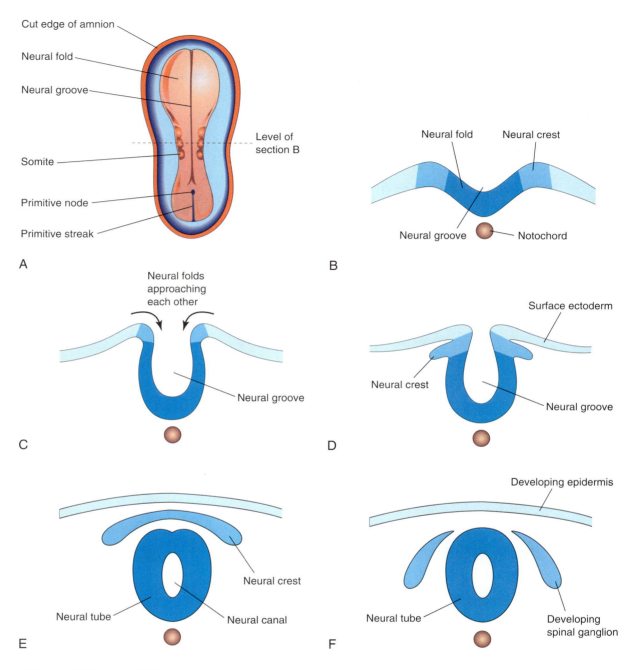

Figure 5–8 **A** to **F,** Diagrammatic transverse sections through progressively older embryos, illustrating the formation of the neural groove, neural tube, and neural crest up to the end of the fourth week.

early formation of the cardiovascular system correlates with the urgent need for transportation of oxygen and nourishment to the embryo from the maternal circulation through the chorion. At the beginning of the third week, blood vessel formation, or **vasculogenesis**, begins in the extraembryonic mesoderm of the umbilical vesicle, connecting stalk, and chorion. Vasculogenesis begins in the chorion (Fig. 5-9A and B). Blood vessels develop approximately 2 days later. At the end of the third week, a **primordial uteroplacental circulation** has developed (Fig. 5-10).

Vasculogenesis and Angiogenesis

Blood vessel formation in the embryo and the extraembryonic membranes during the third week may be summarized as follows (see Fig. 5-9C to F):

Vasculogenesis:

- Mesenchymal cells differentiate into endothelial cell precursors, or **angioblasts** (vessel-forming cells), that aggregate to form isolated angiogenic cell clusters known as **blood islands** (see Fig. 5-9B and C).

Figure 5–9   Successive stages in the development of blood and blood vessels. **A,** The umbilical vesicle (yolk sac) and a portion of the chorionic sac (at approximately 18 days). **B,** Dorsal view of the embryo exposed by removing the amnion. **C** to **F,** Sections of blood islands, showing progressive stages in the development of blood and blood vessels.

- Small cavities appear within the blood islands by the confluence of intercellular clefts.
- Angioblasts flatten to form endothelial cells that arrange themselves around the cavities in the blood islands to form the primordial endothelium.
- The endothelium-lined cavities soon fuse to form networks of endothelial channels.

Angiogenesis:

- Vessels sprout by endothelial budding into adjacent nonvascularized areas and fuse with other vessels.

Blood cells develop from hematopoietic stem cells or from hemangiogenic endothelium or blood vessels as they grow on the umbilical vesicle and allantois at the end of the third week (see Fig. 5-9E and F). Blood formation (**hematogenesis**) does not begin within the embryo until the fifth week. This process occurs first in various parts of the embryonic mesenchyme, chiefly the liver, and later in the spleen, bone marrow, and lymph nodes. Fetal and adult erythrocytes are also derived from hematopoietic progenitor cells (**hemangioblasts**). The mesenchymal cells that surround the primordial endothelial blood vessels differentiate into muscular and connective tissue elements of the vessels.

The **heart and great vessels** form from mesenchymal cells in the heart primordium, or **cardiogenic area** (see Fig. 5-7A and Fig. 5-9B). Paired, endothelium-lined channels—endocardial **heart tubes**—develop during the

Figure 5–10 Endovaginal scan of a 4-week embryo. **A,** A 2-mm secondary umbilical vesicle (*calipers*). **B,** Bright (echogenic) 2.4-mm, 4-week embryo (*calipers*). **C,** Cardiac activity of 116 beats/min demonstrated with motion mode. *Calipers* used to encompass two beats.

third week and fuse to form a **primordial heart tube.** The tubular heart joins with blood vessels in the embryo, connecting stalk, chorion, and umbilical vesicle to form a **primordial cardiovascular system** (Fig. 5-11*C*). By the end of the third week, blood is flowing and the heart begins to beat on day 21 or 22. *The cardiovascular system is the first organ system to reach a primitive functional state.* The embryonic heartbeat can be detected by Doppler ultrasonography (detects motion by monitoring the change in frequency or phase of the returning ultrasound waves) during the fourth week, approximately 6 weeks after the last normal menstrual period (see Fig. 5-10).

DEVELOPMENT OF CHORIONIC VILLI

Shortly after the **primary chorionic villi** appear at the end of the second week, they begin to branch. Early in the third week, mesenchyme grows into the primary villi, forming a core of loose mesenchymal tissue (see Fig. 5-11*A* and *B*). The villi at this stage—**secondary chorionic villi**—cover the entire surface of the chorionic sac (see Fig. 5-9*A* and *B*). Some mesenchymal cells in the villi soon differentiate into both capillaries and blood cells (see Fig. 5-11*C* and *D*). When capillaries are present, the villi are called **tertiary chorionic villi.**

The capillaries in the chorionic villi fuse to form **arteriocapillary networks,** which soon become connected with the embryonic heart through vessels that differentiate from the mesenchyme of the chorion and connecting stalk. *By the end of the third week, embryonic blood begins to flow slowly through the capillaries in the chorionic villi.* Oxygen and nutrients in the maternal blood in the **intervillous space** diffuse through the walls of the villi and enter the embryo's blood (see Fig. 5-11*C*). Carbon dioxide and waste products diffuse from blood in the fetal capillaries through the wall of the villi into the maternal blood. Concurrently, cytotrophoblastic cells of the chorionic villi proliferate and extend through the syncytiotrophoblast to form a **cytotrophoblastic shell,** which gradually surrounds the chorionic sac and attaches it to the endometrium (see Fig. 5-11*C*).

Villi that attach to the maternal tissues through the cytotrophoblastic shell are called **stem chorionic villi** (anchoring villi). The villi that grow from the sides of the stem villi are **branch chorionic villi** (terminal villi). It is through the walls of the branch villi that the main exchange of material between the blood of the mother and the embryo takes place. The branch villi are bathed in continually changing maternal blood in the **intervillous space** (see Fig. 5-11*C*).

SACROCOCCYGEAL TERATOMA

Remnants of the primitive streak may persist and give rise to a large tumor known as a **sacrococcygeal teratoma** (Fig. 5-12). Because it is derived from pluripotent primitive streak cells, the tumor contains tissues derived from all three germ layers in incomplete stages of differentiation. Sacrococcygeal teratomas are the most common tumors in newborn infants and have an incidence of approximately 1 in 27,000 neonates. These tumors are usually surgically excised promptly, and the prognosis is good.

ABNORMAL NEURULATION

Disturbance of neurulation may result in severe abnormalities of the brain and spinal cord (see Chapter 16). **Neural tube defects** are among the most common congenital anomalies. Meroencephaly (anencephaly), or partial absence of the brain, is the most severe defect. Available evidence suggests that the primary disturbance affects the neuroectoderm. Failure of the neural folds to fuse and form the neural tube in the brain region results in meroencephaly, and in the lumbar region, spina bifida cystica (see Chapter 16, Fig. 16-9).

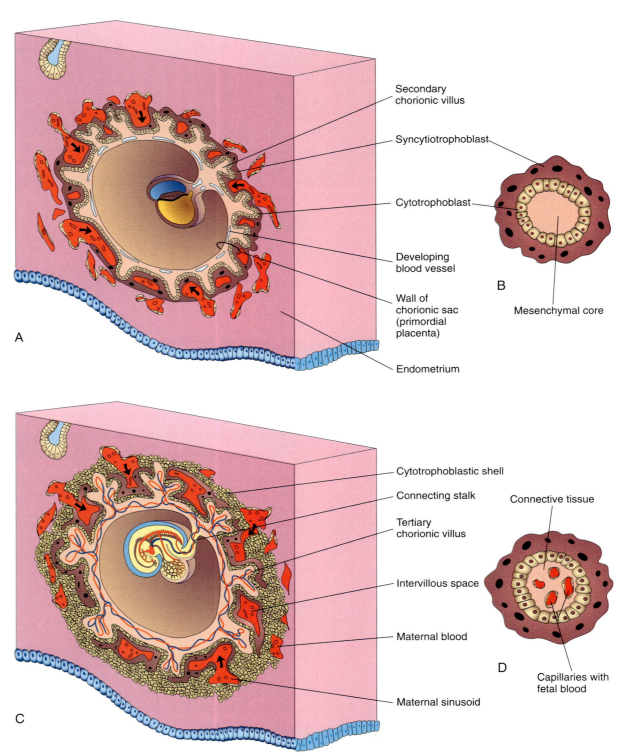

Figure 5–11 Illustrations of the development of the secondary chorionic villi into the tertiary chorionic villi. **A,** Sagittal section of an embryo (at approximately 16 days). **B,** Section of a secondary chorionic villus. **C,** Section of an embryo (at approximately 21 days). **D,** Section of a tertiary chorionic villus. By the end of the third week, a primordial uteroplacental circulation has developed.

Figure 5–12   A female infant with a large sacrococcygeal teratoma that developed from remnants of the primitive streak.

Figure 5–13   Ultrasound image demonstrating a complete hydatidiform mole. Note numerous small cystic spaces. The "cluster of grapes sign" is a typical feature of a molar pregnancy.

ABNORMAL GROWTH OF TROPHOBLAST

Sometimes the embryo dies and the chorionic villi do not complete their development; that is, they do not become vascularized to form tertiary villi. These degenerating villi may form cystic swellings, called **hydatidiform moles** (Fig. 5-13). These moles exhibit variable degrees of trophoblastic proliferation and produce excessive amounts of human chorionic gonadotropin. In 3% to 5% of such cases, these moles develop into malignant trophoblastic lesions, called **choriocarcinomas.** These tumors invariably metastasize (spread) by way of the blood to various sites, such as the lungs, vagina, liver, bone, intestine, and brain.

CLINICALLY ORIENTED QUESTIONS

1. Can drugs and other agents cause birth defects of the embryo if they are present in the mother's blood during the third week? If so, what organs would be most susceptible?

2. Are there increased risks for the embryo associated with pregnancies in women older than 40 years of age? If so, what are they?

The answers to these questions are at the back of this book.

CHAPTER

Fourth to Eighth Weeks of Human Development

All major external and internal structures are established during the fourth to eighth weeks. By the end of this **period**, the main organ systems have begun to develop. Exposure of embryos to **teratogens** (e.g., drugs and viruses) during this period may cause **major birth defects** (see Chapter 19). As the tissues and organs form, the shape of the embryo changes so that, by the eighth week, the embryo has a distinctly human appearance.

▶ FOLDING OF EMBRYO

5 A significant event in the establishment of body form is folding of the **trilaminar embryonic disc** into a somewhat cylindrical embryo (Fig. 6-1). Folding results from rapid growth of the embryo, particularly the brain and spinal cord. Folding at the cranial and caudal ends and at the sides of the embryo occurs simultaneously. Concurrently, a relative constriction occurs at the junction of the embryo and the umbilical vesicle. Head and tail folds cause the cranial and caudal regions to move ventrally as the embryo elongates (see Fig. 6-1A_2 to D_2).

Reconstructions made of the surface ectoderm and all organs and cavities within human embryos at representative stages of development have revealed new findings on the movements that occur from one stage to the next. Movement is caused by biokinetic forces acting on specific tissues. This has been shown to take place simultaneously at every level of magnification from the cell membrane all the way to the surface of the embryo. The movements and forces bring about differentiation that begins on the outside of the cell, and then moves to the inside to react with the nucleus.

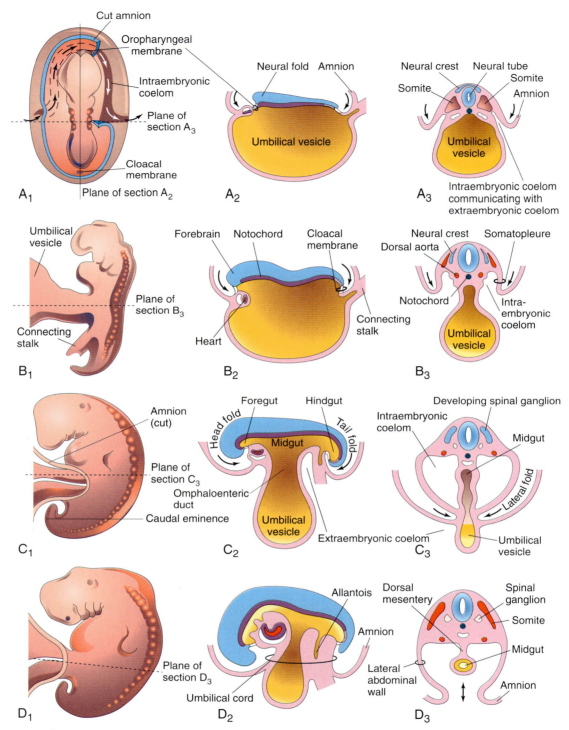

Figure 6–1   Folding of embryos during the fourth week. **A₁,** Dorsal view of an embryo early in the fourth week. Three pairs of somites are visible. The continuity of the intraembryonic coelom and extraembryonic coelom is shown on the right side by removal of a part of the embryonic ectoderm and mesoderm. **B₁, C₁,** and **D₁,** Lateral views of embryos at 22, 26, and 28 days, respectively. **A₂, B₂, C₂,** and **D₂,** Sagittal sections at the plane shown in **A₁. A₃, B₃, C₃,** and **D₃,** Transverse sections at the levels indicated in **A₁** to **D₁.**

Head and Tail Folds

By the beginning of the fourth week, the neural folds in the cranial region form the **primordium of the brain**. Later, the developing forebrain grows cranially beyond the oropharyngeal membrane and overhangs the developing heart. Concomitantly, the **primordial heart** and the **oropharyngeal membrane** move onto the ventral surface of the embryo (Fig. 6-2).

Folding of the caudal end of the embryo results primarily from growth of the distal part of the neural tube, the **primordium of the spinal cord**. As the embryo grows, the tail region projects over the **cloacal membrane**, the future site of the anus (Fig. 6-3*B*). During folding, part of the endodermal germ layer is incorporated into the embryo as the **hindgut** (see Fig. 6-3*C*). The terminal part of the hindgut soon dilates to form the **cloaca** (see Fig. 6-3*C*). The **connecting stalk** (primordium of the umbilical cord) is now attached to the ventral surface of the embryo, and the **allantois**—an endodermal diverticulum of the umbilical vesicle—is partially incorporated into the embryo (see Fig. 6-1*D₂* and Fig. 6-3*C*).

Lateral Folds

Folding of the sides of the developing embryo results from growth of the somites, which produces right and left **lateral folds** (see Fig. 6-1*A₃* to *D₃*). The lateral abdominal body wall folds toward the median plane, rolling the edges of the embryonic disc ventrally and forming a roughly cylindrical embryo. During lateral (longitudinal) folding, part of the endoderm of the umbilical vesicle is incorporated into the embryo as the **foregut**, the primordium of the pharynx (see Fig. 6-2*C*). The foregut lies between the brain and heart, and the oropharyngeal membrane separates the foregut from the **stomodeum**, the primordium of the mouth. As the abdominal wall forms by fusion of the lateral folds, part of the endoderm germ layer is incorporated into the embryo as the **midgut**.

Initially, there is a wide connection between the midgut and the umbilical vesicle (see Fig. 6-1*C₂*). After lateral folding, the connection is reduced to an **omphaloenteric duct**, formerly called the yolk stalk (see Fig. 6-1*C₂*). As the **umbilical cord** forms from the connecting stalk, ventral fusion of the lateral folds reduces the region of communication between the intraembryonic and extraembryonic coelomic cavities (see Fig. 6-1*C₂*). As the amniotic cavity expands and obliterates most of the *extraembryonic coelom*, the amnion forms the epithelial covering of the umbilical cord (see Fig. 6-1*D₂*).

▶ GERM LAYER DERIVATIVES

5 The three germ layers (ectoderm, mesoderm, and endoderm) formed during gastrulation give rise to the primordia of all tissues and organs (Fig. 6-4). The cells of each germ layer divide, migrate, aggregate, and differentiate in rather precise patterns as they form the various organ systems (organogenesis).

CONTROL OF EMBRYONIC DEVELOPMENT

Embryonic development results from genetic plans in the chromosomes. Knowledge of the genes that control human development is increasing (see Chapter 20). Most developmental processes depend on a precisely coordinated interaction of genetic and environmental factors. Several control mechanisms guide differentiation and ensure synchronized development, such as **tissue interactions**, regulated migration of cells and cell colonies, controlled proliferation, and apoptosis (programmed cell death). Each system of the body has its own developmental pattern, and most processes of morphogenesis are regulated by complex molecular mechanisms.

Embryonic development is essentially a process of growth and increasing complexity of structure and function. **Growth is achieved by mitosis**, together with the production of extracellular **matrices**, whereas complexity is achieved through morphogenesis and differentiation. The cells that make up the tissues of very early embryos are **pluripotential**; that is, depending on the circumstances, they are able to follow more than one pathway of development. This broad developmental potential becomes progressively restricted as tissues acquire the specialized features necessary for increased sophistication of structure and function. Such restriction presumes that choices must be made to achieve tissue diversification.

Most evidence indicates that these choices are determined not as a consequence of cell lineage, but rather in response to cues from the immediate surroundings, including the adjacent tissues. As a result, the architectural precision and coordination that are often required for normal function of an organ appear to be achieved by the interaction of its constituent parts during development.

The **interaction of tissues** during development is a recurring theme in embryology. The interactions that lead to a change in the course of development of at least one of the interactants are called **inductions**. Numerous examples of such inductive interactions can be found in the literature; for example, during the *development of the eye*, the optic vesicle induces the development of the lens from the surface ectoderm of the head. When the optic vesicle is absent, the eye does not develop. Moreover, if the optic vesicle is removed and placed in association with surface ectoderm that is not usually involved in eye development, lens formation can be induced. Clearly then, the development of a lens depends on the ectoderm acquiring an association with a second tissue. In the presence of the neuroectoderm of the optic vesicle, the surface ectoderm of the head follows a pathway of development that it would not otherwise have taken. Similarly, many of the morphogenetic tissue movements that play such important roles in shaping the embryo also provide for the changing tissue associations that are fundamental to *inductive tissue interactions*.

The fact that one tissue can influence the *developmental pathway* adopted by another tissue presumes that a signal passes between the two interactants. Analysis of the molecular defects in mutant strains that show abnormal tissue interactions during embryonic development and studies of the development of embryos with targeted

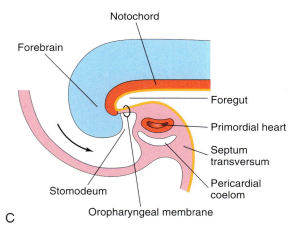

Figure 6–2   Folding of cranial end of the embryo. **A,** Dorsal view of an embryo at 21 days. **B,** Sagittal section of the cranial part of the embryo at the plane in **A,** showing the ventral movement of the heart. **C,** Sagittal section of an embryo at 26 days. Note that the septum transversum, heart, pericardial coelom, and oropharyngeal membrane have moved to the ventral surface of the embryo.

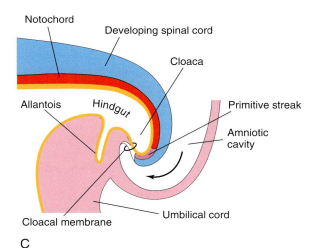

Figure 6–3   Folding of caudal end of the embryo. **A,** Lateral view of a 4-week embryo. **B,** Sagittal section of the caudal part of the embryo at the beginning of the fourth week. **C,** Similar section at the end of the fourth week. Note that part of the umbilical vesicle is incorporated into the embryo as the hindgut and that the terminal part of the hindgut has dilated to form the cloaca. Observe also the change in position of the primitive streak, allantois, cloacal membrane, and connecting stalk.

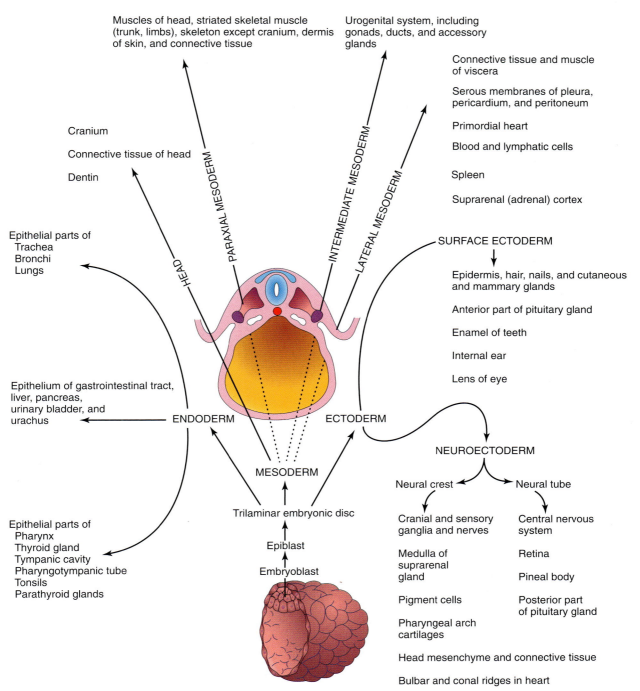

Muscles of head, striated skeletal muscle (trunk, limbs), skeleton except cranium, dermis of skin, and connective tissue

Urogenital system, including gonads, ducts, and accessory glands

Connective tissue and muscle of viscera

Serous membranes of pleura, pericardium, and peritoneum

Primordial heart

Blood and lymphatic cells

Spleen

Suprarenal (adrenal) cortex

Cranium

Connective tissue of head

Dentin

PARAXIAL MESODERM

INTERMEDIATE MESODERM

LATERAL MESODERM

HEAD

SURFACE ECTODERM

Epidermis, hair, nails, and cutaneous and mammary glands

Anterior part of pituitary gland

Enamel of teeth

Internal ear

Lens of eye

Epithelial parts of
    Trachea
    Bronchi
    Lungs

Epithelium of gastrointestinal tract, liver, pancreas, urinary bladder, and urachus

ENDODERM

ECTODERM

NEUROECTODERM

MESODERM

Trilaminar embryonic disc

Epiblast

Embryoblast

Neural crest

Neural tube

Epithelial parts of
    Pharynx
    Thyroid gland
    Tympanic cavity
    Pharyngotympanic tube
    Tonsils
    Parathyroid glands

Cranial and sensory ganglia and nerves

Central nervous system

Medulla of suprarenal gland

Retina

Pigment cells

Pineal body

Posterior part of pituitary gland

Pharyngeal arch cartilages

Head mesenchyme and connective tissue

Bulbar and conal ridges in heart

Figure 6–4 Illustration of derivatives of the three germ layers: ectoderm, endoderm, and mesoderm. Cells from these layers contribute to the formation of different tissues and organs; for example, the endoderm forms the epithelial lining of the gastrointestinal tract and the mesoderm gives rise to connective tissues and muscles.

gene mutations have begun to reveal the *molecular mechanisms of induction*. The mechanism of signal transfer appears to vary with the specific tissues involved. In some cases, the signal appears to take the form of a diffusible molecule that passes from the inductor to the reacting tissue. In other instances, the message appears to be mediated through a nondiffusible extracellular matrix that is secreted by the inductor and that comes into contact with the reacting tissue. In still other cases, the signal appears to require physical contact between the inducing tissue and the responding tissue. Regardless of the mechanism of intercellular transfer involved, the signal is translated into an intracellular message that influences the genetic activity of the responding cells.

To be competent to respond to an inducing stimulus, the cells of the reacting system must express the appropriate receptor for the specific inducing signal molecule, the components of the particular intracellular signal transduction pathway, and the transcription factors that mediate the particular response. Experimental evidence suggests that the acquisition of competence by the responding tissue is often dependent on its previous interactions with other tissues. For example, the lens-forming response of the head ectoderm to the stimulus provided by the optic vesicle appears to be dependent on a previous association of the head ectoderm with the anterior neural plate (see Chapter 20).

ESTIMATION OF EMBRYONIC AGE

Estimates of the age of *recovered* embryos (e.g., after spontaneous abortion) are determined from their external characteristics and measurements of their length (Table 6-1). *Size alone may be an unreliable criterion* because some embryos undergo a progressively slower rate of growth before death. The appearance of the developing limbs is a very helpful criterion for estimating embryonic age. Because embryos are straight in the third and early fourth weeks (Fig. 6-5A), their measurements indicate the greatest length. The sitting height, or *crown–rump length*, is used to estimate the age of older embryos (see Fig. 6-5B and C). Standing height, or *crown–heel length*, is sometimes measured during weeks 14 to 18 (see Fig. 6-5D). The *Carnegie Embryonic Staging System* is used internationally for comparison (see Table 6-1).

HIGHLIGHTS OF THE FOURTH TO EIGHTH WEEKS

The criteria for estimating developmental stages in human embryos are listed in Table 6-1.

ULTRASONOGRAPHIC EXAMINATION OF EMBRYOS

Most women seeking obstetrical care have at least one ultrasonographic examination during their pregnancy for one or more of the following reasons:
* Estimation of gestational age for confirmation of clinical dating
* Evaluation of embryonic growth when intrauterine growth restriction is suspected
* Guidance during chorionic villus or amniotic fluid sampling
* Suspected ectopic pregnancy
* Possible uterine abnormality
* Detection of birth defects

The size of an embryo in a pregnant woman can be estimated using ultrasonographic measurements. *Transvaginal* or *endovaginal ultrasonography* permits accurate measurement of crown–rump length in early pregnancy (Fig. 6-6).

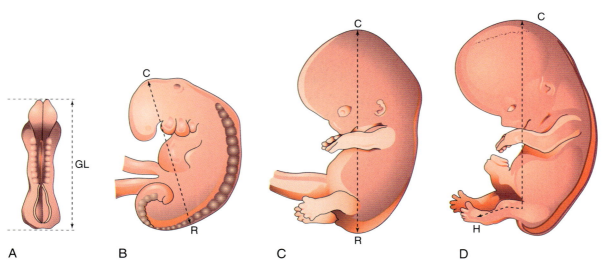

Figure 6–5 Methods used to measure the length of embryos. **A,** Greatest length *(GL)*. **B** and **C,** Crown–rump length. **D,** Crown–heel length.

Table 6–1   Criteria for Estimating Developmental Stages in Human Embryos

AGE (days)	FIGURE REFERENCE	CARNEGIE STAGE	NUMBER OF SOMITES	LENGTH (mm)*	MAIN EXTERNAL CHARACTERISTICS†
20–21	6-1A₁	9	1–3	1.5–3.0	Flat embryonic disc. Deep neural groove and prominent neural folds. Head fold is evident.
22–23	6-8A, C	10	4–12	2.0–3.5	Embryo is straight or slightly curved. Neural tube is forming or has formed opposite somites, but is widely open at the rostral and caudal neuropores. First and second pairs of pharyngeal arches are visible.
24–25	6-9A	11	13–20	2.5–4.5	Embryo is curved owing to head and tail folds. Rostral neuropore is closing. Otic placodes are present. Optic vesicles have formed.
26–27	6-7B 6-10A	12	21–29	3.0–5.0	Upper limb buds appear. Rostral neuropore is closed. Caudal neuropore is closing. Three pairs of pharyngeal arches are visible. Heart prominence is distinct. Otic pits are present.
28–30	6-6 6-11A	13	30–35	4.0–6.0	Embryo has C-shaped curve. Caudal neuropore is closed. Four pairs of pharyngeal arches are visible. Lower limb buds appear. Otic vesicles are present. Lens placodes are distinct.
31–32	6-12A	14	‡	5.0–7.0	Lens pits and nasal pits are visible. Optic cups are present.
33–36		15		7.0–9.0	Hand plates have formed; digital rays are present. Lens vesicles are present. Nasal pits are prominent. Cervical sinuses are visible.
37–40		16		8.0–11.0	Foot plates have formed. Pigment is visible in the retina. Auricular hillocks are developing.
41–43	6-13A	17		11.0–14.0	Digital rays are clearly visible in hand plates. Auricular hillocks outline the future auricle of the external ear. Cerebral vesicles are prominent.
44–46		18		13.0–17.0	Digital rays are clearly evident in foot plates. Elbow region is visible. Eyelids are forming. Notches are between the digital rays in the hands. Nipples are visible.
47–48		19		16.0–18.0	Limbs extend ventrally. Trunk is elongating and straightening. Midgut herniation is prominent.
49–51		20		18.0–22.0	Upper limbs are longer and are bent at the elbows. Fingers are distinct but webbed. Notches are between the digital rays in the feet. Scalp vascular plexus appears.
52–53		21		22.0–24.0	Hands and feet approach each other. Fingers are free and longer. Toes are distinct but webbed. Stubby caudal eminence (tail) is present.
54–55		22		23.0–28.0	Toes are free and longer. Eyelids and auricles of the external ears are more developed.
56	6-14A	23		27.0–31.0	Head is more rounded and shows human characteristics. External genitalia still have undifferentiated appearance. Midgut herniation is still present. Caudal eminence has disappeared.

*The embryonic lengths indicate the usual range. In stages 9 and 10, the measurement is greatest length; in subsequent stages, crown–rump measurements are given.
†Based on O'Rahilly R, Müller F: Developmental Stages in Human Embryos. Washington, DC, Carnegie Institute of Washington, 1987; and Gasser RF: Digitally Reproduced Embryonic Morphology DVDs. Computer Imaging Laboratory, Cell Biology and Anatomy. New Orleans, LA, Louisiana State University Health Sciences Center, 2002–2006.
‡At this stage and subsequent stages, the number of somites is difficult to determine and so is not a useful criterion.

Fourth Week

Major changes in body form occur during the fourth week. At the beginning, the embryo is almost straight. In the fourth week the somites produce conspicuous surface elevations and the **neural tube** is open at the rostral and caudal neuropores (Fig. 6-7A and Fig. 6-8C and D). By 24 days, the *pharyngeal arches* have appeared (see Fig. 6-7A to C). The embryo is now slightly curved because of the head and tail folds. **The early heart produces a large ventral prominence and pumps blood** (Fig. 6-9 and Fig. 6-10). The rostral neuropore is closing at 24 days (see Fig. 6-9B).

At 26 days, the **forebrain** produces a prominent elevation of the head and the long, curved **caudal eminence** (tail-like structure) is present (see Fig. 6-10B). At 28 days, **upper limb buds** are recognizable as small swellings on the

Figure 6–6   Endovaginal scan of embryos. **A,** Endovaginal scan of a 5-week embryo (crown–rump length [CRL] 10 mm [*calipers*]) surrounded by the amniotic membrane (*arrow*). **B,** Coronal scan of a 7-week embryo (CRL 22 mm [*calipers*]). Amnion seen anterior (*arrow*). Umbilical vesicle (yolk sac) anterior.

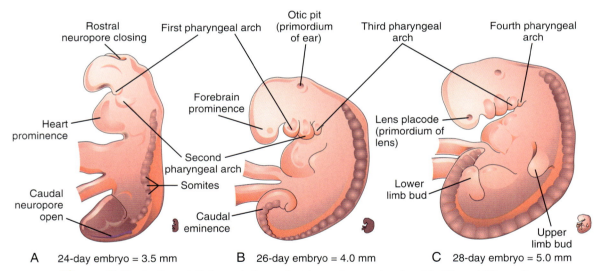

A   24-day embryo = 3.5 mm   **B**   26-day embryo = 4.0 mm   **C**   28-day embryo = 5.0 mm

Figure 6–7   **A, B,** and **C,** Lateral views of older embryos, showing 16, 27, and 33 somites, respectively. The rostral neuropore is normally closed by 25 to 26 days, and the caudal neuropore is usually closed by the end of the fourth week.

ventrolateral body walls (Fig. 6-11*A* and *B*). At 26 days, the **otic pits** (primordia of internal ears) are also visible (see Fig. 6-10*B*). Ectodermal thickenings called **lens placodes**, indicating the future lenses of the eyes, are visible on the sides of the head. The fourth pair of pharyngeal arches and the **lower limb buds** are visible by the end of the fourth week (see Fig. 6-7*C* and Fig. 6-12). By the end of the fourth week, the **caudal neuropore** is usually closed (see Fig. 6-10). Rudiments of many organ systems, especially the *cardiovascular system*, are established.

Fifth Week

Changes in body form are minor during the fifth week compared with those that occurred during the fourth week. **Growth of the head exceeds that of other regions** (see Fig. 6-12*A* and *B*), which is caused mainly by the rapid development of the brain and facial prominences. The face soon contacts the heart prominence. The *mesonephric ridges* indicate the site of the *mesonephric kidneys* (see Fig. 6-12*B*), which are the primordia of the permanent kidneys (see Fig. 6-12*A* and *B*).

Figure 6–8 **A,** Dorsal view of a five-somite embryo at Carnegie stage 10, approximately 22 days. Observe the neural folds and neural groove. The neural folds in the cranial region have thickened to form the primordium of the brain. **B,** Drawing of the structures shown in **A.** Most of the amniotic and chorionic sacs have been cut away to expose the embryo. **C,** Dorsal view of an older embryo at Carnegie stage 10, approximately 23 days. The neural folds have fused opposite the somites to form the neural tube (primordium of spinal cord in this region). The neural tube is in open communication with the amniotic cavity at the cranial and caudal ends through the rostral and caudal neuropores, respectively. **D,** Diagram of the structures shown in **C.** The amniotic fluid provides a buoyant medium that supports the delicate tissues of the early embryo.

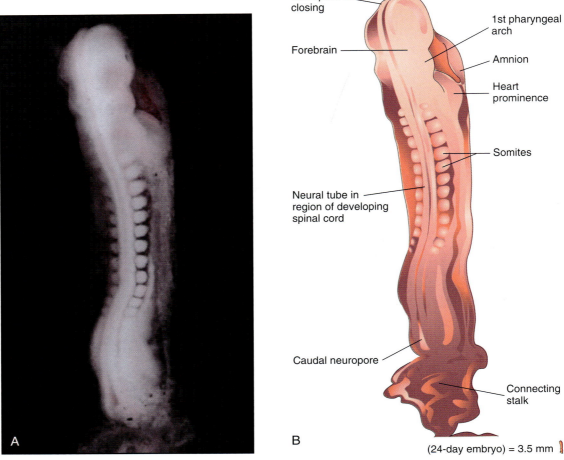

Figure 6–9   **A,** Dorsal view of a 13-somite embryo at Carnegie stage 11, approximately 24 days. The rostral neuropore is closing, but the caudal neuropore is wide open. **B,** Illustration of the structures shown in **A.** The embryo is curved because of folding of the cranial and caudal ends.

Sixth Week

Embryos in the sixth week show spontaneous movements, such as twitching of the trunk and limbs. Embryos at this stage show reflex responses to touch. The primordia of the digits (fingers)—the **digital rays**—begin to develop in the hand plates (Fig. 6-13A and B). Development of the lower limbs occurs 4 to 5 days later than that of the upper limbs.

Several small swellings—**auricular hillocks**—develop and contribute to the formation of the *auricle of the external ear*. The eyes are now obvious largely because retinal pigment has formed. The head is much larger relative to the trunk and is bent over the large **heart prominence**. This head position results from bending in the cervical (neck) region. The trunk then begins to straighten. During the sixth week, the intestines enter the extraembryonic coelom in the proximal part of the umbilical cord. This **umbilical herniation** is a normal event in the embryo, occurring because the abdominal cavity is too small at this stage to accommodate the rapidly growing intestines (see Chapter 12, Fig. 12-11C).

Seventh Week

The limbs undergo considerable change during the seventh week. Notches appear between the digital rays in the **hand plates**, partially separating the future digits. Communication between the primordial gut and the umbilical vesicle is now reduced to a relatively slender duct, the *omphaloenteric duct* (see Fig. 6-1C$_2$).

Eighth Week

At the beginning of this final week of the embryonic period, the digits of the hand are separated, but noticeably webbed (see Fig. 6-13B). Notches are clearly visible between the digital rays of the feet. The **scalp vascular plexus** has appeared and forms a characteristic band around the head. At the end of the fetal period, the digits have lengthened and are separated (Fig. 6-14A and B). *Coordinated limb movements first occur during this week.* Primary ossification begins in the femur. All evidence of the tail-like caudal eminence has disappeared by the end of the eighth week.

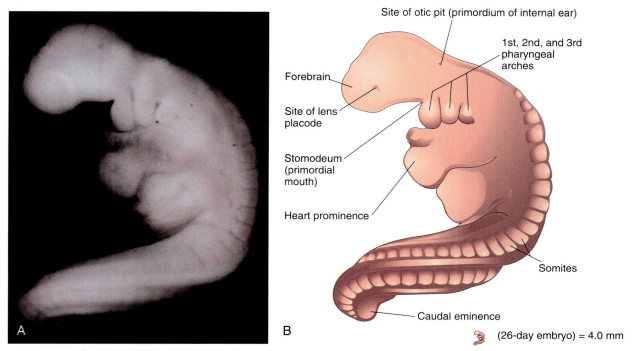

Figure 6–10 **A,** Lateral view of a 27-somite embryo at Carnegie stage 12, approximately 26 days. The embryo is curved, especially its tail-like caudal eminence. Observe the lens placode (primordium of lens of eye). The otic pit indicates early development of the internal ear. **B,** Illustration of the structures shown in **A.** The rostral neuropore is closed, and three pairs of pharyngeal arches are present. (**A,** *From Nishimura H, Semba H, Tanimura T, Tanaka O: Prenatal Development of the Human with Special Reference to Craniofacial Structures: An Atlas. Washington, DC, National Institutes of Health, 1977.*)

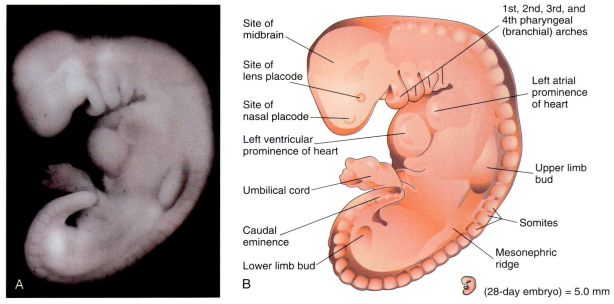

Figure 6–11 **A,** Lateral view of an embryo at Carnegie stage 13, approximately 28 days. The primordial heart is large and is divided into a primordial atrium and a ventricle. The rostral and caudal neuropores are closed. **B,** Drawing indicating the structures shown in **A.** The embryo has a characteristic C-shaped curvature, four pharyngeal arches, and upper and lower limb buds. (**A,** *From Nishimura H, Semba H, Tanimura T, Tanaka O: Prenatal Development of the Human with Special Reference to Craniofacial Structures: An Atlas. Washington, DC, National Institutes of Health, 1977.*)

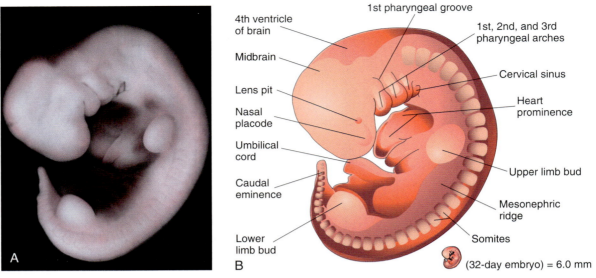

Figure 6–12 **A,** Lateral view of an embryo at Carnegie stage 14, approximately 32 days. The second pharyngeal arch has overgrown the third arch, forming the *cervical sinus*. The mesonephric ridge indicates the site of the mesonephric kidney, an interim functional kidney. **B,** Illustration of the structures shown in **A.** The upper limb buds are paddle-shaped, whereas the lower limb buds are flipper-like. (**A,** *From Nishimura H, Semba H, Tanimura T, Tanaka O: Prenatal Development of the Human with Special Reference to Craniofacial Structures: An Atlas. Washington, DC, National Institutes of Health, 1977.*)

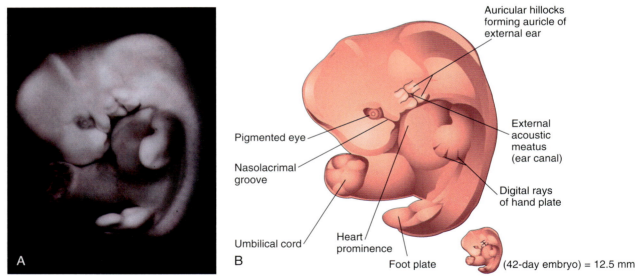

Figure 6–13 **A,** Lateral view of an embryo at Carnegie stage 17, approximately 42 days. Digital rays are visible in the hand plate, indicating the future site of the digits (fingers). **B,** Illustration of the structures shown in **A.** The eye, auricular hillocks, and external acoustic meatus are now obvious. (*From Moore KL, Persaud TVN, Shiota K: Color Atlas of Clinical Embryology, 2nd ed. Philadelphia, Saunders, 2000.*)

The hands and feet each approach each other ventrally. At the end of the eighth week, the embryo has visually distinct human characteristics; however, the head is still disproportionately large, constituting almost half of the embryo (see Fig. 6-14). The neck region is established and the eyelids are closing. By the end of the eighth week, the eyelids begin to unite by epithelial fusion. The intestines are still in the proximal portion of the umbilical cord (see Chapter 12, Fig. 12-11C). The auricles of the external ears begin to assume their final shape, but are still low-set

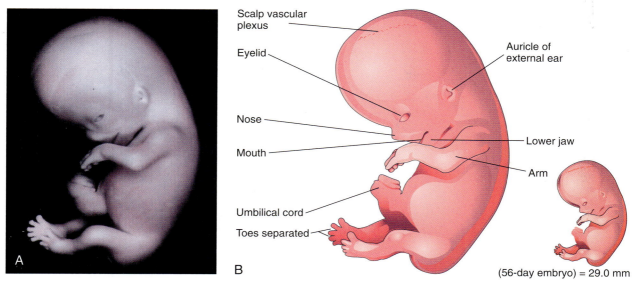

Scalp vascular plexus
Eyelid
Nose
Mouth
Umbilical cord
Toes separated
Auricle of external ear
Lower jaw
Arm

(56-day embryo) = 29.0 mm

A

B

Figure 6–14 **A,** Lateral view of an embryo at Carnegie stage 23, approximately 56 days (end of embryonic period). **B,** Illustration of the structures shown in **A.** (**A,** *From Nishimura H, Semba H, Tanimura T, Tanaka O: Prenatal Development of the Human with Special Reference to Craniofacial Structures: An Atlas. Washington, DC, National Institutes of Health, 1977.*)

on the head. Although sex differences exist in the appearance of the external genitalia, they are not distinctive enough to permit accurate sex identification.

 CLINICALLY ORIENTED QUESTIONS

1. There is little apparent difference between an 8-week embryo and a 9-week fetus. Why do embryologists give them different names?

2. When does the embryo become a human being?

3. Can the sex of embryos be determined by ultrasonography? What other methods can be used to determine sex?

The answers to these questions are at the back of this book.

Fetal Period:
The Ninth Week to Birth

D evelopment during the fetal period is concerned primarily with body growth and differentiation of tissues, organs, and systems. **Rudimentary organ systems** were formed during the embryonic period. The rate of body growth during the fetal period is rapid, and fetal weight gain is phenomenal during the terminal weeks (Table 7-1). Ultrasonographic measurements of the **crown–rump length (CRL)** can be used to determine fetal size and probable age (Fig. 7-1). The intrauterine period may be divided into days, weeks, or months (Table 7-2), but confusion arises if it is not stated whether the age is calculated from the **last normal menstrual period (LNMP)** or from the **fertilization age**. *Unless otherwise stated, fetal age in this book is calculated from the estimated time of fertilization, and months refer to calendar months.* Clinically, the gestational period is divided into **three trimesters**, each lasting 3 months. Various measurements and external characteristics are useful for estimating fetal age (see Table 7-1). Measurement of the CRL is the method of choice for estimating fetal age until the end of the *first trimester*.

Table 7–1 Criteria for Estimating Fertilization Age during the Fetal Period

AGE (weeks)	CROWN–RUMP LENGTH (mm)*	FOOT LENGTH (mm)*	FETAL WEIGHT (g)†	MAIN EXTERNAL CHARACTERISTICS
Previable Fetus				
9	50	7	8	Eyelids are closing or have closed. Head is rounded. External genitalia are still not distinguishable as male or female. Intestinal herniation is present.
10	61	9	14	Intestine is in the abdomen. Early fingernail development.
12	87	14	45	Sex is distinguishable externally. Well-defined neck.
14	120	20	110	Head is erect. Lower limbs are well developed. Early toenail development.
16	140	27	200	Auricles of the ears stand out from the head.
18	160	33	320	Vernix caseosa covers the skin. Fetal movement (quickening) is felt by the mother.
20	190	39	460	Head and body hair (lanugo) are visible.
Viable Fetus‡				
22	210	45	630	Skin is wrinkled and red.
24	230	50	820	Fingernails are present. Lean body.
26	250	55	1000	Eyes are partially open. Eyelashes are present.
28	270	59	1300	Eyes are open. Most fetuses have scalp hair. Skin is slightly wrinkled.
30	280	63	1700	Toenails are present. Body is filling out. Testes are descending.
32	300	68	2100	Fingernails extend to fingertips. Skin is smooth.
36	340	79	2900	Body is usually plump. Lanugo is almost absent. Toenails extend to the toe tips. Flexed limb; firm grasp.
38	360	83	3400	Prominent chest; breasts protrude. Testes in the scrotum or palpable in the inguinal canals. Fingernails extend beyond fingertips.

*These measurements are averages, and dimensional variations increase with age.

†These weights refer to fetuses that have been fixed for approximately 2 weeks in 10% formalin. Fresh specimens usually weigh approximately 5% less.

‡There is no sharp limit of development, age, or weight at which a fetus automatically becomes viable or beyond which survival is ensured, but experience has shown that it is uncommon for an infant to survive if its weight is less than 500 g or if its fertilization age or developmental age is less than 22 weeks.

Figure 7–1 Endovaginal scan of a 9-week fetus with a crown–rump length of 41.7 mm *(calipers)*. Chorionic cavity *(CC)* has low-level echoes normally, while the amniotic cavity *(AC)* is echo-free.

HIGHLIGHTS OF FETAL PERIOD

There is no formal staging system for the fetal period; however, it is helpful to consider the main changes that occur in periods of 4 to 9 weeks.

Nine to Twelve Weeks

At the beginning of the ninth week, *the head constitutes half of the CRL of the fetus* (see Fig. 7-1). Subsequently, growth in body length accelerates rapidly so that, by the end of 12 weeks, the CRL has almost doubled (see Table 7-1).

At 9 weeks, the face is broad, the eyes are widely separated, the ears are low set, and the eyelids are fused. Early in the ninth week, the legs are short and the thighs are relatively small. By the end of 12 weeks, the upper limbs have almost reached their final relative lengths, but the lower limbs are still slightly shorter than their final relative lengths.

The ***external genitalia*** of males and females are not fully developed until the end of the 12th week. Intestinal

Table 7–2 Comparison of Gestational Time Units

	CALENDAR			LUNAR
REFERENCE POINT	DAYS	WEEKS	MONTHS	MONTHS
Fertilization	266	38	8.75	9.5
Last normal menstrual period	280	40	9.25	10

Figure 7–2 An 11-week fetus that was spontaneously aborted (×1.5). Its chorionic and amniotic sacs have been removed. Note that the head is relatively large.

coils are clearly visible in the proximal end of the umbilical cord until the middle of the 10th week. By the 11th week, *the intestines have returned to the abdomen* (Fig. 7-2). Urine formation begins between the 9th and 12th weeks, and urine is discharged through the urethra into the amniotic fluid. The fetus reabsorbs some of this fluid after swallowing it. Fetal waste products in blood are transferred to the maternal circulation by passing across the placental membrane (see Chapter 8).

Thirteen to Sixteen Weeks

Growth is very rapid during this period (Fig. 7-3 and Fig. 7-4; see Table 7-1). By 16 weeks, the head is relatively small compared with that of the 12-week fetus, and the lower limbs have lengthened. *Limb movements*, which

first occur at the end of the embryonic period, become coordinated by the 14th week, but they are too slight to be felt by the mother. However, these movements are visible during ultrasonographic examinations.

By the beginning of the 16th week, the developing bones are clearly visible on ultrasound images. *Slow eye movements* occur at 14 weeks. Scalp hair patterning is also determined during this period. By 16 weeks, the ovaries are differentiated and contain *primordial ovarian follicles* that have **oogonia** (primordial germ cells). The eyes face anteriorly rather than anterolaterally.

Seventeen to Twenty Weeks

Growth slows down during this period, but the fetus still increases its CRL by approximately 50 mm (see Fig. 7-3 and Fig. 7-5; see Table 7-1). *Fetal movements—quickening—*are commonly felt by the mother. The skin is now covered with a greasy material—**vernix caseosa.** It consists of dead epidermal cells and a fatty secretion from the *fetal sebaceous glands.* The vernix caseosa protects the delicate fetal skin from abrasions, chapping, and hardening that could result from exposure to the amniotic fluid. Fetuses are usually completely covered with fine, downy hair—*lanugo*—that helps to hold the vernix on the skin.

Eyebrows and head hair are also visible. *Brown fat* forms during weeks 17 through 20 and is the site of heat production, particularly in the neonate. This specialized adipose tissue, found chiefly at the neck, posterior to the sternum, produces heat by oxidizing fatty acids.

By 18 weeks, the **fetal uterus** is formed and canalization of the vagina has begun. By 20 weeks, the testes have begun to descend, but they are still located on the posterior abdominal wall.

Twenty-One to Twenty-Five Weeks

Substantial weight gain occurs during this period, and the fetus is better proportioned. The skin is usually wrinkled and more translucent. The skin is pink to red because blood is visible in the capillaries. At 21 weeks, rapid eye movements begin, and *blink-startle responses* have been reported at 22 to 23 weeks. *Fingernails* are present by 24 weeks. Also by 24 weeks, the secretory epithelial cells (type II pneumocytes) in the interalveolar walls of the lung have begun to secrete **surfactant,** a surface-active lipid that maintains the patency of the developing alveoli of the lungs (see Chapter 11). Although a 22- to 25-week fetus born prematurely may survive initially if given intensive care support; however, the fetus may die because its respiratory system is still immature. Fetuses born

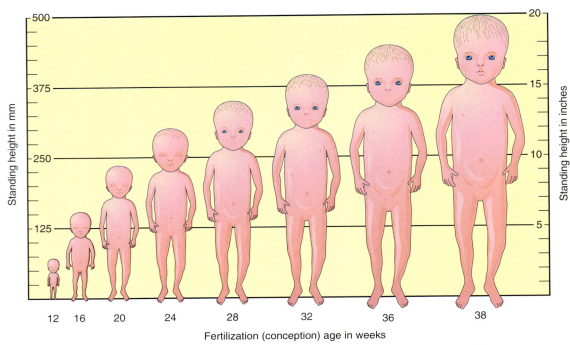

Figure 7–3   Diagram drawn to scale illustrating the changes in size of human fetuses.

Figure 7–4   A 13-week fetus. **A,** An enlarged photograph of the head and shoulders (×2). **B,** Actual size.

before 26 weeks of gestation have a high risk of neuro-developmental (functional) disability.

Twenty-Six to Twenty-Nine Weeks

During this period, fetuses usually survive if born prematurely and given intensive care because the lungs have developed sufficiently to provide adequate gas exchange.

In addition, the central nervous system has matured to the stage at which it can direct rhythmic breathing movements and control body temperature. The highest neonatal mortality occurs in low-birth-weight infants weighing 2500 g or less. *The eyelids are open at 26 weeks* and lanugo and head hair are well developed. Toenails are visible and considerable subcutaneous fat is now present, smoothing out many of the skin wrinkles.

Figure 7–5 **A,** A 17-week fetus (actual size). Fetuses at this age are unable to survive if born prematurely, mainly because the respiratory system is immature. **B,** Magnetic resonance imaging scan of an 18-week-old normal fetus (20 weeks' gestational age). (**A,** *From Moore KL, Persaud TVN, Shiota K: Color Atlas of Clinical Embryology, 2nd ed. Philadelphia, Saunders, 2000.*)

Thirty to Thirty-Eight Weeks

The *pupillary light reflex of the eyes* can be elicited at 30 weeks. Usually, by the end of this period, the skin is pink and smooth and the upper and lower limbs have a chubby appearance. Fetuses born at 32 weeks usually survive. Fetuses at 35 weeks have a firm grasp and exhibit a spontaneous orientation to light. As term approaches (37–38 weeks), the nervous system is sufficiently mature to carry out some integrative functions. Most fetuses during this "finishing period" are plump (Fig. 7-6). At 36 weeks, the circumferences of the head and abdomen are approximately equal. Growth slows as the time of birth approaches (Fig. 7-7). Most fetuses weigh approximately 3400 g at term (Fig. 7-8). A fetus adds approximately 14 g of fat daily during the last weeks of gestation. The chest is prominent, and the breasts protrude slightly in both sexes.

Expected Date of Delivery

The expected date of delivery of a fetus is 266 days, or 38 weeks, after fertilization (i.e., 280 days or 40 weeks after the LNMP) (see Table 7-2). Approximately 12% of babies are born 1 to 2 weeks after the expected time of birth.

FACTORS INFLUENCING FETAL GROWTH

The fetus requires substrates for growth and production of energy. Gases and nutrients pass freely to the fetus from the mother through the **placental membrane** (see

Figure 7–6 A healthy male neonate at 36 weeks' gestational age.

Chapter 8). **Glucose** is a primary source of energy for fetal metabolism and growth; **amino acids** are also required. **Insulin** is required for the metabolism of glucose and is secreted by the fetal pancreas. Insulin, human growth hormone, and some small polypeptides (e.g., insulin-like growth factor I) are believed to stimulate fetal growth.

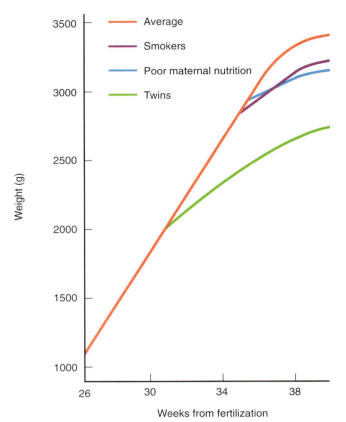

Figure 7–7 Graph showing the rate of fetal growth during the last trimester. After 36 weeks, the average growth rate deviates from the straight line. The decline, particularly after full term (38 weeks), probably reflects inadequate fetal nutrition caused by placental changes. Other factors affecting fetal growth rate (smoking, maternal malnutrition, twins) are also shown. (*Modified from Gruenwald P: Growth of the human fetus. I. Normal growth and its variation. Am J Obstet Gynecol 94:1112, 1966.*)

Many factors—maternal, fetal, and environmental—may affect prenatal growth. **In general, factors operating throughout pregnancy, such as *cigarette smoking* and *consumption of alcohol*,** tend to produce **intrauterine growth restriction** (IUGR) and small neonates, whereas factors operating during the last trimester (e.g., maternal malnutrition) usually produce underweight neonates with normal length and head size. Severe maternal malnutrition resulting from a poor-quality diet is known to cause reduced fetal growth (see Fig. 7-7).

Neonates (newborns) resulting from twin, triplet, and other multiple pregnancies usually weigh considerably less than infants resulting from a single pregnancy (see Fig. 7-7). It is evident that the total requirements of two or more fetuses exceed the nutritional supply available from the placenta during the third trimester.

Repeated cases of IUGR in one family indicate that recessive genes may be the cause of the abnormal growth. In recent years, structural and numeric chromosomal aberrations have also been shown to be associated with cases of restricted fetal growth. IUGR is pronounced in neonates with trisomy 21 (Down syndrome) (see Chapter 19).

Figure 7–8 Full-term female neonate weighing 3.3 kg (7.2 lb). Note the fatty vernix caseosa covering part of her body.

Lower birth weight has been shown to be a risk factor for many adult diseases, including hypertension, diabetes, and cardiovascular disease. Higher birth weight resulting from gestational diabetes is associated with adult obesity and diabetes.

PROCEDURES FOR ASSESSING FETAL STATUS

Ultrasonography

Ultrasonography is the primary imaging modality in the evaluation of the fetus because of its wide availability, quality of images, low cost, and lack of known adverse effects (Fig. 7-9). Placental and fetal size, multiple births, abnormalities of placental shape, and abnormal presentations can also be determined. Many developmental anomalies can also be detected prenatally by ultrasonography.

Diagnostic Amniocentesis

Diagnostic amniocentesis is a common invasive prenatal diagnostic procedure (Fig. 7-10*A*) typically performed during the second trimester. For prenatal diagnosis, amniotic fluid is sampled by insertion of a hollow needle through the mother's anterior abdominal and uterine walls and into the amniotic sac. A syringe is then attached to the needle and amniotic fluid is withdrawn. The procedure is relatively devoid of risk, especially when performed by an experienced physician using ultrasonography as a guide for outlining the position of the fetus and placenta.

Chorionic Villus Sampling

Biopsy of chorionic villi (see Fig. 7-10B) is performed to detect chromosomal abnormalities, inborn errors of metabolism, and X-linked disorders. Chorionic villus sampling can be performed as early as 7 weeks after fertilization. The rate of fetal loss is approximately 1%,

Figure 7–9 Ultrasonogram (axial scan) of a 25-week fetus showing the facial profile.

slightly more than the risk associated with amniocentesis (0.5%). The major advantage of chorionic villus sampling over amniocentesis is that it allows fetal chromosomal sampling to be performed several weeks earlier.

Cell Cultures

Fetal sex and chromosomal aberrations can also be determined by studying the sex chromosomes in cultured fetal cells obtained during amniocentesis. The cultures are commonly performed when an autosomal abnormality, such as occurs in Down syndrome, is suspected. Inborn errors of metabolism and enzyme deficiencies in fetuses can also be detected by studying cell cultures.

Percutaneous Umbilical Cord Blood Sampling

For chromosomal analysis, blood samples may be obtained from the umbilical vein by **percutaneous umbilical cord blood sampling (PUBS)**. Ultrasonographic scanning is used to outline the location of the vessels. PUBS is often performed approximately 20 weeks after the LNMP to obtain samples for chromosomal analysis when ultrasound or other examinations have shown characteristics of birth defects.

Magnetic Resonance Imaging

When fetal treatment, such as surgery, is planned, computed tomography and **magnetic resonance imaging (MRI)** may be used. MRI has the advantage of not requiring ionizing radiation to produce images. These studies

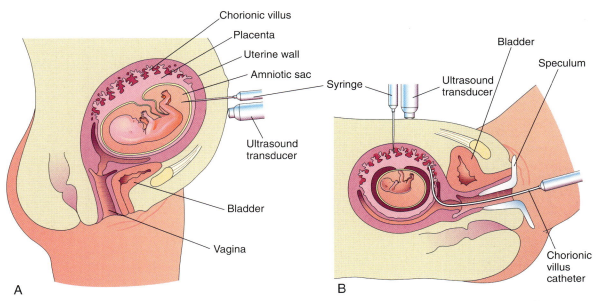

A

B

Figure 7–10 **A,** Illustration of the technique of amniocentesis. Using ultrasonographic guidance, a needle is inserted through the mother's abdominal and uterine walls into the amniotic sac. A syringe is attached and amniotic fluid is withdrawn for diagnostic purposes. **B,** Illustration of chorionic villus sampling. Two sampling approaches are shown—one through the anterior abdominal wall and amniotic sac using a needle, and one through the vagina and cervical canal using a malleable chorionic villus catheter.

can provide additional information about a fetal abnormality detected by ultrasound.

Fetal Monitoring

Continuous fetal heart rate monitoring in high-risk pregnancies is routine and provides information about the oxygenation of the fetus. *Fetal distress*, as indicated by an abnormal heart rate or rhythm, suggests that the fetus is in jeopardy.

Alpha-Fetoprotein Assay

Alpha fetoprotein (AFP), a glycoprotein that is synthesized in the fetal liver and umbilical vesicle, escapes from the fetal circulation into the amniotic fluid in fetuses with an open neural tube defects, such as spina bifida with myeloschisis (see Chapter 19). AFP can also enter the amniotic fluid from open ventral wall defects, as occurs with gastroschisis and omphalocele (see Chapter 13). AFP can also be measured in maternal serum.

Noninvasive Prenatal Diagnosis

Down syndrome (trisomy 21) is the most commonly known of the chromosomal disorders, and children born with this condition have varying degrees of intellectual disability. Noninvasive screening for trisomy 21 is based on the isolation of fetal cells in maternal blood and the detection of cell-free fetal DNA and RNA. Compared to amniocentesis and chorionic villus biopsy, the results are available earlier and there are fewer complications. The methodology of this DNA-based diagnostic test continues to evolve and be refined to improve its reliability.

NEONATAL PERIOD

The neonatal period pertains to the first 4 weeks after birth. The *early neonatal period* is from birth to 7 days.

The **neonate** (newborn) is not a miniature adult, and an extremely preterm infant is not the same as full-term infant. The *late neonatal period* is from 7 to 28 days. The umbilical cord usually drops off 7 to 8 days after birth, the end of the early neonatal period.

At birth, the head of a neonate is large in proportion to the rest of its body. Thereafter, the head grows more slowly than the trunk (torso) of the body. Usually a neonate loses about 10% of its birth weight 3 to 4 days after birth, owing to the loss of excess extracellular fluid and discharge of *meconium*, the first greenish intestinal material ejected from the rectum.

When the neonate's hand is touched, it will usually grasp a finger. If the mother holds the baby close to her chest, the baby will search (root) for her breast to find the nipple and feed. Neonates are born with full visual capacity to see objects and colors about 8 to 15 inches away; however, they are extremely nearsighted. Some *preterm neonates' eyes* are crossed because the eye muscles are not fully developed. A gentle stroke on the baby's cheek makes the baby turn toward the touch with its mouth open.

CLINICALLY ORIENTED QUESTIONS

1. Do mature embryos move at all? Can a first-trimester fetus move its limbs? If so, can the mother feel her baby kicking at this time?

2. Some reports suggest that vitamin supplementation around the time of conception will prevent neural tube defects, such as spina bifida. Is there scientific proof to support this statement?

3. Can the needle injure the fetus during amniocentesis? Is there a risk of inducing an abortion or causing maternal or fetal infection?

The answers to these questions are at the back of this book.

8

Placenta and Fetal Membranes

T he fetal part of the placenta and fetal membranes separate the embryo or fetus from the **endometrium**—the inner layer of the uterine wall. The chorion, amnion, umbilical vesicle, and allantois constitute the fetal membranes. An interchange of substances (e.g., nutrients and oxygen) occurs between the maternal and fetal blood through the placenta. The vessels in the umbilical cord connect the placental circulation with the fetal circulation.

PLACENTA

The placenta is the primary site of nutrient and gas exchange between the mother and fetus. The placenta is a **fetomaternal organ** that has two components:

- A **fetal part** that develops from part of the chorionic sac
- A **maternal part** that is derived from the endometrium, the mucous membrane comprising the inner layer of the uterine wall

The placenta and umbilical cord form a *transport system* for substances passing between the mother and fetus. Nutrients and oxygen pass from the maternal blood through the placenta to the fetal blood, and waste materials and carbon dioxide pass from the fetal blood through the placenta to the maternal blood. *The placenta and fetal membranes perform the following functions and activities:* protection, nutrition, respiration, excretion of waste products, and hormone production. Shortly after birth, the placenta and fetal membranes are expelled from the uterus as the ***afterbirth (extruded waste products).***

Decidua

The *decidua* is the endometrium of the uterus in a pregnant woman. It is the functional layer of the endometrium that separates from the remainder of the uterus after ***parturition*** (childbirth). The **three regions of the decidua** are named according to their relation to the implantation site (Fig. 8-1):

- **Decidua basalis**—the part of the decidua deep to the conceptus (embryo and membranes) that forms the maternal part of the placenta
- **Decidua capsularis**—the superficial part of the decidua overlying the conceptus
- **Decidua parietalis**—the remaining intervening parts of the decidua

In response to increasing ***progesterone levels*** in the maternal blood, the connective tissue cells of the decidua enlarge to form pale-staining **decidual cells**. These cells enlarge as glycogen and lipid accumulate in their cytoplasm. The cellular and vascular changes in the decidua that result from pregnancy are referred to as the **decidual reaction**. Many decidual cells degenerate near the chorionic sac in the region of the syncytiotrophoblast and, together with maternal blood and uterine secretions, provide a rich source of nutrition for the embryo. *Decidual regions, clearly recognizable during ultrasonography, are important in diagnosing early pregnancy.*

Development of Placenta

Early placental development is characterized by the rapid proliferation of the trophoblast and development of the chorionic sac and chorionic villi. By the end of the third week, the anatomical arrangements necessary for physiologic exchanges between the mother and embryo have been established. By the end of the fourth week, a complex vascular network develops in the placenta, allowing maternal-embryonic exchanges of gases, nutrients, and metabolic waste products.

Chorionic villi cover the entire chorionic sac until the beginning of the eighth week (see Fig. 8-1*D* and Fig. 8-2). As this sac grows, the villi associated with the decidua capsularis are compressed, reducing the blood supply to them. These villi soon degenerate, producing a relatively avascular bare area, the **smooth chorion** (see Fig. 8-1*D*). As these villi disappear, those associated with the decidua basalis rapidly increase in number, branch profusely, and enlarge (Fig. 8-3). This bushy part of the chorionic sac is the **villous chorion**, or **chorion frondosum** (see Fig. 8-1*E* and Fig. 8-4).

Homeobox genes (HLX *and* DLX3*) expressed on the trophoblast and blood vessels help to regulate the development of the placenta.*

ULTRASONOGRAPHY OF CHORIONIC SAC

The size of the chorionic sac is useful in determining the gestational age of embryos in patients with uncertain menstrual histories. Growth of the chorionic sac is extremely rapid between the 5th and 10th weeks of development. Modern ultrasound devices permit detection of the chorionic sac when it has a median diameter of 2 to 3 mm (see Fig. 8-4). Chorionic sacs with this diameter indicate a gestational age of approximately 18 days after fertilization.

Fetomaternal Junction

The *fetal part of the placenta* (villous chorion) is attached to the *maternal part of the placenta* (decidua basalis) by the **cytotrophoblastic shell**, the external layer of trophoblastic cells on the maternal surface of the placenta (Fig. 8-5). The chorionic villi attach firmly to the decidua basalis through the cytotrophoblastic shell and anchor the chorionic sac to the decidua basalis. **Endometrial arteries and veins** pass freely through gaps in the cytotrophoblastic shell and open into the *intervillous space* (see Fig. 8-5).

The **shape of the placenta** is determined by the shape of the persistent area of chorionic villi (see Fig. 8-1*F*). Usually this is a circular area, giving the placenta a discoid shape. As the chorionic villi invade the decidua basalis during placental formation, decidual tissue is eroded to enlarge the intervillous space. This erosion produces several wedge-shaped areas of decidua—**placental septa**—that project toward the **chorionic plate** (see Fig. 8-5). The placental septa divide the fetal part of the placenta into irregular convex areas—**cotyledons** (see Fig. 8-3). Each cotyledon consists of two or more **stem villi** and many **branch villi**.

The **decidua capsularis**, the layer overlying the implanted chorionic sac, forms a capsule over the external surface of the sac (see Fig. 8-1*A* to *D*). As the conceptus enlarges, the decidua capsularis bulges into the uterine cavity and becomes greatly attenuated. Eventually, parts of the **decidua capsularis** make contact and fuse with the **decidua parietalis**, thereby slowly obliterating the uterine cavity (see Fig. 8-1*E* and *F*). By 22 to 24 weeks, reduced blood supply to the decidua capsularis causes it to degenerate and disappear.

Intervillous Space

This space of the placenta contains maternal blood, which is derived from the lacunae that developed in the syncytiotrophoblast during the second week of development (see Chapter 4, Fig. 4-1*B*). The large, blood-filled space results from the coalescence and enlargement of the **lacunar networks**. The intervillous space is divided into compartments by the ***placental septa***; however, free communication occurs between the compartments because the septa do not reach the **chorionic plate** (see Fig. 8-5), the part of the chorion associated with the placenta.

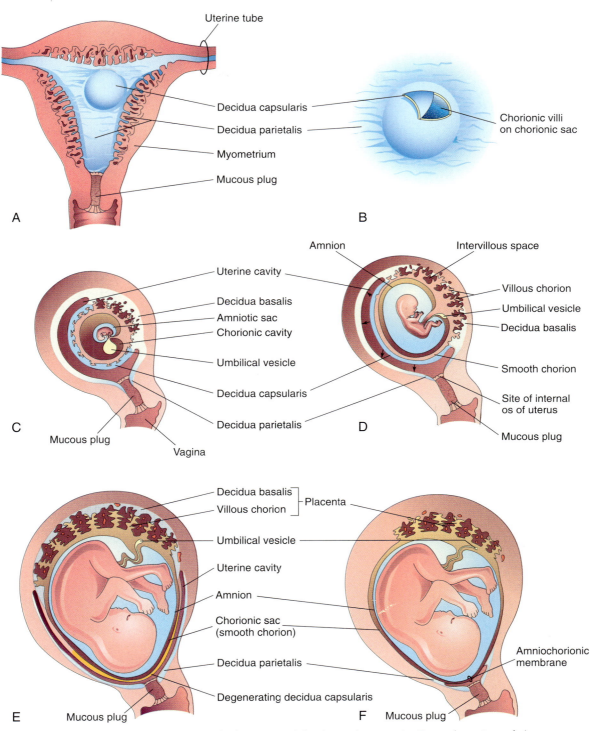

Figure 8–1 Development of placenta and fetal membranes. **A,** Coronal section of the uterus showing elevation of the decidua capsularis and the expanding chorionic sac at 4 weeks. **B,** Enlarged illustration of the implantation site. The chorionic villi were exposed by cutting an opening in the decidua capsularis. **C** to **F,** Sagittal sections of the gravid (pregnant) uterus from the 5th to 22nd weeks, showing the changing relationship of the fetal membranes to the decidua. In **F,** the amnion and chorion are fused with each other and with the decidua parietalis, thereby obliterating the uterine cavity.

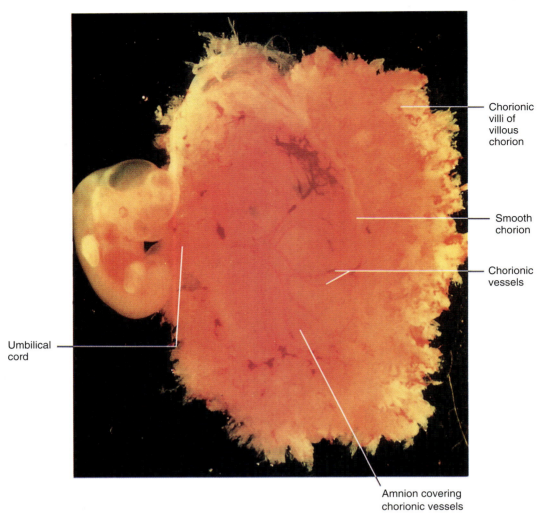

Chorionic
villi of
villous
chorion

Smooth
chorion

Chorionic
vessels

Umbilical
cord

Amnion covering
chorionic vessels

Figure 8–2   Lateral view of a spontaneously aborted embryo at Carnegie stage 14, approximately 32 days. The chorionic and amniotic sacs have been opened to show the embryo.

Maternal blood enters the intervillous space from the **spiral arteries** in the decidua basalis (see Fig. 8-5); these arteries pass through gaps in the cytotrophoblastic shell and discharge blood into the **intervillous space**. This large space is drained by endometrial veins that also penetrate the cytotrophoblastic shell. The numerous **branch villi**, arising from **stem villi**, are continuously showered with maternal blood as it circulates through the intervillous space. The blood in this space carries oxygen and nutritional materials that are necessary for fetal growth and development. The maternal blood also contains fetal waste products, such as carbon dioxide, salts, and products of protein metabolism.

Amniochorionic Membrane

The amniotic sac enlarges faster than the chorionic sac. As a result, the amnion and smooth chorion soon fuse to form the **amniochorionic membrane** (see Fig. 8-1F). This composite membrane fuses with the decidua capsularis and, after disappearance of this part of the decidua, adheres to the decidua parietalis. *It is the amniochorionic membrane that ruptures during labor.* Preterm rupture of this membrane is the most common event leading to premature labor. When the amniochorionic membrane ruptures, the amniotic fluid escapes through the cervix and vagina.

Placental Circulation

The many *branch chorionic villi* of the placenta provide a large surface area where materials (e.g., oxygen, and nutrients) are exchanged across the very thin **placental membrane** interposed between the fetal and maternal circulations (Fig. 8-6B and C). It is through the branch villi that the main exchange of material between the mother and the fetus takes place. The placental membrane consists of extrafetal tissues.

Fetoplacental Circulation

Poorly oxygenated blood leaves the fetus and passes through the **umbilical arteries** (see Fig. 8-5 and Fig. 8-7). At the attachment of the umbilical cord to the placenta, these arteries divide into a number of radially disposed

Figure 8–3   A human chorionic sac containing a 13-week fetus that aborted spontaneously. The villous chorion is where chorionic villi persist and form the fetal part of the placenta. In situ, the cotyledons were attached to the decidua basalis and the intervillous space was filled with maternal blood.

Figure 8–4   Endovaginal axial scan of a gravid uterus showing a 3-week chorionic sac *(arrow)* in the posterior endometrium (decidua). There is a bright (echogenic) ring of chorionic villi *(open arrows)* around the sac. *M,* Myometrium.

chorionic arteries that branch freely in the **chorionic plate** before entering the chorionic villi (see Fig. 8-5). The blood vessels form an extensive **arteriocapillary venous system** within the chorionic villi (see Fig. 8-6*A*), which brings the fetal blood extremely close to the maternal

blood (see Fig. 8-7). This system provides a very large surface area for the exchange of metabolic and gaseous products between the maternal and fetal blood. *Normally, no intermingling of fetal and maternal blood occurs.* The well-oxygenated fetal blood in the fetal capillaries passes into thin-walled veins that follow the chorionic arteries to the site of attachment of the umbilical cord, where they converge to form the **umbilical vein**. This large vessel carries oxygen-rich blood to the fetus (see Fig. 8-5).

Maternal-Placental Circulation

The maternal blood enters the intervillous space through 80 to 100 **spiral endometrial arteries** in the decidua basalis (see Fig. 8-5). The entering blood is at considerably higher pressure than that in the intervillous space, so the blood spurts toward the **chorionic plate**. As the pressure dissipates, the blood flows slowly around the branch villi, allowing an exchange of metabolic and gaseous products with the fetal blood. The blood eventually returns through the endometrial veins to the maternal circulation (see Fig. 8-7). Reductions of uteroplacental circulation result in **fetal hypoxia** (decreased level of oxygen) and **intrauterine growth restriction**. The intervillous space of the mature placenta contains approximately 150 ml of blood that is replenished three or four times each minute.

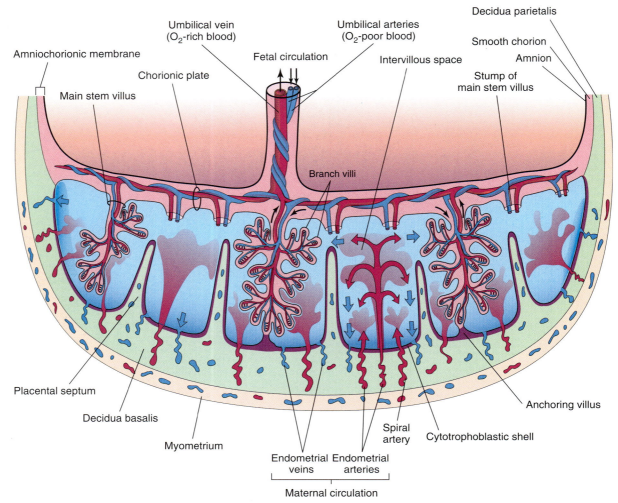

Figure 8–5 Illustration of a transverse section through a full-term placenta, showing (1) the relation of the villous chorion (fetal part of placenta) to the decidua basalis (maternal part of placenta); (2) the fetal placental circulation; and (3) the maternal-placental circulation. Maternal blood flows into the intervillous spaces in funnel-shaped spurts from the spiral arteries, and exchanges occur with the fetal blood as the maternal blood flows around the branch villi. The inflowing arterial blood pushes venous blood out of the intervillous space and into the endometrial veins. Note that the umbilical arteries carry poorly oxygenated fetal blood (shown in *blue*) to the placenta and that the umbilical vein carries oxygenated blood (shown in *red*) to the fetus. Only one stem villus is shown in each cotyledon, but the stumps of those that have been removed are indicated. *Arrows* indicate direction of maternal (*red* and *blue*) and fetal (*black*) blood flow.

Placental Membrane

The membrane consists of the extrafetal tissues that separate the maternal and fetal blood. Until about 20 weeks, *the placental membrane consists of four layers* (see Fig. 8-6B and C): syncytiotrophoblast, cytotrophoblast, connective tissue of the villus, and endothelium of the fetal capillaries. After the 20th week, microscopic changes occur in the branch villi that result in the cytotrophoblast becoming attenuated in many villi.

Eventually, cytotrophoblastic cells disappear over large areas of the villi, leaving only thin patches of syncytiotrophoblast. As a result, the placental membrane at full term consists of only three layers in most places (see Fig. 8-6C). In some areas, the placental membrane becomes markedly thinned. At these sites, the syncytiotrophoblast comes in direct contact with the endothelium of the fetal capillaries to form a *vasculosyncytial placental membrane.*

Only a few substances, endogenous or exogenous, are unable to pass through the placental membrane. In this regard, the membrane acts as a true barrier only when the molecule or organism has a certain size, configuration, and charge. *Most drugs and other substances in the maternal plasma pass through the placental membrane and are found in the fetal plasma* (see Fig. 8-7).

During the third trimester, numerous nuclei in the syncytiotrophoblast of the villi aggregate to form **syncytial knots**—*nuclear aggregations* (see Fig. 8-6C). These knots

Figure 8–6 **A,** Illustration of a stem chorionic villus showing its arteriocapillary-venous system. The arteries carry poorly oxygenated fetal blood and waste products from the fetus, whereas the vein carries oxygenated blood and nutrients to the fetus. **B** and **C,** Sections through a branch villus at 10 weeks' gestation and at full term, respectively. The placental membrane, composed of extrafetal tissues, separates the maternal blood in the intervillous space from the fetal blood in the capillaries in the villi. Note that the placental membrane becomes very thin at full term. Hofbauer cells **(B)** are believed to be phagocytic cells.

regularly break off and are carried from the intervillous space into the maternal circulation. Some knots may lodge in capillaries of the maternal lungs, where they are rapidly destroyed by local enzyme action. Toward the end of pregnancy, **fibrinoid material** forms on the surfaces of villi (see Fig. 8-6C).

Functions of Placenta

The placenta has many functions:

- Metabolism (e.g., synthesis of glycogen)
- Transport of gases and nutrients as well as drugs and infectious agents
- Protection by maternal antibodies
- Excretion of waste products
- Endocrine synthesis and secretion (e.g., human chorionic gonadotropin)

Placental Metabolism

The placenta synthesizes glycogen, cholesterol, and fatty acids, which serve as sources of nutrients and energy for the embryo or fetus. Many of the metabolic activities of the placenta are critical for two of its other major activities: transport and endocrine secretion.

Placental Transport

The large surface area of the placental membrane facilitates the transport of substances in both directions between the placenta and the maternal blood. Almost all materials are transported across the placental membrane by one of the following **four main transport mechanisms:** simple diffusion, facilitated diffusion, active transport, and pinocytosis.

Passive transport by simple diffusion is usually characteristic of substances moving from areas of higher to lower concentration until equilibrium is established. *Facilitated diffusion* requires a transporter but no energy. *Active transport* against a concentration gradient requires energy. This mechanism of transport may involve carrier molecules that temporarily combine with the substances to be transported. *Pinocytosis* is a form of endocytosis in which the material being engulfed is a small amount of extracellular fluid. Some proteins are transferred very slowly through the placenta by pinocytosis.

Transfer of Gases. Oxygen, carbon dioxide, and carbon monoxide cross the placental membrane by simple diffusion. *Interruption of oxygen transport for several minutes endangers the survival of the embryo or fetus.* The efficiency of the placental membrane approaches that

Figure 8–7   Transport across the placental membrane. The extrafetal tissues, across which transport of substances between the mother and fetus occurs, collectively constitute the placental membrane. *IgG*, Immunoglobulin G; *IgM*, immunoglobulin M; *IgS*, immunoglobulin S.

of the lungs for gas exchange. The quantity of oxygen reaching the fetus is generally flow-limited, rather than diffusion-limited. **Fetal hypoxia** results primarily from factors that diminish either uterine blood flow or fetal blood flow through the placenta. Nitrous oxide, an inhalation analgesic and anesthetic, also readily crosses the placenta.

Nutritional Substances. *Nutrients constitute the bulk of substances transferred from the mother to the embryo or fetus. Water* is rapidly exchanged by simple diffusion and in increasing amounts as pregnancy advances. *Glucose* produced by the mother and placenta is quickly transferred to the embryo or fetus by facilitated diffusion mediated primarily by GLUT-1—an insulin-independent glucose carrier. Maternal cholesterol, triglycerides, and phospholipids are transferred. Although free fatty acids are transported, the amount transferred appears to be relatively small with a preference toward long-chain polyunsaturated fatty acids. *Amino acids* cross the placenta to the fetus in high concentrations by active transport. *Vitamins* cross the placental membrane and are essential for normal development. A maternal protein, *transferrin*, crosses the placental membrane and carries iron to the embryo or fetus. The placental surface contains special receptors for this protein.

Hormones. *Protein hormones* such as insulin and pituitary hormones do not reach the embryo or fetus in significant amounts, except for a slow transfer of thyroxine and triiodothyronine. Unconjugated *steroid hormones* cross the placental membrane relatively freely. **Testosterone** and certain synthetic progestins also cross the placenta (see Chapter 19).

Electrolytes. These compounds are freely exchanged in significant quantities, each at its own rate. When a mother receives intravenous fluids with electrolytes, they also pass to the fetus and affect the fetal water and electrolyte status.

Drugs and Drug Metabolites. Most drugs and drug metabolites cross the placenta by simple diffusion. **Drugs taken by the mother can affect the embryo or fetus, directly or indirectly,** by interfering with maternal or placental metabolism. **Some drugs cause major birth defects** (see Chapter 19). *Fetal drug addiction* may occur after maternal use of drugs such as heroin, and *neonates may experience withdrawal symptoms.* Most drugs used for the management of labor readily cross the placental membrane. Depending on the dose and timing in relation to delivery, these drugs may cause respiratory depression of the neonate. Neuromuscular blocking agents such as succinylcholine, which might be used during operative obstetrics, cross the placenta in only very small amounts. All sedatives and analgesics affect the fetus to some degree. Inhaled anesthetics can also cross the placental membrane and affect fetal breathing if used during parturition.

Infectious Agents. Cytomegalovirus, rubella, and coxsackieviruses, as well as viruses associated with variola, varicella, measles, and poliomyelitis, may pass through the placental membrane and cause *fetal infection*. In some cases, as with the **rubella virus**, severe birth defects may result (see Chapter 19). *Treponema pallidum* can cause fetal syphilis, and *Toxoplasma gondii* can produce destructive changes in the brain and eyes of the fetus.

Placental Protection by Maternal Antibodies

The fetus produces only small amounts of antibodies because of its **immature immune system**. Some passive immunity is conferred on the fetus by placental transfer of maternal antibodies. Only immunoglobulin G is transferred across the placenta (receptor-mediated transcytosis). *Maternal antibodies confer fetal immunity for diseases such as diphtheria, smallpox, and measles;* however, no immunity is acquired to **pertussis** (whooping cough) or **varicella** (chickenpox).

Placental Excretion of Waste Products

Urea, a nitrogenous waste product, and uric acid pass through the placental membrane by simple diffusion. Conjugated bilirubin (which is fat soluble) is easily transported by the placenta and is quickly cleared.

Placental Endocrine Synthesis and Secretion

Using precursors derived from the fetus, the mother, or both, the *syncytiotrophoblast* of the placenta synthesizes protein and steroid hormones. **Protein hormones** synthesized by the placenta include the following:

- Human chorionic gonadotropin (hCG)
- Human chorionic somatomammotropin (human placental lactogen)
- Human chorionic thyrotropin
- Human chorionic corticotropin

The glycoprotein **hCG**, similar to luteinizing hormone, is first secreted by the syncytiotrophoblast during the second week of development. The *hCG maintains the corpus luteum*, preventing the onset of menstrual periods.

HEMOLYTIC DISEASE OF THE NEONATE

Small amounts of fetal blood may pass to the maternal blood through microscopic breaks in the placental membrane. If the fetus is Rh-positive and the mother is Rh-negative, the fetal cells may stimulate the formation of anti-Rh antibody by the mother's immune system. This antibody passes to the fetal blood and causes hemolysis of fetal Rh-positive blood cells and anemia in the fetus. Some fetuses with **hemolytic disease** of the neonate, or **fetal erythroblastosis**, do not make a satisfactory intrauterine adjustment. They may die unless delivered early or given intraperitoneal or intravenous transfusions of packed Rh-negative blood cells to maintain them until after birth. Hemolytic disease of the neonate is relatively uncommon now because $Rh_0(D)$ immune globulin given to the mother usually prevents development of this disease in the fetus.

The concentration of hCG in the maternal blood and urine rises to a maximum by the eighth week and then declines. The placenta also plays a major role in the production of **steroid hormones** (i.e., progesterone and estrogens). *Progesterone is essential for the maintenance of pregnancy.*

Uterine Growth During Pregnancy

The uterus of a nonpregnant woman is in the pelvis. It increases in size during pregnancy to accommodate the growing fetus. As the uterus enlarges, it increases in weight and its walls become thinner. During the first trimester, the uterus expands out of the pelvic cavity, and by 20 weeks, it usually reaches the level of the umbilicus. By 28 to 30 weeks, the uterine fundus reaches the epigastric region, the area between the xiphoid process of the sternum and umbilicus.

PARTURITION

Parturition (childbirth) is the process during which the fetus, placenta, and fetal membranes are expelled from the mother (Fig. 8-8). **Labor is the *sequence of uterine contractions*** that result in dilation of the uterine cervix and delivery of the fetus and placenta from the uterus. The factors that trigger labor are not completely understood, but several hormones are related to the initiation of contractions. The fetal hypothalamus secretes **corticotropin-releasing hormone**, stimulating the pituitary gland to produce **adrenocorticotropic hormone (ACTH)**. ACTH causes the suprarenal cortex to secrete **cortisol**, which is involved in the synthesis of **estrogens**.

Peristaltic contractions of the uterine smooth muscle are elicited by **oxytocin**, which is released by the maternal neurohypophysis of the pituitary gland. This hormone is administered clinically when it is necessary to induce labor. Oxytocin also stimulates the release of **prostaglandins** that, in turn, stimulate myometrial contractility by sensitizing the myometrial cells to oxytocin. Estrogens also increase myometrial contractile activity and stimulate the release of oxytocin and prostaglandins.

Stages of Labor

Labor is a continuous process; however, for clinical purposes it is divided into three stages:

- **Dilation** begins with *progressive dilation of the cervix* (see Fig. 8-8*A* and *B*) and ends with complete dilation of the cervix. During this phase, regular **contractions of the uterus occur** less than 10 minutes apart. The average duration of the first stage is approximately 12 hours for first pregnancies (*primigravidas*) and approximately 7 hours for women who have had a child previously (*multigravidas*).
- **Expulsion** begins when the cervix is fully dilated and ends with delivery of the fetus (see Fig. 8-8*C* to *E*). During this stage, the *fetus descends through the cervix and vagina*. As soon as the fetus is outside the mother, it is called a *neonate*. The average duration of this stage is 50 minutes for primigravidas and 20 minutes for multigravidas.

Uterine wall   Amnion and chorion

A   Cervical canal

Placenta   Vagina

B   Anus

Anterior abdominal wall
Pubis

C

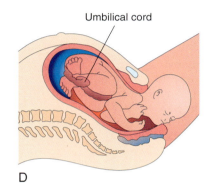

Umbilical cord

D

Figure 8–8   Illustrations of parturition (childbirth). **A** and **B,** The cervix is dilating during the first stage of labor. **C** to **E,** The fetus is passing through the cervix and vagina during the second stage of labor. **F** and **G,** As the uterus contracts during the third stage of labor, the placenta folds and pulls away from the uterine wall. Separation of the placenta results in bleeding and formation of a large hematoma (mass of blood). Pressure on the abdomen facilitates placental separation. **H,** The placenta is expelled and the uterus contracts.

E

F

Hematoma
(blood clot)

Contracted uterus

G

H   Expelled placenta, membranes, and umbilical cord

- **Placental separation** begins as soon as the fetus is born and *ends with the expulsion of the placenta and fetal membranes* (see Fig. 8-8*F* to *H*). A **hematoma** forms deep to the placenta and separates it from the uterine wall. The placenta and fetal membranes are then expelled. Contractions of the uterus constrict the spiral arteries, preventing excessive uterine bleeding. The duration of this stage is approximately 15 minutes. A

retained or **adherent placenta**—one not expelled within 1 hour of delivery—is a cause of *postpartum bleeding.*

Placenta and Fetal Membranes after Birth

The placenta usually has a discoid (disc-like) shape, with a diameter of 15 to 20 cm and a thickness of 2 to 3 cm

Figure 8–9 Placentas and fetal membranes after birth, shown approximately one third their actual size. **A,** Maternal surface, showing cotyledons and grooves around them. Each convex cotyledon consists of a number of main stem villi with their many branch villi. The grooves were occupied by the placental septa when the maternal and fetal parts of the placenta were together (see Fig. 8-5). **B,** Fetal surface showing blood vessels running in the chorionic plate deep to the amnion and converging to form the umbilical vessels at the attachment of the umbilical cord.

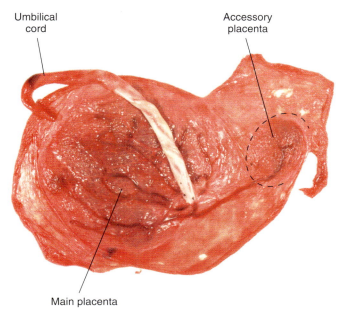

Figure 8–10 Maternal surface of a full-term placenta and an accessory placenta. The umbilical cord is attached to the edge of the fetal surface of the placenta.

PLACENTAL ABNORMALITIES

Abnormal adherence of the chorionic villi to the myometrium of the uterine wall is called *placenta accreta* (Fig. 8-11). When chorionic villi penetrate the myometrium all the way to the perimetrium (peritoneal covering), the abnormality is called *placenta percreta*. Third-trimester bleeding is the most common presenting sign of these placental abnormalities. After birth, the placenta does not separate from the uterine wall, and attempts to remove it may cause severe hemorrhage that is difficult to control. When the blastocyst implants close to or overlying the internal os of the uterus, the abnormality is called *placenta previa*. Late-pregnancy bleeding can result from this placental abnormality. In such cases, the fetus is delivered by cesarean section because the placenta blocks the cervical canal. Magnetic resonance imaging and ultrasonography are used for imaging the placenta in various clinical situations.

(Fig. 8-9). The margins of the placenta are continuous with the ruptured amniotic and chorionic sacs.

Variations in Placental Shape

As the placenta develops, chorionic villi usually persist only where the villous chorion is in contact with the decidua basalis (see Fig. 8-1*E* and *F*). When villi persist elsewhere, several variations in placental shape occur, such as **accessory placenta** (Fig. 8-10). Examination of the placenta, prenatally by ultrasonography or postnatally by gross and microscopic study, may provide clinical information about the causes of placental dysfunction, intrauterine growth restriction, fetal distress and death, and neonatal illness. Postnatal placental examination can also determine whether the expelled placenta is intact. Retention of cotyledons or an accessory placenta in the uterus causes **postpartum uterine hemorrhage**.

Maternal Surface of Placenta

The *cobblestone appearance* of the maternal surface of the placenta is produced by slightly bulging villous areas—the **cotyledons**—which are separated by grooves formerly occupied by **placental septa** (see Fig. 8-9*A*).

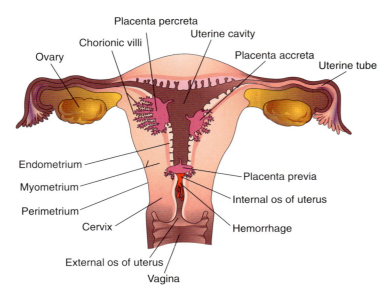

Figure 8–11 Placental abnormalities. In **placenta accreta,** there is abnormal adherence of the placenta to the myometrium (muscle layer). In **placenta percreta**, the placenta has penetrated the full thickness of the myometrium. In **placenta previa**, the placenta overlies the internal os of the uterus, blocking the cervical canal.

ABSENCE OF UMBILICAL ARTERY

In approximately 1 in 200 neonates, only one umbilical artery is present (Fig. 8-12), a condition that may be associated with chromosomal and fetal abnormalities. Absence of an umbilical artery is accompanied by a 15% to 20% incidence of cardiovascular anomalies in the fetus. Absence of an artery results from either agenesis or degeneration of this vessel early in development.

Figure 8–12 Transverse section of the umbilical cord. Note that the cord is covered by a single-layered epithelium derived from the enveloping amnion. It has a core of mucous connective tissue. Observe also that the cord has one umbilical artery and one vein. Usually, there are two arteries.

Fetal Surface of Placenta

The umbilical cord usually attaches near the center of the fetal surface, and its epithelium is continuous with the amnion adhering to the chorionic plate of the placenta (see Fig. 8-9B), giving the fetal surface a smooth texture. The chorionic vessels radiating to and from the umbilical cord are visible through the transparent amnion. The **umbilical vessels** branch on the fetal surface, forming the **chorionic vessels**, which enter the chorionic villi (see Fig. 8-5).

Umbilical Cord

The attachment of the cord to the placenta is usually near the center of the fetal surface of the placenta (see Fig. 8-9B), but it may attach at other locations (see Fig. 8-10). The cord is usually 1 to 2 cm in diameter and 30 to 90 cm in length (see Fig. 8-10). *Doppler ultrasonography* may be used for prenatal diagnosis of the position and structural abnormalities of the cord. Long cords have a tendency to prolapse through the cervix or to coil around the fetus. Prompt recognition of *prolapse of the cord* is important because, during delivery, it may be compressed between the presenting body part of the fetus and the mother's bony pelvis, causing **fetal anoxia.** If the

deficiency of oxygen persists for more than 5 minutes, the fetus's brain may be damaged.

The umbilical cord usually has *two arteries and one vein* surrounded by mucoid connective tissue (*Wharton jelly*). Because the umbilical vessels are longer than the cord, twisting and bending of the cord is common. The cord frequently forms loops, producing *false knots* that are of no significance; however, in approximately 1% of pregnancies, *true knots* form in the umbilical cord. These may tighten and cause fetal death secondary to fetal anoxia (Fig. 8-13C). In most cases, the knots form during labor as a result of the fetus passing through a loop of the cord. Because these knots are usually loose, they have no clinical significance. Simple looping of the cord around the fetus occasionally occurs. In approximately one fifth of all deliveries, the cord is loosely *looped around the neck* without causing increased fetal risk.

AMNION AND AMNIOTIC FLUID

The **amnion** forms a fluid-filled, membranous *amniotic sac* that surrounds the embryo and later the fetus; the sac

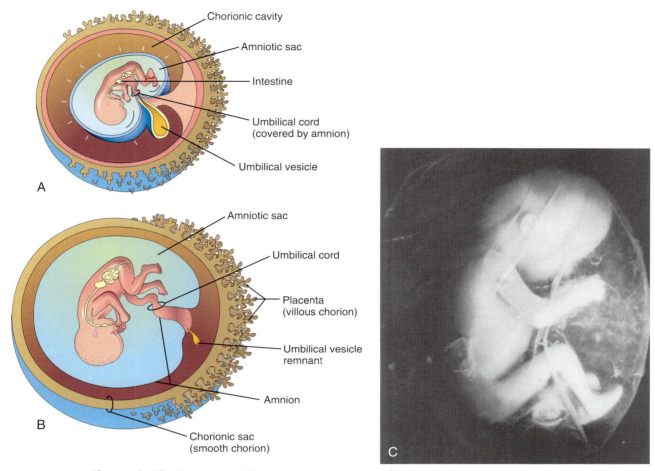

Chorionic cavity
Amniotic sac
Intestine
Umbilical cord
(covered by amnion)
Umbilical vesicle
A

Amniotic sac
Umbilical cord
Placenta
(villous chorion)
Umbilical vesicle
remnant
Amnion
B
Chorionic sac
(smooth chorion)
C

Figure 8–13 Illustrations of how the amnion enlarges, fills the chorionic sac, and envelops the umbilical cord. Observe that part of the umbilical vesicle is incorporated into the embryo as the primordial gut. Formation of the fetal part of the placenta and degeneration of the chorionic villi are also shown. **A,** At 10 weeks. **B,** At 20 weeks. **C,** A 12-week fetus within its amniotic sac (actual size). The fetus and its membranes aborted spontaneously. It was removed from its chorionic sac with the amniotic sac intact. Note that the umbilical cord is looped around the left ankle of the fetus.

contains amniotic fluid (see Fig. 8-13). As the amnion enlarges, it gradually obliterates the chorionic cavity and forms the epithelial covering of the umbilical cord (see Fig. 8-13A and B). **Amniotic fluid** plays a major role in fetal growth and development. Initially cells of the amnion secrete some amniotic fluid. Most fluid is derived from *maternal tissue fluid* by diffusion across the **amniochorionic membrane** from the decidua parietalis (see Fig. 8-5). Later, there is diffusion of fluid through the chorionic plate from blood in the intervillous space of the placenta.

Before **keratinization** (formation of keratin) of the skin occurs, a major pathway for passage of water and solutes in tissue fluid from the fetus to the amniotic cavity is through the skin. Fluid is also secreted by the fetal respiratory and gastrointestinal tracts and enters the amniotic cavity. *Beginning in the 11th week, the fetus contributes to the amniotic fluid by expelling urine into the amniotic cavity.*

The water content of amniotic fluid changes every 3 hours. Large amounts of water pass through the **amniochorionic membrane** into the maternal tissue fluid and into the uterine capillaries. An exchange of fluid with fetal blood also occurs through the **umbilical cord** and at the site where the amnion adheres to the chorionic plate on the fetal surface of the placenta (see Fig. 8-5 and Fig. 8-9B); thus, amniotic fluid is in balance with the fetal circulation.

Amniotic fluid is swallowed by the fetus and absorbed by its respiratory and digestive tracts. It has been estimated that, during the final stages of pregnancy, **the fetus swallows up to 400 ml of amniotic fluid daily**. The fluid is absorbed by the gastrointestinal tract and passes into the fetal bloodstream. The waste products cross the placental membrane and enter the maternal blood in the **intervillous space**. Excess water in the fetal blood is excreted by the fetal kidneys and returned to the amniotic sac through the fetal urinary tract.

Virtually all of the fluid in the amniotic cavity is water, in which undissolved material (such as desquamated fetal epithelial cells) is suspended. Amniotic fluid contains approximately equal portions of dissolved organic compounds and inorganic salts. Half of the organic constituents are protein; the other half is composed of carbohydrates, fats, enzymes, hormones, and pigments. As pregnancy advances, the composition of the amniotic fluid changes as fetal urine is added. Because fetal urine enters the amniotic fluid, fetal enzyme systems, amino acids, hormones, and other substances can be studied by examining fluid removed by **amniocentesis**. Studies of cells in the amniotic fluid permit the detection of chromosomal abnormalities.

Significance of Amniotic Fluid

The embryo floats freely in the amniotic sac. Amniotic fluid has critical functions in the development of the embryo and fetus:

- Permits uniform external growth of the embryo
- Acts as a barrier to infection
- Permits fetal lung development
- Prevents adherence of the amnion to the embryo
- Cushions the embryo against injuries by distributing impacts that the mother may receive
- Helps to control embryonic body temperature by maintaining a relatively constant temperature
- Enables the fetus to move freely, thereby aiding muscular development (e.g., in the limbs)
- Assists in maintaining homeostasis of fluid and electrolytes

DISORDERS OF AMNIOTIC FLUID VOLUME

A low volume of amniotic fluid—*oligohydramnios*—results, in some cases, from placental insufficiency, with *diminished placental blood flow*. Preterm rupture of the amniochorionic membrane is the most common cause of oligohydramnios. In the presence of **renal agenesis** (failure of kidney formation), the lack of fetal urine in the amniotic fluid is the main cause of oligohydramnios. A similar decrease in amniotic fluid occurs with obstructive **uropathy** (urinary tract obstruction). Complications of oligohydramnios include fetal abnormalities (pulmonary hypoplasia, facial defects, and limb defects) caused by fetal compression by the uterine wall.

A high volume of amniotic fluid is termed *polyhydramnios*. Most cases of polyhydramnios (60%) are idiopathic (of unknown cause); 20% of cases are caused by maternal factors, whereas 20% are fetal in origin. Polyhydramnios may be associated with severe anomalies of the central nervous system, such as **meroencephaly** (anencephaly) (see Chapter 16). With other birth defects, such as esophageal atresia, amniotic fluid accumulates because it cannot pass to the fetal stomach and the intestines for absorption.

UMBILICAL VESICLE

The umbilical vesicle can be observed sonographically early during the fifth week of gestation. At 32 days, the umbilical vesicle is large (see Fig. 8-1C). By 10 weeks, the umbilical vesicle has shrunk to a pear-shaped remnant approximately 5 mm in diameter (see Fig. 8-13A). By 20 weeks, the umbilical vesicle is very small (see Fig. 8-13B).

Significance of Umbilical Vesicle

The umbilical vesicle is nonfunctional as far as yolk storage is concerned (hence the name change from yolk sac to umbilical vesicle), but the presence of the vesicle is essential for several reasons:

- It has a role in the *transfer of nutrients* to the embryo during the second and third weeks before the utero-placental circulation is established.
- *Blood cells* first develop in the well-vascularized, extra-embryonic mesoderm covering the wall of the umbilical vesicle beginning in the third week (see Chapter 5), and continue to develop there until hematopoietic activity begins in the liver during the sixth week.
- During the fourth week, the dorsal part of the umbilical vesicle is incorporated into the embryo as the *primordial gut* (see Chapter 6, Fig. 6-1). Its endoderm, derived from the epiblast, gives rise to *the epithelium of the trachea, bronchi, lungs, and alimentary canal*.
- *Primordial germ cells* appear in the endodermal lining of the wall of the umbilical vesicle in the third week and subsequently migrate to the developing gonads—testis or ovary (see Chapter 13). The cells differentiate into spermatogonia in males and oogonia in females.

ALLANTOIS

The allantois is not functional in human embryos; however, it is important for three reasons:

- Blood cell formation occurs in its wall during the third to fifth weeks of development.

PREMATURE RUPTURE OF FETAL MEMBRANES

Premature rupture of the amniochorionic membrane is the most common event leading to premature labor and delivery and the most common complication resulting in oligohydramnios. Loss of amniotic fluid removes the major protection the fetus has against infection. Rupture of the membrane may cause various fetal birth defects that constitute the **amniotic band syndrome**, or *amniotic band disruption complex* (Fig. 8-14). These birth defects are associated with a variety of abnormalities, ranging from constriction of digits (fingers) to major scalp, craniofacial, and visceral defects. The cause of these defects is probably related to constriction by encircling amniotic bands (see Fig. 8-14).

Chorion

Fibrous bands of disrupted amnion

Fetal surface of placenta

Umbilical cord

Figure 8–14 A fetus with amniotic band syndrome, showing amniotic bands constricting the left arm.

- Its blood vessels become the umbilical vein and arteries.
- The intraembryonic portion of the allantois runs from the umbilicus to the urinary bladder, with which it is continuous (see Chapter 13, Fig. 13-11*E*). As the bladder enlarges, the allantois involutes to form a thick tube, the **urachus** (see Chapter 13, Fig. 13-11*G*). After birth, the urachus becomes a fibrous cord, the median umbilical ligament, which extends from the apex of the urinary bladder to the umbilicus.

MULTIPLE PREGNANCIES

Multiple pregnancies (gestations) are associated with higher risks of chromosomal anomalies, fetal morbidity, and fetal mortality than single gestations. The risks are progressively greater as the number of fetuses increases. In North America, *twins* naturally occur approximately once in every 85 pregnancies, *triplets* approximately once in every 90^2 pregnancies, *quadruplets* approximately once in every 90^3 pregnancies, and *quintuplets* approximately once in every 90^4 pregnancies.

Twins and Fetal Membranes

Twins that originate from two zygotes are **dizygotic (DZ) twins**—fraternal twins (Fig. 8-15), whereas twins that originate from one zygote are **monozygotic (MZ) twins**—identical twins (Fig. 8-16). The fetal membranes and placentas vary according to the origin of the twins. *Approximately two thirds of twins are dizygotic, and the rate of DZ twinning increases with maternal age.* The study of twins is important in human genetics because it is useful for comparing the effects of genes and environment on development. If an abnormal condition does not show a simple genetic pattern, comparison of its incidence in MZ and DZ twins may show that heredity is involved.

Dizygotic Twins

Because they result from the fertilization of two oocytes by two sperms, DZ twins may be of the same sex or different sexes. For the same reason, they are no more alike genetically than brothers or sisters born at different times. *DZ twins always have two amnions and two chorions* (see Fig. 8-15*A*), but the chorions and placentas may be fused (see Fig. 8-15*B*). DZ twinning shows a hereditary tendency. The recurrence risk in families with one set of DZ twins is approximately triple that of the general population. The incidence of DZ twinning shows considerable racial variation, ranging from 1 in 500 in Asian populations, to 1 in 125 in white populations, to as high as 1 in 20 in some African populations.

Monozygotic Twins

Because they result from the fertilization of one oocyte and develop from one zygote (see Fig. 8-16), *MZ twins are of the same sex, are genetically identical, and are similar in physical appearance.* Physical differences between MZ twins are environmentally induced, such as by anastomosis of the placental vessels, resulting in differences in blood supply from the placenta (Fig. 8-17). MZ twinning usually begins in the blastocyst stage,

TWIN TRANSFUSION SYNDROME

Twin transfusion syndrome occurs in 10% to 15% of **monochorionic-diamniotic MZ twins.** Arterial blood may be preferentially shunted from one twin through arteriovenous anastomoses in the placenta into the venous circulation of the other twin. The donor twin is small, pale, and anemic (see Fig. 8-17), whereas the recipient twin is large and polycythemic (i.e., having a higher than normal red blood cell count). The placenta shows similar abnormalities; the part of the placenta supplying the anemic twin is pale, whereas the part supplying the polycythemic twin is dark red. In lethal cases, death results from anemia in the donor twin and from congestive heart failure in the recipient twin.

Figure 8–15 Dizygotic twins developing from two zygotes. The relationship of the fetal membranes and placentas are shown for instances in which the blastocysts implant separately **(A)** and the blastocysts implant close together **(B)**. In both cases, there are two amnions and two chorions.

ESTABLISHING ZYGOSITY OF TWINS

Establishment of the zygosity of twins is important, particularly because of the introduction of tissue and organ transplantation (e.g., bone marrow transplants). **Twin zygosity** is now determined by molecular testing. Any two people who are not MZ twins are virtually certain to show differences in some of the large number of DNA markers that can be studied.

Late division of the early embryonic cells (i.e., division of the embryonic disc during the second week) results in MZ twins with one amniotic sac and one chorionic sac. A

monochorionic-monoamniotic twin placenta is associated with a fetal mortality rate approaching 50%. The umbilical cords are frequently so entangled that circulation of the blood through their vessels ceases, and one or both fetuses die.

Ultrasonography plays an important role in the diagnosis of twin pregnancies and the management of various conditions that may complicate MZ twinning, such as intrauterine growth restriction, intrauterine fetal distress, and premature labor.

Two amnions

One placenta
One chorionic sac
Two amniotic sacs

Two inner
cell masses

Zygote

Two-cell
stage

Single placenta

Anastomosis of placental vessels
and arteriovenous communication
between circulatory systems of twins

Figure 8–16 Illustrations of how approximately 65% of monozygotic twins develop from one zygote by division of the inner cell mass. These twins always have separate amnions, a single chorionic sac, and a common placenta. If there is anastomosis of the placental vessels, one twin may receive most of the nutrition from the placenta (see Fig. 8-17).

Figure 8–17 Monozygotic, monochorionic-diamniotic twins. Note the wide discrepancy in size resulting from an uncompensated arteriovenous anastomosis of the placental vessels. Blood was shunted from the smaller twin to the larger one, producing the twin transfusion syndrome.

Figure 8–18 Illustrations of how approximately 35% of monozygotic twins develop from one zygote. Separation of the blastomeres may occur at any point from the two-cell stage to the morula stage, producing two identical blastocysts. Each embryo subsequently develops its own amniotic and chorionic sacs. The placentas may be separate or fused. In most cases, there is a single placenta resulting from secondary fusion, whereas in fewer cases, there are two placentas. In the latter cases, examination of the placenta suggests that they are dizygotic twins. This explains why some monozygotic twins are incorrectly classified as dizygotic twins at birth.

approximately at the end of the first week, and results from division of the embryoblast into two embryonic primordia (see Fig. 8-16). Subsequently, two embryos, each in its own amniotic sac, develop within one chorionic sac and share a common placenta, a **monochorionic-diamniotic twin placenta**. Uncommonly, early separation of the embryonic blastomeres (e.g., during the two- to eight-cell stage) results in MZ twins with two amnions, two chorions, and two placentas that may or may not be fused (Fig. 8-18). In such cases, it is impossible to determine, from the membranes alone, whether the twins are monozygotic or dizygotic.

Other Types of Multiple Births

Triplets may be derived from:

- One zygote and be identical
- Two zygotes and consist of identical twins and a singleton

CONJOINED TWINS

If the embryonic disc does not divide completely, various types of conjoined (MZ) twins may form. The terminology used to describe the twins is based on the regions of the body that are attached; for example, *thoracopagus* indicates anterior union of the thoracic regions. In some cases, the twins are connected to each other by skin only or by cutaneous and other tissues, such as fused livers. Some conjoined twins can be separated successfully by surgery. The incidence of conjoined twins is 1 in 50,000 to 1 in 100,000 births.

- Three zygotes and be of the same sex or of different sexes, in which case the infants are no more similar than infants from three separate pregnancies

Similar combinations occur in quadruplets, quintuplets, sextuplets, and septuplets.

CLINICALLY ORIENTED QUESTIONS

1. What is meant by the term *stillbirth*? Do older women have more stillborn infants?

2. A fetus was born dead, reportedly because of a "cord accident." What does this mean? Do these "accidents" always kill the infant? If not, what birth defects may be present?

3. What is the scientific basis of the home pregnancy tests that are sold in drugstores?

4. What is the proper name for what laypeople sometimes refer to as the *bag of water*? Does premature rupture of the "bag" induce the birth of the fetus? What is meant by a *dry birth*?

5. What does *fetal distress* mean? How is the condition recognized? What causes the distress?

6. Is twinning more common in older mothers? Is twinning hereditary?

The answers to these questions are at the back of this book.

Body Cavities, Mesenteries, and Diaphragm

E arly in the fourth week of development, the **intraembryonic coelom**—the primordium of the body cavities—appears as a horseshoe-shaped cavity (Fig. 9-1*A*). The bend in this cavity at the cranial end of the embryo represents the **future** *pericardial cavity,* and its limbs indicate the future *pleural and peritoneal cavities.* The distal part of each limb of the intraembryonic coelom is continuous with the **extraembryonic coelom** at the lateral edges of the embryonic disc (see Fig. 9-1*B*). This communication is important because most of the midgut normally herniates through this communication into the umbilical cord. The intra-embryonic coelom provides room for the abdominal organs to develop and move. During embryonic lateral folding, the limbs of the coelom are brought together on the ventral aspect of the embryo (Fig. 9-2*A* to *F*).

▶ EMBRYONIC BODY CAVITY

The **intraembryonic coelom** becomes *the embryonic body cavity,* which is divided into three well-defined body cavities during the fourth week (see Fig. 9-2 and Fig. 9-4): a *pericardial cavity,* two *pericardioperitoneal canals* connecting the pericardial and peritoneal cavities, and a large *peritoneal cavity.* These body cavities are lined by the mesothelium—a parietal wall derived from the somatic mesoderm and a visceral wall derived from the splanchnic mesoderm (Fig. 9-3*E*). The mesothelium forms the major portion of the peritoneum.

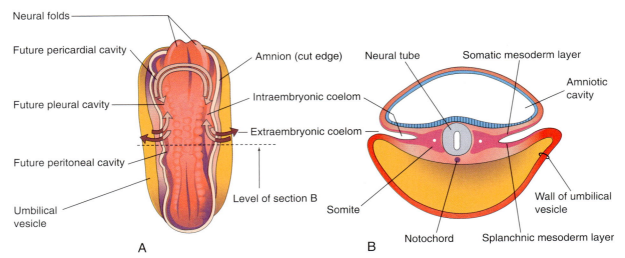

Figure 9–1 **A,** Dorsal view of a 22-day embryo, showing the outline of the horseshoe-shaped intraembryonic coelom. The amnion has been removed and the coelom is shown as if the embryo were translucent. The continuity of the intraembryonic coelom, as well as the communication of its right and left limbs with the extraembryonic coelom, is indicated by *arrows.* **B,** Transverse section through the embryo at the level shown in **A.**

The **peritoneal cavity** is connected to the extraembryonic coelom at the umbilicus (Fig. 9-4C and D). The peritoneal cavity loses its connection with the extraembryonic coelom during the 10th week as the intestines return to the abdomen from the umbilical cord (see Chapter 12).

During formation of the head fold, the heart and **pericardial cavity** are relocated ventrocaudally, anterior to the foregut (see Fig. 9-2A, B, D, and E). As a result, the pericardial cavity opens into the **pericardioperitoneal canals**, which pass dorsal to the foregut (see Fig. 9-4B and D). After embryonic folding, the caudal parts of the foregut, midgut, and hindgut are suspended in the peritoneal cavity from the dorsal abdominal wall by the **dorsal mesentery** (see Fig. 9-2F and Fig. 9-3B to E).

Mesenteries

A mesentery is a double layer of peritoneum that begins as an extension of the visceral peritoneum that covers an organ. The mesentery connects the organ to the body wall and conveys its vessels and nerves. Transiently, the dorsal and ventral mesenteries divide the peritoneal cavity into right and left halves (see Fig. 9-3C). The ventral mesentery soon disappears (see Fig. 9-3E), except where it is attached to the caudal part of the foregut (primordium of stomach and proximal part of duodenum). The peritoneal cavity then becomes a continuous space (see Fig. 9-3A and Fig. 9-4D). The arteries supplying the primordial gut—*celiac arterial trunk* (foregut), the *superior mesenteric artery* (midgut), and *inferior mesenteric artery* (hindgut)—pass between the layers of the dorsal mesentery (see Fig. 9-3C).

Division of Embryonic Body Cavity

Each pericardioperitoneal canal lies lateral to the proximal part of the foregut (future esophagus) and dorsal to

the **septum transversum**—a thick plate of mesoderm that occupies the space between the thoracic cavity and the **omphaloenteric duct** (see Fig. 9-4A and B).

The septum transversum is the **primordium of the central tendon of the diaphragm**. Partitions form in each pericardioperitoneal canal, separating the pericardial cavity from the pleural cavities, and the pleural cavities from the peritoneal cavity (see Fig. 9-3A). Because of the growth of the **bronchial buds** (primordia of bronchi and lungs) into the *pericardioperitoneal canals* (Fig. 9-5A), a pair of membranous ridges is produced in the lateral wall of each canal. The cranial ridges—the *pleuropericardial folds*—are located superior to the developing lungs, and the caudal ridges—the *pleuroperitoneal folds*—are located inferior to the lungs.

Pleuropericardial Membranes

As the **pleuropericardial folds** enlarge, they form partitions that separate the pericardial cavity from the pleural cavities. These partitions—**pleuropericardial membranes**—contain the **common cardinal veins** (see Fig. 9-5A and B), which drain the venous system into the sinus venosus of the primordial heart (see Chapter 14). Initially the bronchial buds are small relative to the heart and pericardial cavity (see Fig. 9-5). They grow laterally from the caudal end of the trachea into the **pericardioperitoneal canals** (future pleural canals). As the **primordial pleural cavities** expand ventrally around the heart, they extend into the body wall, splitting the mesenchyme into two layers: (1) an outer layer that becomes the thoracic wall and (2) an inner layer (pleuropericardial membrane) that becomes the fibrous pericardium, the outer layer of the pericardial sac that encloses the heart (see Fig. 9-5C and D).

The *pleuropericardial membranes* project into the cranial ends of the **pericardioperitoneal canals** (see Fig. 9-5B). With subsequent growth of the common cardinal

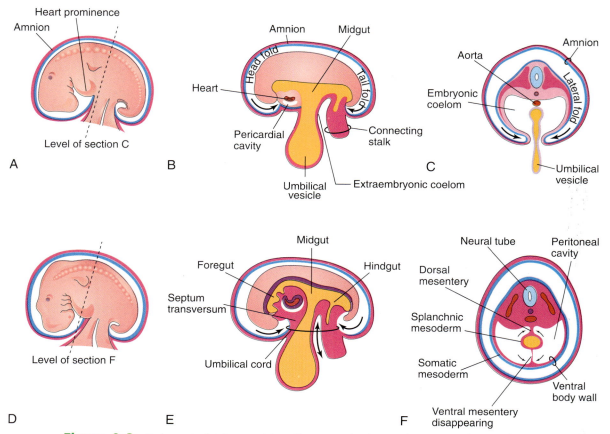

Figure 9–2 Embryonic folding and its effects on the intraembryonic coelom and other structures. **A,** Lateral view of an embryo (approximately 26 days). **B,** Schematic sagittal section of the embryo, showing the head and tail folds. **C,** Transverse section at the level shown in **A,** indicating how fusion of the lateral folds gives the embryo a cylindrical form. **D,** Lateral view of an embryo (approximately 28 days). **E,** Schematic sagittal section of the embryo, showing the reduced communication between the intraembryonic and extraembryonic coeloms (*double-headed arrow*). **F,** Transverse section, as indicated in **D,** showing the formation of the ventral body wall and the disappearance of the ventral mesentery. The *arrows* indicate the junction of the somatic and splanchnic layers of the mesoderm. The somatic mesoderm will become the parietal peritoneum lining the abdominal wall, and the splanchnic mesoderm will become the visceral peritoneum covering the organs (e.g., stomach).

veins, positional displacement of the heart, and expansion of the pleural cavities, the pleuropericardial membranes become mesentery-like folds extending from the lateral thoracic wall. By the seventh week, the pleuropericardial membranes fuse with the mesenchyme ventral to the esophagus, separating the pericardial cavity from the pleural cavities (see Fig. 9-5C). The primordial mediastinum consists of a mass of mesenchyme that extends from the sternum to the vertebral column, separating the developing lungs (see Fig. 9-5D). The right pleuropericardial opening closes slightly earlier than the left one and produces a larger pleuropericardial membrane.

Pleuroperitoneal Membranes

As the **pleuroperitoneal folds** enlarge, they project into the pericardioperitoneal canals. Gradually, the folds become membranous, forming the **pleuroperitoneal membranes** (Fig. 9-6B and C). Eventually, these membranes separate the pleural cavities from the peritoneal cavity. The *pleuroperitoneal membranes* are produced as the developing lungs and pleural cavities expand and invade the body wall. They are attached dorsolaterally to the abdominal wall and their crescentic free edges initially project into the caudal ends of the **pericardioperitoneal canals**.

During the sixth week, the pleuroperitoneal membranes extend ventromedially until their free edges fuse with the dorsal mesentery of the esophagus and the septum transversum (see Fig. 9-6C). This membrane separates the pleural cavities from the peritoneal cavity. *Closure of the pleuroperitoneal openings* is completed by the migration of **myoblasts** (primordial muscle cells) into the pleuroperitoneal membranes (see Fig. 9-6D and E). The pleuroperitoneal opening on the right side closes slightly before the left one.

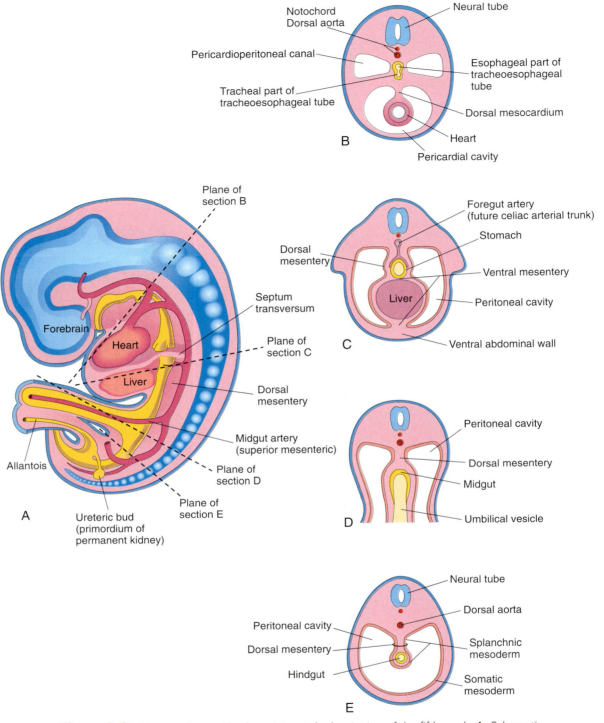

Figure 9–3 Mesenteries and body cavities at the beginning of the fifth week. **A,** Schematic sagittal section. Note that the dorsal mesentery serves as a pathway for the arteries that supply the developing gut. Nerves and lymphatics also pass between the layers of this mesentery. **B to E,** Transverse sections through the embryo at the levels shown in **A.** The ventral mesentery disappears except in the region of the terminal esophagus, stomach, and first part of the duodenum. Note that the right and left parts of the peritoneal cavity, which are separate in **C,** are continuous in **E.**

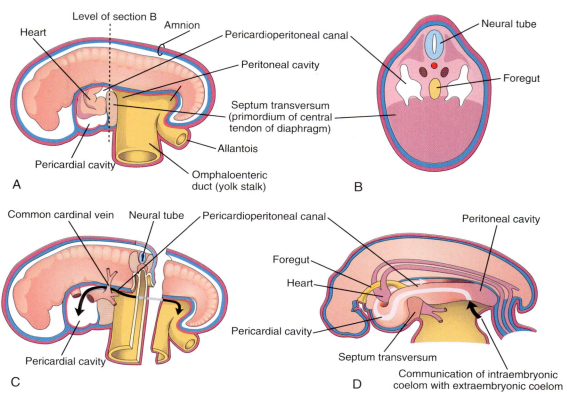

Figure 9–4 Illustration of an embryo (approximately 24 days). **A,** The lateral wall of the pericardial cavity has been removed to show the primordial heart. **B,** Transverse section of the embryo, showing the relationship of the pericardioperitoneal canals to the septum transversum and foregut. **C,** Lateral view of the embryo, with the heart removed. The embryo has also been sectioned transversely to show the continuity of the intraembryonic and extraembryonic coeloms (*arrow*). **D,** Illustration of the pericardioperitoneal canals that arise from the dorsal wall of the pericardial cavity and pass on each side of the foregut to join the peritoneal cavity. The *arrow* shows the communication of the extraembryonic coelom with the intraembryonic coelom and the continuity of the intraembryonic coelom at this stage.

◉ DEVELOPMENT OF DIAPHRAGM

6   The diaphragm is a dome-shaped, musculotendinous partition that separates the thoracic and abdominal cavities. It is a composite structure that develops from four embryonic components (see Fig. 9-6):

- Septum transversum
- Pleuroperitoneal membranes
- Dorsal mesentery of esophagus
- Muscular ingrowth from lateral body walls

Septum Transversum

This transverse septum, which is composed of mesodermal tissue, is the **primordium of the central tendon of the diaphragm** (see Fig. 9-6D and E). The septum transversum grows dorsally from the ventrolateral body wall and forms a semicircular shelf that separates the heart from the liver. After the head folds ventrally during the fourth week, the septum transversum forms a thick, incomplete connective tissue partition between the pericardial and abdominal cavities (see Fig. 9-4). The septum transversum expands and fuses with the mesenchyme ventral to the esophagus and the pleuroperitoneal membranes (see Fig. 9-6C).

Pleuroperitoneal Membranes

These membranes fuse with the dorsal mesentery of the esophagus and the septum transversum (see Fig. 9-6C). This fusion completes the partition between the thoracic and abdominal cavities and forms the **primordial diaphragm**. The pleuroperitoneal membranes represent relatively small portions of the neonate's diaphragm (see Fig. 9-6E).

Dorsal Mesentery of Esophagus

The septum transversum and pleuroperitoneal membranes fuse with the dorsal mesentery of the esophagus. This mesentery becomes the median portion of the diaphragm. The **crura of the diaphragm**—a pair of diverging muscle bundles that cross in the median plane anterior to the aorta (see Fig. 9-6E)—develop from myoblasts (primordial muscle cells) that grow into the dorsal mesentery of the esophagus.

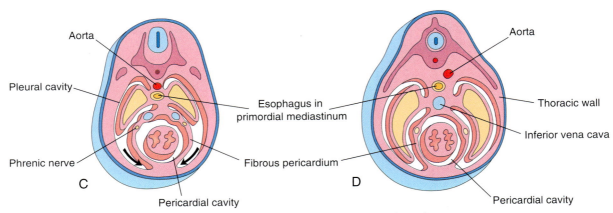

Figure 9–5 Transverse sections through an embryo cranial to the septum transversum, showing successive stages in the separation of the pleural cavities from the pericardial cavity. Growth and development of the lungs, expansion of the pleural cavities, and formation of the fibrous pericardium are also shown. **A,** At 5 weeks. The *arrows* indicate the communications between the pericardioperitoneal canals and the pericardial cavity. **B,** At 6 weeks. The *arrows* indicate the development of the pleural cavities as they expand into the body wall. **C,** At 7 weeks. Expansion of the pleural cavities ventrally (*arrows*) around the heart is evident. The pleuropericardial membranes are now fused in the median plane with each other, and with the mesoderm ventral to the esophagus. **D,** At 8 weeks. Continued expansion of the lungs and pleural cavities and formation of the fibrous pericardium and the thoracic wall are shown.

Muscular Ingrowth from Lateral Body Walls

During the 9th to 12th weeks, the lungs and pleural cavities enlarge, "burrowing" into the lateral body walls (see Fig. 9-5). During this process, the tissue of the body wall is split into two layers:

● An external layer that becomes part of the definitive abdominal wall
● An internal layer that contributes to the peripheral parts of the diaphragm, external to the parts derived from the pleuroperitoneal membranes (see Fig. 9-6*D* and *E*)

Further extension of the developing pleural cavities into the lateral body walls forms the right and left **costodiaphragmatic recesses** (Fig. 9-7), establishing the characteristic dome-shaped configuration of the diaphragm.

Positional Changes and Innervation of the Diaphragm

During the fourth week of development, the septum transversum lies opposite the third to fifth cervical somites. During the fifth week, myoblasts from these somites migrate into the developing diaphragm, bringing their nerve fibers with them. Consequently, the **phrenic nerves** that supply motor innervation to the diaphragm arise from the ventral primary rami of the third, fourth, and fifth cervical spinal nerves, which join together on each side to form a phrenic nerve. The phrenic nerves also supply sensory fibers to the superior and inferior surfaces of the right and left domes of the diaphragm.

Rapid growth of the dorsal part of the embryo's body results in an *apparent descent of the diaphragm.* By the sixth week, the developing diaphragm is at the level of the thoracic somites. The phrenic nerves now have a descending course. By the beginning of the eighth week, the

Figure 9–6 Development of the diaphragm. **A,** Lateral view of an embryo at the end of the fifth week (actual size), indicating the level of **B** to **D** sections. **B** to **E** show the developing diaphragm as viewed inferiorly. **B,** Transverse section, showing the unfused pleuroperitoneal membranes. **C,** Similar section at the end of the sixth week, after fusion of the pleuroperitoneal membranes with the other two diaphragmatic components. **D,** Transverse section of a 12-week embryo, after ingrowth of the fourth diaphragmatic component from the body wall. **E,** View of the diaphragm of a neonate, indicating the embryologic origin of its components.

POSTEROLATERAL DEFECT OF DIAPHRAGM

Posterolateral defect of the diaphragm is the only relatively common congenital anomaly involving the diaphragm (Fig. 9-8A). This diaphragmatic defect occurs in approximately 1 in 3000 neonates and is associated with **congenital diaphragmatic hernia (CDH)**—herniation of abdominal contents into the thoracic cavity.

CDH is the *most common cause of pulmonary hypoplasia*. CDH can lead to life-threatening respiratory difficulties. If severe lung hypoplasia is present, some primordial alveoli may rupture, causing air to enter the pleural cavity (*pneumothorax*). Usually unilateral, CDH results from defective formation or fusion of the pleuroperitoneal membrane with the other three parts of the diaphragm (see Fig. 9-6B). This birth defect produces a large opening in the posterolateral region of the diaphragm. If a pleuroperitoneal canal is still open when the intestines return to the abdomen from the umbilical cord in the 10th week, some intestine and other viscera may pass into the thorax and compress the lungs. Often the stomach, spleen, and most of the intestines herniate (see Fig. 9-8B and C). The defect usually occurs on the left side, and it is likely related to the earlier closure of the right pleuroperitoneal opening. *Chromosomal abnormalities and gene mutations, including those of the zinc finger factor GATA6, have been implicated in cases of CDH.* Ultrasonography and magnetic resonance imaging can provide a *prenatal diagnosis* of CDH.

dorsal part of the diaphragm lies at the level of the first lumbar vertebra. The phrenic nerves in the embryo enter the diaphragm by passing through the pleuropericardial membranes. For this reason, the phrenic nerves subsequently lie on the fibrous pericardium of the heart, which is derived from the pleuropericardial membranes (see Fig. 9-5C and D). The costal border of the diaphragm receives sensory fibers from the lower intercostal nerves because of the origin of the peripheral part of the diaphragm from the lateral body walls (see Fig. 9-6D and E).

EVENTRATION OF DIAPHRAGM

In the relatively uncommon condition of **diaphragmatic eventration**, half of the diaphragm has defective musculature, causing it to balloon into the thoracic cavity as an aponeurotic (membranous) sheet, forming a **diaphragmatic pouch** (see Fig. 9-8A). Consequently, the abdominal viscera are displaced superiorly into the pocket-like outpouching of the diaphragm. This birth defect results mainly from failure of the muscular tissue from the body wall to extend into the pleuroperitoneal membrane on the affected side.

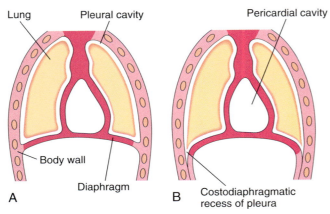

Figure 9–7   **A** and **B**, Extension of the pleural cavities into the body walls to form the peripheral parts of the diaphragm, the costodiaphragmatic recesses, and the characteristic dome-shaped configuration of the diaphragm.

RETROSTERNAL (PARASTERNAL) HERNIA

Herniations may occur through the **sternocostal hiatus**, the opening for the superior epigastric vessels in the retrosternal area. The hiatus is located between the sternal and costal parts of the diaphragm. Herniation of the intestine into the pericardial sac may occur or, conversely, part of the heart may descend into the peritoneal cavity in the epigastric region. Large birth defects are commonly associated with **body wall defects** in the umbilical region (e.g., omphalocele; see Chapter 12).

Figure 9–8   **A,** This "window view" overlooking the thorax and the abdomen shows the herniation of the intestine into the thorax through a posterolateral defect in the left side of the diaphragm. Note that the left lung is compressed and hypoplastic. **B,** Diaphragmatic hernia. Note the herniation of the stomach and small intestine into the thorax through a posterolateral defect in the left side of the diaphragm, similar to that shown in **A.** Note that the heart is pushed to the right side of the thorax. **C,** Radiograph showing a diaphragmatic hernia on the left side. Note the loops of small intestine in the thoracic cavity and the displacement of the heart into the right thoracic cavity.

CLINICALLY ORIENTED QUESTIONS

1. Is it possible for an infant to be born with a defect that results in its stomach and liver being located in its chest? How might this occur?

2. A male neonate had respiratory distress and was diagnosed with CDH. Is this a common birth defect? What would determine whether this infant would survive? Can diaphragmatic defects be operated on before birth?

3. Do the lungs develop normally in infants who are born with a CDH?

4. A man underwent routine chest radiography approximately 1 year ago and was told that a small part of his small intestine was in his chest. Is it possible for him to have a CDH without being aware of it? Would his lung on the affected side be normal?

The answers to these questions are at the back of this book.

Pharyngeal Apparatus, Face, and Neck

T he **pharyngeal apparatus** consists of *pharyngeal arches, pharyngeal pouches, pharyngeal grooves,* and *pharyngeal membranes* (Fig. 10-1). These embryonic structures contribute to the formation of the face and neck.

PHARYNGEAL ARCHES

These arches begin to develop early in the fourth week as **neural crest cells** migrate into the future head and neck regions (see Chapter 6, Fig. 6-4). Initially, each pharyngeal arch consists of a core of **mesenchyme** (embryonic connective tissue) and is covered externally by ectoderm and internally by endoderm (see Fig. 10-1*D* and *E*). The first pair of arches, the primordium of the jaws, appears as surface elevations lateral to the developing pharynx. Other arches soon appear as obliquely disposed, rounded ridges on each side of the future head and neck regions. By the end of the fourth week, four pairs of arches are visible externally (see Fig. 10-1*A*). The fifth and sixth arches are rudimentary and are not visible on the surface of the embryo. The arches are separated from each other by the **pharyngeal grooves** (clefts). Like the arches, the grooves are numbered in a craniocaudal sequence.

The arches support the lateral walls of the primordial pharynx, which is derived from the cranial part of the foregut. The **stomodeum** (primordial mouth) initially appears as a slight depression of the surface ectoderm (see Fig. 10-1*A*). It is separated from the cavity of

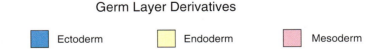

Germ Layer Derivatives

- Ectoderm
- Endoderm
- Mesoderm

Figure 10–1   Illustrations of the pharyngeal apparatus. **A,** Lateral view showing the development of four pharyngeal arches. **B** and **C,** Ventral (facial) views showing the relationship of the pharyngeal arches to the stomodeum. **D,** Frontal section through the cranial region of an embryo. **E,** Horizontal section showing the arch components and the floor of the primordial pharynx. **F,** Sagittal section of the cranial region of an embryo, showing the openings of the pharyngeal pouches in the lateral wall of the primordial pharynx.

the primordial pharynx by a bilaminar membrane—the **oropharyngeal membrane**—composed of fused ectoderm and endoderm. The oropharyngeal membrane ruptures at approximately 26 days (see Fig. 10-1*B* and *C*), bringing the primordial pharynx and foregut into communication with the amniotic cavity. The arches contribute extensively to the formation of the face, nasal cavities, mouth, larynx, pharynx, and neck (see Fig. 10-2 and Fig. 10-23).

The **first arch** develops two prominences (see Fig. 10-1*B* and Fig. 10-2): the smaller *maxillary prominence* and the larger *mandibular prominence*. The **second arch**

(hyoid) makes a major contribution to the formation of the hyoid bone (see Fig. 10-4*B*).

Pharyngeal Arch Components

A typical arch has the following components (Fig. 10-3*A* and *B*):

- An *arch artery* (aortic arch artery) that arises from the truncus arteriosus of the primordial heart and courses around the primordial pharynx to enter the dorsal aorta

Second pharyngeal groove

Third pharyngeal arch

Cervical sinus

Second pharyngeal arch

Heart

Maxillary prominence

Mandibular prominence

Stomodeum

Figure 10–2   A Carnegie stage 13, 4½-week human embryo.

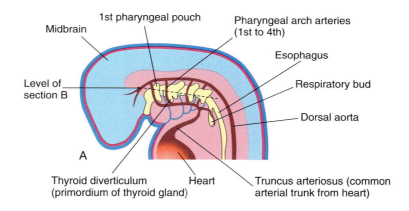

Midbrain

1st pharyngeal pouch

Pharyngeal arch arteries (1st to 4th)

Esophagus

Level of section B

Respiratory bud

Dorsal aorta

A

Thyroid diverticulum (primordium of thyroid gland)

Heart

Truncus arteriosus (common arterial trunk from heart)

1st arch

2nd arch

Cartilages

Nerve

Muscle

B

1st pharyngeal membrane

2nd pharyngeal pouch

3rd pharyngeal arch artery

3rd pharyngeal pouch

4th pharyngeal arch

Germ Layer Derivatives

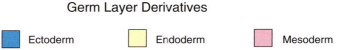

Ectoderm   Endoderm   Mesoderm

Figure 10–3   **A,** Illustration of the pharyngeal pouches and pharyngeal arch arteries. **B,** Horizontal section through the embryo showing the floor of the primordial pharynx and illustrating the germ layer origin of the pharyngeal arch components.

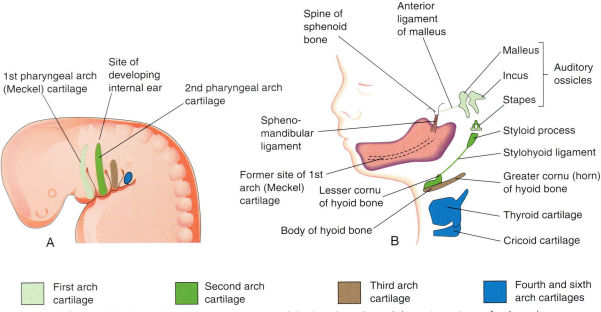

Figure 10–4 **A,** Schematic lateral view of the head, neck, and thoracic regions of a 4-week embryo, showing the location of the cartilages in the pharyngeal arches. **B,** Similar view of a 24-week fetus, showing the adult derivatives of the arch cartilages. Note that the mandible is formed by intramembranous ossification of mesenchymal tissue surrounding the first arch cartilage.

- A *cartilaginous rod* that forms the skeleton of the arch
- A *muscular component* that is the primordium of the muscles in the head and neck
- A *nerve* that supplies the mucosa and muscles derived from each arch

Derivatives of Pharyngeal Arch Arteries

The transformation of the arch arteries into the adult arterial pattern of the head and neck is described in the section on the pharyngeal arch artery derivatives in Chapter 14.

Derivatives of Pharyngeal Arch Cartilages

The dorsal end of the **first arch cartilage** becomes ossified to form two middle ear bones, the **malleus** and **incus** (Fig. 10-4 and Table 10-1). The middle section of the cartilage regresses, but its *perichondrium* forms the **anterior ligament of the malleus** and **sphenomandibular ligament** (see Fig. 10-4*B*). Ventral parts of the first arch cartilage form the horseshoe-shaped primordium of the mandible. Each half of the mandible forms lateral to and in close association with its cartilage. The cartilage disappears as the mandible develops around it by *intramembranous ossification* (see Chapter 15).

The dorsal end of the **second arch cartilage** contributes to the **stapes** of the middle ear and the **styloid process** of the temporal bone. The part of the cartilage between the **styloid process** and the hyoid bone regresses; its perichondrium forms the **stylohyoid ligament**. The ventral end of the second arch cartilage ossifies to form the lesser cornu of the **hyoid bone**.

The **third arch cartilage** ossifies to form the greater cornu of the hyoid bone. (The body of the hyoid forms

from the hypopharyngeal eminence—see Development of Tongue.) The **fourth and sixth arch cartilages** fuse to form the **laryngeal cartilages**, except for the epiglottis. The epiglottic and thyroid cartilages appear to develop from neural crest cells (see Fig. 10-21*A* to *C*). The cricoid cartilage develops from mesoderm.

Derivatives of Pharyngeal Arch Muscles

The muscular components of the arches form various muscles in the head and neck; for example, the musculature of the first arch forms the **muscles of mastication** and others (Fig. 10-5*A* and *B* and Table 10-1).

Derivatives of Pharyngeal Arch Nerves

Each arch is supplied by its own cranial nerve (CN). The *special visceral efferent (branchial) components* of the cranial nerves supply muscles derived from the pharyngeal arches (Fig. 10-6*A* and Table 10-1). Because the mesenchyme from the pharyngeal arches contributes to the dermis and mucous membranes of the head and neck, these areas are supplied with the *special visceral afferent nerves*. The facial skin is supplied by the fifth cranial nerve (CN V, or **trigeminal nerve**); however, only the caudal two branches (*maxillary* and *mandibular*) supply derivatives of the first pharyngeal arch (see Fig. 10-6*B*). CN V is the principal sensory nerve of the head and neck and is the motor nerve for the muscles of mastication. Its sensory branches innervate the face, teeth, and mucous membranes of the nasal cavities, palate, mouth, and tongue (see Fig. 10-6*C*). The seventh cranial nerve (CN VII, or **facial nerve**), the ninth cranial nerve (CN IX, or **glossopharyngeal nerve**), and the 10th cranial nerve (CN X, or **vagus nerve**) supply the second, third, and caudal

Table 10–1 Structures Derived from Pharyngeal Arch Components*

ARCH	NERVE	MUSCLES	SKELETAL STRUCTURES	LIGAMENTS
First (mandibular)	Trigeminal[†] (CN V)	Muscles of mastication[‡] Mylohyoid and anterior belly of digastric Tensor tympani Tensor veli palatini	Malleus Incus	Anterior ligament of malleus Sphenomandibular ligament
Second (hyoid)	Facial (CN VII)	Muscles of facial expression[§] Stapedius Stylohyoid Posterior belly of digastric	Stapes (portion) Styloid process Lesser cornu of hyoid bone	Stylohyoid ligament
Third	Glossopharyngeal (CN IX)	Stylopharyngeus	Greater cornu of hyoid bone	
Fourth and sixth[∥]	Superior laryngeal branch of vagus (CN X) Recurrent laryngeal branch of vagus (CN X)	Cricothyroid Levator veli palatini Constrictors of pharynx Intrinsic muscles of larynx Striated muscles of esophagus	Thyroid cartilage Cricoid cartilage Arytenoid cartilage Corniculate cartilage Cuneiform cartilage	

*The derivatives of the pharyngeal arch arteries are described in Chapter 14.
[†]The ophthalmic division of the fifth cranial nerve (CN V) does not supply any pharyngeal arch components.
[‡]Temporalis, masseter, medial, and lateral pterygoids.
[§]Buccinator, auricularis, frontalis, platysma, and orbicularis oris and oculi.
[∥]The fifth pharyngeal arch regresses. The cartilaginous components of the fourth and sixth arches fuse to form the cartilages of the larynx.

Figure 10–5 A, Lateral view of the head, neck, and thoracic regions of a 4-week embryo showing the muscles derived from the pharyngeal arches. The *arrow* shows the pathway taken by myoblasts from the occipital myotomes to form the tongue musculature. **B,** The head and neck regions of a 20-week fetus, showing the muscles derived from the pharyngeal arches. Parts of the platysma and sternocleidomastoid muscles have been removed to show the deeper muscles. Note that myoblasts from the second arch migrate from the neck to the head, where they give rise to the muscles of facial expression. These muscles are supplied by the facial nerve (cranial nerve VII), the nerve of the second pharyngeal arch.

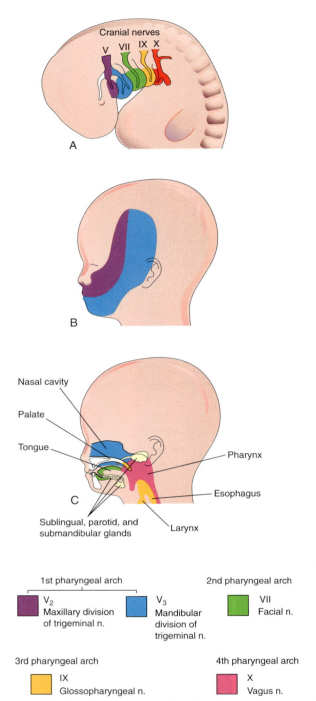

Cranial nerves
V   VII   IX   X

A

B

Nasal cavity

Palate

Tongue

Pharynx

Esophagus

C

Sublingual, parotid, and submandibular glands

Larynx

1st pharyngeal arch

V₂
Maxillary division of trigeminal n.

V₃
Mandibular division of trigeminal n.

2nd pharyngeal arch

VII
Facial n.

3rd pharyngeal arch

IX
Glossopharyngeal n.

4th pharyngeal arch

X
Vagus n.

Figure 10–6 **A,** Lateral view of the head, neck, and thoracic regions of a 4-week embryo, showing the cranial nerves that supply the pharyngeal arches. **B,** The head and neck regions of a 20-week fetus, showing the superficial distribution of the two caudal branches of the first arch nerve (cranial nerve V). **C,** Sagittal section of the fetal head and neck, showing the deep distribution of the sensory fibers of the nerves to the teeth and mucosa of the tongue, pharynx, nasal cavity, palate, and larynx.

(fourth to sixth) arches, respectively. The superior laryngeal branch of the vagus nerve supplies the fourth arch, whereas its recurrent laryngeal branch supplies the sixth arch. The nerves of the second to sixth pharyngeal arches (see Fig. 10-6*A*) innervate the mucous membranes of the tongue, pharynx, and larynx (see Fig. 10-6*C*).

PHARYNGEAL POUCHES

The primordial pharynx widens cranially where it joins the *stomodeum*, and narrows caudally, where it joins the *esophagus* (see Fig. 10-3*A*). The endoderm of the pharynx lines the internal aspects of the pharyngeal arches and passes into the **pharyngeal pouches** (see Fig. 10-1*D* and *E* and Fig. 10-7*A*). The pairs of pouches develop in a craniocaudal sequence between the arches. The first pair of pouches, for example, lies between the first and second pharyngeal arches. Four pairs of pouches are well defined; the fifth pair is absent or rudimentary. The endoderm of the pouches contacts the ectoderm of the pharyngeal grooves, and together they form the double-layered **pharyngeal membranes** (see Fig. 10-3*B*). *Expression of the Tbx2 gene in the pharyngeal pouches is essential for the formation of the pharyngeal arches and pouches.*

Derivatives of Pharyngeal Pouches 7

The **first pouch** gives rise to the **tubotympanic recess** (see Fig. 10-7*B*). The first pharyngeal membrane contributes to the formation of the **tympanic membrane** (eardrum) (see Fig. 10-7*C*). The cavity of the tubotympanic recess gives rise to the **tympanic cavity** and **mastoid antrum**. The connection of the *tubotympanic recess* with the pharynx forms the **pharyngotympanic tube** (auditory tube).

The **second pouch** is largely obliterated as the **palatine tonsil** develops (see Figs. 10-7*C* and Fig. 10-8). A part of this pouch remains as the **tonsillar sinus (fossa)**. The endoderm of the second pouch proliferates and grows into the underlying mesenchyme. The central parts of these buds break down, forming **tonsillar crypts (pit-like depressions)**. The pouch endoderm forms the surface epithelium and the lining of the crypts. Lymphoid infiltration occurs approximately in the seventh month, while germinal centers are not apparent until the neonatal period.

The **third pouch** expands and develops a solid, bulbar, dorsal part and a hollow, elongate ventral part (see Fig. 10-7*B*). The connection between the pouch and pharynx is reduced to a narrow duct that soon degenerates. By the sixth week of development, the epithelium of each bulbar dorsal part begins to differentiate into an **inferior parathyroid gland**. The epithelium of the elongated ventral parts of the third pair of pouches proliferates, obliterating their cavities. These parts come together in the median plane to form the **thymus**. The primordia of the thymus and parathyroid glands lose their connections with the pharynx. Later, the inferior parathyroid glands separate from the thymus and lie on the dorsal surface of the thyroid gland, whereas the thymus descends into the superior mediastinum (see Fig. 10-7*C* and Fig. 10-8). The mesenchyme surrounding the thymic primordium is derived from *neural crest cells*.

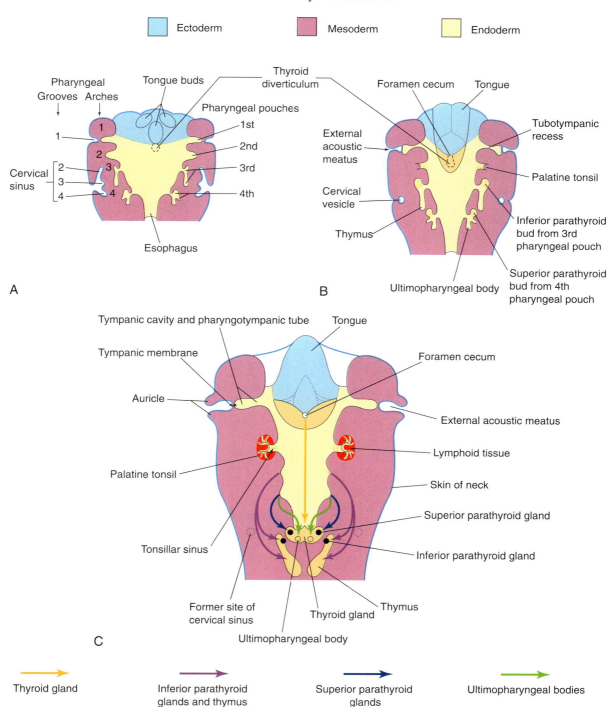

Germ Layer Derivatives

Ectoderm   Mesoderm   Endoderm

Figure 10–7 Schematic horizontal sections of the embryo showing the adult derivatives of the pharyngeal pouches. **A,** At 5 weeks. Note that the second pharyngeal arch grows over the third and fourth arches, burying the second to fourth pharyngeal grooves in the cervical sinus. **B,** At 6 weeks. **C,** At 7 weeks. Note the migration of the developing thymus, parathyroid, and thyroid glands into the neck.

Figure 10–8 A sagittal section of the head, neck, and upper thoracic regions of a 20-week fetus, showing the adult derivatives of the pharyngeal pouches and the descent of the thyroid gland into the neck.

AURICULAR SINUSES AND CYSTS

Small auricular sinuses and cysts are usually located in a triangular area of skin anterior to the auricle of the external ear (Fig. 10-9D); however, they may occur in other sites around the auricle or in its lobule (earlobe). Although some sinuses and cysts are remnants of the first pharyngeal groove, others represent ectodermal folds sequestered during formation of the auricle from the auricular hillocks (swellings that contribute to the auricle).

The dorsal part of each **fourth pouch** develops into a **superior parathyroid gland**, which lies on the dorsal surface of the thyroid gland (see Fig. 10-7B). The parathyroid glands derived from the third pouches descend with the thymus and are carried to a more inferior position than the parathyroid glands that are derived from the fourth pouches (see Fig. 10-8). The elongated ventral part of each fourth pouch develops into the **ultimopharyngeal body**, which fuses with the thyroid gland, giving rise to the **parafollicular cells (C cells)** of the thyroid gland. These cells produce **calcitonin**, a hormone involved in the regulation of calcium. C cells differentiate from **neural crest cells** that migrate from the pharyngeal arches into the fourth pair of pharyngeal pouches.

If the **fifth pharyngeal pouch** develops, it is rudimentary and becomes part of the fourth pharyngeal pouch.

▶ PHARYNGEAL GROOVES

7   The head and neck regions of the embryo exhibit four grooves (clefts) on each side during the fourth and fifth

CERVICAL (BRANCHIAL) SINUSES

Cervical sinuses are uncommon, and almost all that open externally on the side of the neck result from failure of the second pharyngeal groove and cervical sinus to obliterate (see Fig. 10-9B and Fig. 10-10A). The sinus typically opens along the anterior border of the sternocleidomastoid muscle in the inferior third of the neck. Anomalies of the other grooves occur in approximately 5% of cases.

External cervical sinuses are commonly detected during infancy because of the discharge of mucous material from their orifices in the neck. These *lateral cervical sinuses* are bilateral in approximately 10% of cases and are commonly associated with auricular sinuses.

Internal cervical sinuses open into the pharynx and are very rare. Almost all of these sinuses result from persistence of the proximal part of the second pharyngeal pouch, so they usually open into the tonsillar sinus or near the palatopharyngeal arch (see Fig. 10-9B and D). Normally, this pouch disappears as the palatine tonsil develops; its normal remnant is the tonsillar sinus.

CERVICAL (BRANCHIAL) FISTULA

An abnormal canal that opens internally into the tonsillar sinus and externally on the side of the neck is a *cervical fistula*. This rare birth defect results from persistence of parts of the second pharyngeal groove and pouch (see Fig. 10-9C and D and Fig. 10-10B). The fistula ascends from its opening in the neck, through the subcutaneous tissue and platysma muscle, to reach the tonsillar sinus.

CERVICAL (BRANCHIAL) CYSTS

The third and fourth pharyngeal arches are buried in the cervical sinus (see Fig. 10-7A). Remnants of parts of the cervical sinus, the second groove, or both may persist and form a spherical or elongated cyst (see Fig. 10-9D). Cervical cysts often do not become apparent until late childhood or early adulthood, when they produce a slowly enlarging, painless swelling in the neck (Fig. 10-11). The cysts enlarge because of accumulation of fluid and cellular debris derived from desquamation of their epithelial linings (Fig. 10-12).

CERVICAL (BRANCHIAL) VESTIGES

Normally the pharyngeal cartilages disappear, except for the parts that form ligaments or bones; however, in unusual cases, cartilaginous or bony remnants of the pharyngeal arch cartilages appear under the skin on the side of the neck. These are usually found anterior to the inferior third of the sternocleidomastoid muscle (see Fig. 10-9D).

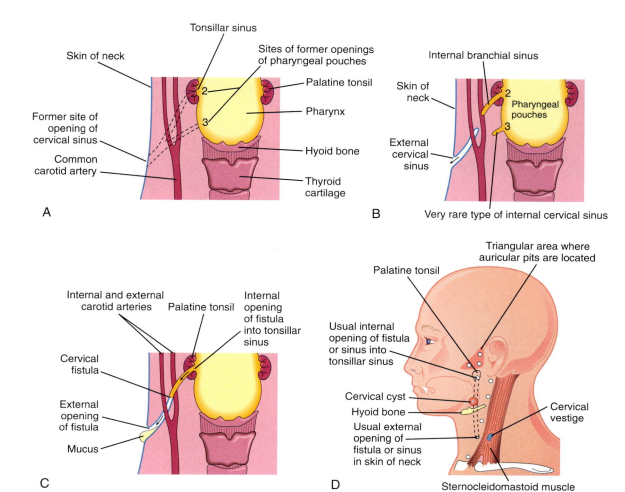

Figure 10–9 **A,** The adult pharyngeal and neck regions, indicating the former sites of openings of the cervical sinus and pharyngeal pouches (2 and 3). The *broken lines* indicate possible courses of cervical fistulas. **B,** The embryologic basis for various types of cervical sinus. **C,** Illustration of a cervical fistula resulting from the persistence of parts of the second pharyngeal groove and the second pharyngeal pouch. **D,** Possible sites of cervical cysts and openings of the cervical sinuses and fistulas. A cervical vestige is also shown.

FIRST PHARYNGEAL ARCH SYNDROME

Abnormal development of the first pharyngeal arch results in various congenital anomalies of the eyes, ears, mandible, and palate that together constitute *first pharyngeal arch syndrome* (Fig. 10-13). This syndrome is believed to result from insufficient migration of neural crest cells into the first arch during the fourth week. There are two main clinical manifestations of first arch syndrome:

* **Treacher Collins syndrome** (mandibulofacial dysostosis), is most often caused by an autosomal dominant gene defect (*TCOF1*), and results in underdevelopment of the zygomatic bones of the face—**malar hypoplasia**. Characteristic features of the syndrome include

down-slanting palpebral fissures, birth defects of the lower eyelids, deformed external ears, and sometimes defects of the middle and internal ears.

* **Pierre Robin sequence** consists of hypoplasia of the mandible, cleft palate, and defects of the eye and ear. Many cases of this syndrome are sporadic; however, some appear to have a genetic basis. In *Robin morphogenetic complex*, the proposed initiating defect is a small mandible (micrognathia), which results in posterior displacement of the tongue and obstruction to full closure of the palatine processes, resulting in bilateral cleft palate (see Fig. 10-33).

Figure 10–11   A swelling in a boy's neck produced by a cervical cyst. These large cysts often lie free in the neck, just inferior to the angle of the mandible, but they may develop anywhere along the anterior border of the sternocleidomastoid muscle, as in this case.

Figure 10–10   **A,** A child's neck showing a catheter inserted into the external opening of a cervical (branchial) sinus. The catheter allows definition of the length of the tract, which facilitates surgical excision. **B,** A fistulogram of a complete cervical fistula. The radiograph was taken after injection of a contrast medium to show the course of the fistula through the neck.

Figure 10–12   A large cervical cyst (B) shown by computed tomography of the neck region of a woman who had a "lump" in the neck, similar to that shown in Figure 10-11. The low-density cyst is anterior to the right sternocleidomastoid muscle (s) at the level of the hyoid bone (h). The normal appearance of the left carotid sheath (c) is shown for comparison with the compressed sheath on the right side. (*From McNab T, McLennan MK, Margolis M: Radiology rounds. Can Fam Physician 41:1673, 1995.*)

weeks (see Fig. 10-1A). These grooves separate the pharyngeal arches externally. Only one pair of grooves contributes to structures; the first pair persists as the **external acoustic meatus** (ear canal) (see Fig. 10-7C). The other grooves lie in a slit-like depression—the **cervical sinus**—and are usually obliterated with it as the neck develops (see Fig. 10-7A and B). Birth defects of the *second* pharyngeal groove are the most common of such defects.

PHARYNGEAL MEMBRANES

7   These membranes form where the epithelia of the grooves and pouches approach each other. The membranes appear

Figure 10–13 An infant with first arch syndrome, a pattern of birth defects resulting from insufficient migration of the neural crest cells into the first pharyngeal arch. Note the deformed auricle of the external ear, preauricular appendage, defect in the cheek between the auricle and the mouth, hypoplasia of the mandible, and macrostomia (large mouth).

in the floors of the grooves during the fourth week (see Fig. 10-1*D* and 10-3*B*). Only one pair of membranes contributes to the formation of adult structures; the first membrane becomes the **tympanic membrane** (see Fig. 10-7*C*).

DEVELOPMENT OF THYROID GLAND

The **thyroid gland** *is the first endocrine gland to develop.* It begins to form at approximately 24 days from a median endodermal thickening in the floor of the primordial pharynx. This thickening soon forms a small outpouching—the **thyroid primordium** (Fig. 10-14*A*). As the embryo and tongue grow, the developing thyroid gland descends in the neck, passing ventral to the developing hyoid bone and the laryngeal cartilages. For a short time, it is connected to the tongue by the **thyroglossal duct** (see Fig. 10-14*A* and *B*). As a result of rapid cell proliferation, the lumen of the thyroid diverticulum soon obliterates and divides into right and left lobes, which are connected by the **thyroid isthmus** of the thyroid gland.

By 7 weeks, the thyroid gland has assumed its definitive shape and has usually reached its final site in the neck (see Fig. 10-14*C*). By this time, the **thyroglossal duct** has usually degenerated and disappeared. The proximal opening of the thyroglossal duct persists as a small pit—the **foramen cecum** in the dorsum of the tongue (see Fig. 10-7*C*). A **pyramidal lobe** of the thyroid gland extends superiorly from the isthmus in approximately 50% of

DiGEORGE SYNDROME

Infants with DiGeorge syndrome are born without a thymus and parathyroid glands. The disease is characterized by *congenital hypoparathyroidism* (hypocalcemia); increased susceptibility to infections (from immune deficiency—specifically, defective T-cell function); palate abnormalities; micrognathia (airway obstruction due to retropositioned tongue); low-set, notched ears; nasal clefts; and cardiac abnormalities (birth defects of the arch of the aorta and heart). *DiGeorge syndrome* occurs when the third and fourth pharyngeal pouches do not differentiate into the thymus and parathyroid glands. The facial birth defects result primarily from abnormal development of the first pharyngeal arch components during formation of the face and ears. *DiGeorge syndrome commonly involves a microdeletion (22q11.2 region), mutation of the* HIRA, UFDIL, *and* Tbx1 *genes, and neural crest cell defects.* The incidence of DiGeorge syndrome is 1 in 2000 to 4000 births.

ECTOPIC PARATHYROID GLANDS

The parathyroids are highly variable in number and location. They may be found anywhere near or within the thyroid gland or the thymus (Fig. 10-15). The superior glands are more constant in position than the inferior ones. Occasionally, an inferior parathyroid gland does not descend and remains near the bifurcation of the common carotid artery. In other cases, it may accompany the thymus into the thorax.

ABNORMAL NUMBER OF PARATHYROID GLANDS

In unusual cases, there may be more than four parathyroid glands. **Supernumerary parathyroid glands** probably result from division of the primordia of the original glands. Absence of a parathyroid gland results from failure of one of the primordia to differentiate, or from atrophy of a gland early in development.

people. This lobe may be attached to the hyoid bone by fibrous tissue, smooth muscle, or both.

During the 11th week, **colloid** begins to appear in the **thyroid follicles**; thereafter, iodine concentration and the synthesis of thyroid hormones can be demonstrated. By 20 weeks, the levels of fetal thyroid-stimulating hormone and thyroxine begin to increase, reaching adult levels by 35 weeks.

DEVELOPMENT OF TONGUE

Near the end of the fourth week, a median triangular elevation appears in the floor of the primordial pharynx,

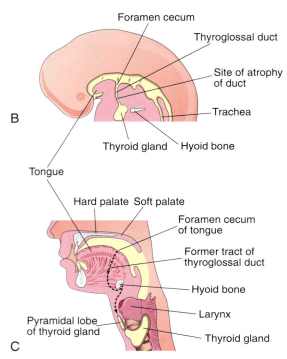

Figure 10–14   Development of the thyroid gland. **A** and **B,** Schematic sagittal sections of the head and neck regions at 5 and 6 weeks, showing successive stages in the development of the thyroid gland. **C,** Similar section of an adult head and neck, showing the path taken by the thyroid gland during its embryonic descent (indicated by the former tract of the thyroglossal duct).

THYROGLOSSAL DUCT CYSTS AND SINUSES

A remnant of the thyroglossal duct may persist and form a cyst in the tongue or in the anterior part of the neck, usually just inferior to the hyoid bone (Fig. 10-16). The swelling produced by a *thyroglossal duct cyst* usually develops as a painless, progressively enlarging, movable median mass (Fig. 10-17). The cyst may contain some thyroid tissue. After infection of a cyst, perforation of the skin occurs in some cases, forming a **thyroglossal duct sinus** that usually opens in the median plane of the neck, anterior to the laryngeal cartilages (Fig. 10-18A).

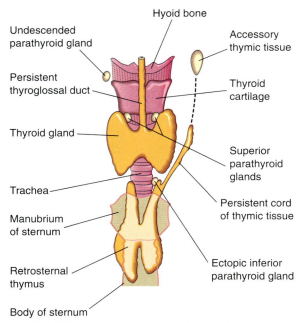

Figure 10–15   Anterior view of the thyroid gland, thymus, and parathyroid glands, showing various possible congenital anomalies that may occur.

ECTOPIC THYROID GLAND

Infrequently, an **ectopic thyroid gland** is located along the normal route of its descent from the tongue (see Fig. 10-14*B*). In 90% of cases this is represented by **lingual thyroid glandular tissue**. Incomplete descent of the thyroid gland results in a **sublingual thyroid gland** that appears high in the neck, at or just inferior to the hyoid bone (Fig. 10-19 and Fig. 10-20). In 70% of cases, an ectopic sublingual thyroid gland is the only thyroid tissue present.

It is clinically important to differentiate an ectopic thyroid gland from a thyroglossal duct cyst, or from accessory thyroid tissue, to prevent *inadvertent surgical removal of the thyroid gland* because this may be the only thyroid tissue present. Failure to recognize the thyroid gland may leave the person permanently dependent on thyroid medication.

just rostral to the foramen cecum (Fig. 10-21*A*). This swelling—the **median lingual swelling** (tongue bud)—is the first indication of tongue development. Soon, two oval **lateral lingual swellings (distal tongue buds)** develop on each side of the median tongue swelling. The three lingual swellings result from the proliferation of mesenchyme in the ventromedial parts of the first pair of pharyngeal arches. The lateral lingual swellings rapidly increase in size, merge with each other, and overgrow the median tongue swelling.

The merged lateral swellings form the anterior two thirds (oral part) of the tongue (see Fig. 10-21C). The plane of fusion of the lateral swellings is indicated superficially by the midline groove of the tongue and internally by the fibrous **lingual septum**. The median lingual swelling forms no recognizable part of the adult tongue.

Formation of the posterior third (pharyngeal part) of the tongue is indicated by two elevations that develop caudal to the foramen cecum (see Fig. 10-21A):

- The **copula** forms by fusion of the ventromedial parts of the second pair of pharyngeal arches.
- The **hypopharyngeal eminence** develops caudal to the copula from mesenchyme in the ventromedial parts of the third and fourth pairs of pharyngeal arches.

As the tongue develops, the copula is gradually overgrown by the hypopharyngeal eminence and disappears

Figure 10–16 Computed tomography scan of a thyroglossal duct cyst in a child. The cyst is located in the neck anterior to the thyroid cartilage (see also Fig. 10-4B).

(see Fig. 10-21B and C). As a result, the pharyngeal part of the tongue develops from the rostral part of the **hypopharyngeal eminence**. The line of fusion of the anterior and posterior parts of the tongue is roughly indicated by a V-shaped groove—the *terminal sulcus* (see Fig. 10-21C). Cranial neural crest cells migrate into the developing tongue and give rise to its connective tissue and vasculature. Most of the tongue muscles are derived from myoblasts (myogenic progenitors) that migrate from the occipital somites (see Fig. 10-5A). The **hypoglossal nerve (CN XII)** accompanies the myoblasts during their migration and innervates the tongue muscles as they develop. *The molecular mechanisms involved in the development of the tongue include myogenic regulating factors, the paired box genes Pax3 and Pax7, as well as the transforming growth factor β (TGF-β), fibroblast growth factor (FGF), and sonic hedgehog (SHH) genes.*

CONGENITAL LINGUAL CYSTS AND FISTULAS

Cysts in the tongue may be derived from remnants of the thyroglossal duct (see Fig. 10-14A). They may enlarge and produce pharyngeal pain, dysphagia (difficulty in swallowing), or both. Fistulas may also arise as a result of persistence of the lingual parts of the thyroglossal duct; such fistulas open through the *foramen cecum* into the oral cavity.

ANKYLOGLOSSIA

The lingual frenulum normally connects the inferior surface of the tongue to the floor of the mouth (Fig. 10-22). **Ankyloglossia** (tongue-tie) occurs in approximately 1 in 300 North American infants, but is usually of no functional significance. A short frenulum usually stretches with time, making surgical correction of the anomaly unnecessary.

Figure 10–17 Computed tomography scans. **A,** The level of the thyrohyoid membrane and the base of the epiglottis. **B,** The level of the thyroid cartilage, which is calcified. A thyroglossal duct cyst extends cranially to the margin of the hyoid bone.

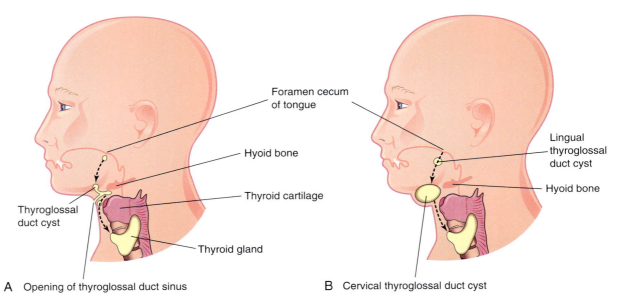

A Opening of thyroglossal duct sinus   **B** Cervical thyroglossal duct cyst

Figure 10–18 **A,** Sketch of the head and neck, showing the possible locations of thyroglossal duct cysts. A thyroglossal duct sinus is also illustrated. The *broken line* indicates the course taken by the duct during the descent of the developing thyroid gland from the foramen cecum to its final position in the anterior part of the neck. **B,** Similar sketch showing lingual and cervical thyroglossal duct cysts. Most thyroglossal duct cysts are located just inferior to the hyoid bone.

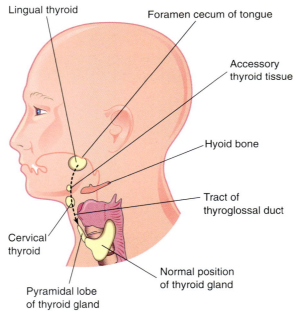

Figure 10–19 The head and neck, showing the usual sites of ectopic thyroid tissue. The *broken line* indicates the path followed by the thyroid gland during its descent, as well as the former tract of the thyroglossal duct.

Lingual Papillae and Taste Buds

Lingual papillae appear by the end of the eighth week. The **vallate** and **foliate papillae** appear first, close to the terminal branches of the glossopharyngeal nerve (CN IX). The **fungiform** papillae appear later, near the terminations of the chorda tympani branch of the facial nerve.

The long and numerous papillae are called **filiform papillae** because of their thread-like shape. They develop during the early fetal period (10–11 weeks). They contain afferent nerve endings that are sensitive to touch.

Taste buds develop during weeks 11 to 13 by inductive interaction between the epithelial cells of the tongue and invading gustatory nerve cells from the chorda tympani, glossopharyngeal, and vagus nerves. **Facial responses** can be induced by bitter-tasting substances at 26 to 28 weeks, indicating that reflex pathways between taste buds and facial muscles are established by this stage.

Nerve Supply of Tongue

The sensory supply to the mucosa of almost the entire anterior tongue (oral part) is from the lingual branch of the mandibular division of the trigeminal nerve (CN V), the nerve of the first pharyngeal arch (see Fig. 10-21C). Although the facial nerve is the nerve of the second pharyngeal arch, its chorda tympani branch supplies the taste buds in the anterior two thirds of the tongue, except for the vallate papillae. Because the second arch component, the **copula** (narrow part connecting two structures), is overgrown by the third arch component, the facial nerve does not supply any of the tongue mucosa, except for the taste buds in the anterior part of the tongue. The vallate papillae in the anterior tongue are innervated by the glossopharyngeal nerve (CN IX) of the third pharyngeal arch (see Fig. 10-21C). The posterior third of the tongue is innervated mainly by the glossopharyngeal nerve (CN IX) of the third pharyngeal arch. The superior laryngeal branch of the vagus nerve (CN X) of the fourth arch supplies a small area of the tongue anterior to the epiglottis (see Fig. 10-21C). All muscles of the tongue are supplied by the hypoglossal nerve (CN XII), except for the

Figure 10–20 **A,** Sublingual thyroid mass in a 5-year-old girl. **B,** Technetium 99m pertechnetate scan showing a sublingual thyroid gland (*) without evidence of functioning thyroid tissue in the anterior part of the neck. *(From Leung AKC, Wong AL, Robson WLLM: Ectopic thyroid gland simulating a thyroglossal duct cyst: a case report. Can J Surg 38:87, 1995.)*

palatoglossus, which is supplied from the pharyngeal plexus by fibers arising from the vagus nerve.

DEVELOPMENT OF SALIVARY GLANDS

During the sixth and seventh weeks, the salivary glands begin as solid epithelial buds from the endoderm of the primordial oral cavity (see Fig. 10-6C). The buds undergo branching morphogenesis and grow into the underlying mesenchyme. The connective tissue in the glands is derived from neural crest cells. All parenchymal (secretory) tissue arises by proliferation of the oral epithelium.

The **parotid glands** are the first to appear (early in the sixth week). They develop from buds that arise from the oral ectodermal lining near the angles of the stomodeum. The buds grow toward the ears, branching to form solid cords with rounded ends. Later, the cords canalize and become ducts by approximately 10 weeks. The rounded ends of the cords differentiate into acini. Secretions begin at 18 weeks. The capsule of the connective tissue develops from the surrounding mesenchyme.

The **submandibular glands** appear late in the sixth week. They develop from endodermal buds in the floor of the stomodeum. Solid cellular processes grow posteriorly, lateral to the developing tongue. Later they branch and differentiate. Acini begin to form at 12 weeks and secretory activity begins at 16 weeks. Growth of the submandibular glands continues after birth, with the formation of mucous acini. Lateral to the developing tongue, a linear groove forms that soon closes over to form the submandibular duct.

The **sublingual glands** appear in the eighth week, approximately 2 weeks later than the other salivary glands (see Fig. 10-6C). They develop from multiple endodermal epithelial buds in the **paralingual sulcus.**

These buds branch and canalize to form 10 to 12 ducts that open independently into the floor of the mouth.

DEVELOPMENT OF FACE

The facial primordia appear around the **stomodeum** early in the fourth week (Fig. 10-23A). Facial development depends on the inductive influence of three organizing areas:

- Forebrain (which establishes a gradient of SHH factor)
- Frontonasal ectoderm
- Developing eye

The **five facial primordia** that appear as prominences around the *stomodeum* (see Fig. 10-23A) are:

- A frontonasal prominence
- Paired maxillary prominences
- Paired mandibular prominences

The maxillary and mandibular prominences are derivatives of the first pair of pharyngeal arches. The prominences are produced by mesenchyme derived from neural crest cells that migrate into the arches during the fourth week of development. These cells are the major source of connective tissue components, including cartilage, bone, and ligaments in the facial and oral regions.

The **frontonasal prominence** (FNP) surrounds the ventrolateral part of the forebrain, which gives rise to the optic vesicles that form the eyes (see Fig. 10-23A and Fig. 10-24). The frontal part of the FNP forms the forehead; the nasal part of the frontonasal prominence forms the rostral boundary of the stomodeum and nose. The **maxillary prominences** form the lateral boundaries of the

Pharyngeal Arch Derivatives of Tongue

■ 1st pharyngeal arch (CN V—mandibular division)
■ 2nd pharyngeal arch (CN VII—chorda tympani)
■ 3rd pharyngeal arch (CN IX—glossopharyngeal)
■ 4th pharyngeal arch (CN X—vagus)

Figure 10–21 *A* and *B*, Schematic horizontal sections through the pharynx showing successive stages in the development of the tongue during the fourth and fifth weeks. *C*, Drawing of an adult tongue, showing the pharyngeal arch derivation of the nerve supply of its mucosa (mucous membrane). *CN*, Cranial nerve.

Figure 10–22 An infant with ankyloglossia (tongue-tie). Note the short frenulum, which extends to the tip of the tongue. Ankyloglossia interferes with protrusion of the tongue and it may make breast-feeding difficult.

stomodeum and the **mandibular prominences** constitute the caudal boundary of the stomodeum (see Fig. 10-23*A* and Fig. 10-24). The lower jaw and the lower lip are the first parts of the face to form. They result from merging of the medial ends of the mandibular prominences. The common "chin dimple" results from incomplete fusion of the prominences.

By the end of the fourth week, bilateral oval thickenings of the surface ectoderm—**nasal placodes**—have developed on the inferolateral parts of the frontonasal prominence (see Fig. 10-24 and Fig. 10-25*A* and *B*). Initially, these placodes are convex, but later, they are stretched to produce a flat depression in each placode. The mesenchyme in the margins of the placodes proliferates, producing horseshoe-shaped elevations—the medial and lateral **nasal prominences** (see Fig. 10-23*B* and Fig. 10-25*D* and *E*). As a result, the nasal placodes lie in depressions—**nasal pits** (see Figs. 10-23*B* and Fig. 10-25*C* and *D*). These pits are the primordia of the anterior nares (nostrils) and nasal cavities (see Fig. 10-25*E*).

Proliferation of mesenchyme in the maxillary prominences causes them to enlarge and grow medially toward each other and the nasal prominences (see Fig. 10-23*B* and *C* and Fig. 10-24). The medial migration of the maxillary prominences moves the medial nasal prominences toward the median plane and each other. *This process is regulated by transcription factor PDGFRa signaling.* Each lateral nasal prominence is separated from the maxillary prominence by a cleft called the **nasolacrimal groove** (see Fig. 10-23*B*).

By the end of the fifth week, **six auricular hillocks**—*primordia of the auricles* (mesenchymal swellings) form around the first pharyngeal groove (three on each side), the primordium of the external acoustic meatus (ear canal). Initially, the external ears are positioned in the neck region; however, as the mandible develops, they ascend to the side of the head at the level of the eyes (see Fig. 10-23*B* and *C*).

By the end of the sixth week, each maxillary prominence has begun to merge with the lateral nasal prominence along the line of the nasolacrimal groove (Fig. 10-26*A* and *B*). This establishes continuity between the side of the nose, formed by the lateral nasal prominence, and the cheek region, formed by the maxillary prominence.

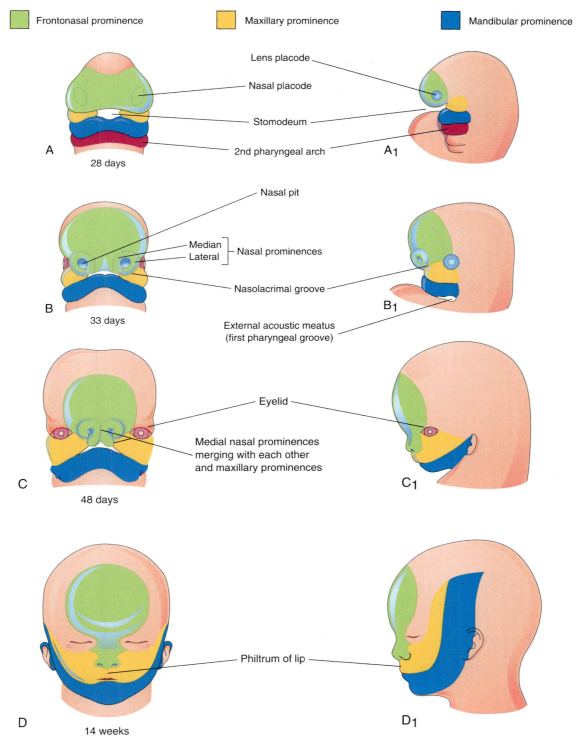

Figure 10–23   **A** to **D₁,** Diagrams illustrating progressive stages in the development of the human face.

The **nasolacrimal duct** develops from a rod-like thickening of ectoderm in the floor of the *nasolacrimal groove*. This thickening gives rise to a solid epithelial cord that separates from the ectoderm and sinks into the mesenchyme. Later, as a result of **apoptosis** (programmed cell death), this cord canalizes to form the nasolacrimal duct. The cranial end of this duct expands to form the *lacrimal sac*. In the late fetal period, the nasolacrimal duct drains into the inferior meatus in the lateral wall of the nasal cavity. The duct usually becomes completely patent (open) after birth.

Between weeks 7 and 10, the **medial nasal prominences** merge with each other and with the maxillary and lateral nasal prominences (see Fig. 10-23C), resulting in

Figure 10–24 Scanning electron micrograph of a ventral view of a human embryo at approximately 33 days (Carnegie stage 15; crown–rump length, 8 mm). Observe the prominent frontonasal prominence *(FNP)* surrounding the telencephalon (forebrain). Also observe the nasal pits *(NP)* located in the ventrolateral regions of the frontonasal prominence. Medial and lateral nasal prominences surround these pits. The wedge-shaped maxillary prominences *(MXP)* form the lateral boundaries of the stomodeum. The fusing mandibular prominences *(MDP)* are located just caudal to the stomodeum. The second pharyngeal arch *(BA2)* is clearly visible and shows overhanging margins. The third pharyngeal arch *(BA3)* is also clearly visible. *(From Hinrichsen K: The early development of morphology and patterns of the face in the human embryo. Adv Anat Embryol Cell Biol 98:1, 1985.)*

disintegration of their contacting surface epithelia. This causes intermingling of the underlying mesenchyme. Merging of the medial nasal and maxillary prominences results in continuity of the upper jaw and lip and separation of the nasal pits from the stomodeum. As the medial nasal prominences merge, they form an **intermaxillary segment** (see Fig. 10-26C to F). The segment gives rise to the:

- Median part (philtrum) of the upper lip
- Premaxillary part of the maxilla and its associated gingiva (gum)
- Primary palate

The lateral parts of the upper lip, most of the maxilla, and the secondary palate form from the **maxillary prominences** (see Fig. 10-23D). These prominences merge laterally with the mandibular prominences. Recent studies indicate that the lower part of the medial nasal prominences appears to have become deeply positioned and covered by medial extensions of the maxillary prominences to form the **philtrum**.

Figure 10–25 Progressive stages in the development of a human nasal sac (primordial nasal cavity). **A,** Ventral view of an embryo at approximately 28 days. **B** to **E,** Transverse sections through the left side of the developing nasal sac.

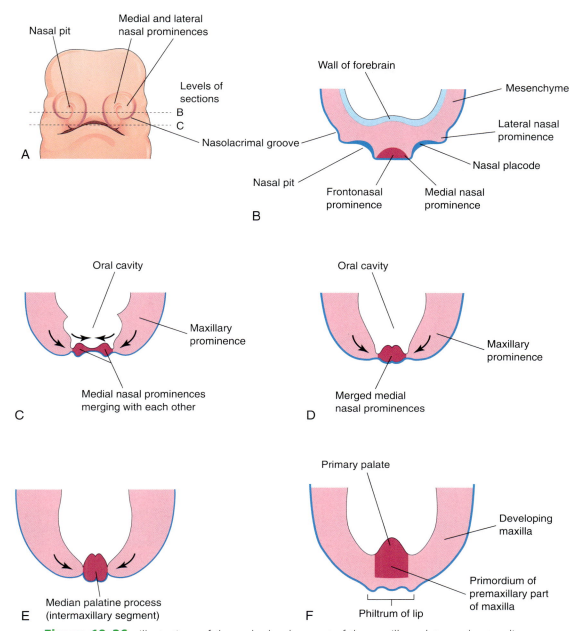

Figure 10–26 Illustrations of the early development of the maxilla, palate, and upper lip. **A,** Facial view of a 5-week embryo. **B** and **C,** Sketches of horizontal sections at the levels shown in **A**. The *arrows* in **C** indicate subsequent growth of the maxillary and medial nasal prominences toward the median plane and merging of the prominences with each other. **D** to **F,** Similar sections of older embryos illustrating merging of the medial nasal prominences with each other and the maxillary prominences to form the upper lip. Recent studies suggest that the upper lip is formed entirely from the maxillary prominences.

The primordial lips and cheeks are invaded by myoblasts from the second pair of pharyngeal arches, which differentiate into the **facial muscles** (see Fig. 10-5 and Table 10-1). The myoblasts from the first pair of arches differentiate into the muscles of mastication. The smallness of the face prenatally results from the following:

- Rudimentary upper and lower jaws
- No erupted deciduous teeth
- Small size of nasal cavities and maxillary sinuses

DEVELOPMENT OF NASAL CAVITIES

As the face develops, the **nasal placodes** become depressed, forming **nasal pits** (see Fig. 10-24 and Fig. 10-25). Proliferation of the surrounding mesenchyme forms the medial and lateral **nasal prominences** and results in deepening of the nasal pits and formation of primordial **nasal sacs**. Each sac grows dorsally, ventral to the developing forebrain (Fig. 10-27A). At first, the nasal sacs are separated from the oral cavity by the **oronasal membrane**.

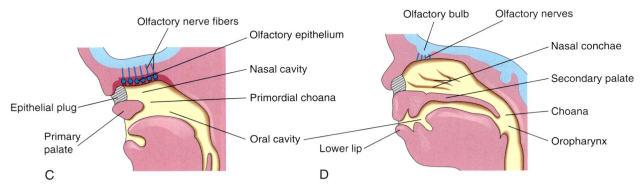

Figure 10–27   Sagittal sections of the head showing development of the nasal cavities. The nasal septum has been removed. **A,** 5 weeks. **B,** 6 weeks, showing breakdown of the oronasal membrane. **C,** 7 weeks, showing the nasal cavity communicating with the oral cavity and development of the olfactory epithelium. **D,** 12 weeks, showing that the palate and lateral wall of the nasal cavity are evident.

This membrane ruptures by the end of the sixth week, bringing the nasal and oral cavities into communication (see Fig. 10-27*B* and *C*). Proliferating epithelial cells (epithelial plug) fills the anterior lumen of the nasal cavity by 7 to 8 weeks. This epithelial plug undergoes apoptosis and by the 17th week, the nasal passages are reopened becoming the nasal vestibule.

The regions of continuity between the nasal and oral cavities are the **primordial choanae** (right or left openings from the nasal cavity into the nasal pharynx), which lie posterior to the primary palate. After the *secondary palate* develops, the choanae are located at the junction of the nasal cavity and pharynx (see Fig. 10-27*D*). While these changes are occurring, the superior, middle, and inferior **nasal conchae** develop as elevations of the lateral walls of the nasal cavities (see Fig. 10-29*E* and *G*). Concurrently, the ectodermal epithelium in the roof of each nasal cavity becomes specialized to form the **olfactory epithelium**. Some epithelial cells differentiate into olfactory receptor cells. The axons of these cells constitute the **olfactory nerves**, which grow into the olfactory bulbs of the brain (see Fig. 10-27*C* and *D*).

Paranasal Sinuses

Some paranasal sinuses, such as the **maxillary sinuses**, begin to develop during late fetal life; the remainder of

POSTNATAL DEVELOPMENT OF PARANASAL SINUSES

Most of the paranasal sinuses are rudimentary or absent in neonates. The *maxillary sinuses* are small at birth. They grow slowly until puberty and are not fully developed until all of the permanent teeth have erupted in early adulthood.

No **frontal** or **sphenoid sinuses** are present at birth. The **ethmoid cells** (sinuses) are small before 2 years, and they do not begin to grow rapidly until 6 to 8 years. At approximately 2 years, the two most anterior ethmoid cells grow into the frontal bone, forming a frontal sinus on each side. Usually, the frontal sinuses are visible on radiographs by 7 years. The two most anterior ethmoid cells grow into the frontal bone at approximately 2 years, forming a frontal sinus on each side. The two most posterior ethmoid cells grow into the sphenoid bone at approximately 2 years of age, forming two sphenoidal sinuses. Growth of the paranasal sinuses is important in altering the size and shape of the face during infancy and childhood and in adding resonance to the voice during adolescence.

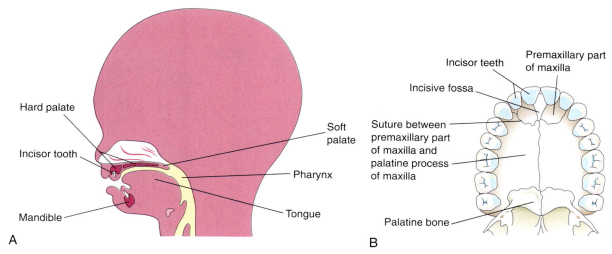

Figure 10–28 **A,** Sagittal section of the head of a 20-week fetus, illustrating the location of the palate. **B,** The bony palate and alveolar arch of a young adult. The suture between the premaxillary part of the maxilla and the fused palatal processes of the maxillae is usually visible in the crania (skulls) of young persons. The suture is not visible in the hard palates of most dried crania because they are usually from old adults.

them develop after birth. They form from outgrowths (diverticula) of the walls of the nasal cavities, becoming pneumatic (air-filled) extensions of the nasal cavities in the adjacent bones. The original openings of the diverticula persist as the orifices of the adult sinuses.

▶ DEVELOPMENT OF PALATE

8 The palate develops from two primordia: the primary palate and secondary palate. **Palatogenesis** (a regulated morphogenetic process) begins in the sixth week but is not completed until the 12th week. *Multiple molecular pathways, including* Wnt *and* PRICKLE1, *are involved.* The critical period of pathogenesis is from the end of the sixth week until the beginning of the ninth week.

Primary Palate

Early in the sixth week, the primary palate (**median palatine process**) begins to develop from the deep part of the intermaxillary segment of the maxilla (see Fig. 10-26F and Fig. 10-27). Initially, this segment is a wedge-shaped mass of mesenchyme between the internal surfaces of the maxillary prominences of the developing maxillae. The primary palate forms the **premaxillary part of the maxilla** (Fig. 10-28B). It represents only a small part of the adult hard palate (the part anterior to the incisive fossa).

Secondary Palate

The secondary palate (definitive palate) is the primordium of the hard and soft parts of the palate (see Fig. 10-27D and Fig. 10-28A and B). It begins to develop early in the sixth week from two mesenchymal projections that extend from the internal aspects of

the maxillary prominences. Initially, these structures—**lateral palatine processes** (palatal shelves)—project inferomedially on each side of the tongue (Fig. 10-29A to C). As the jaws develop, they pull the tongue away from its root, and, as a result, it is brought lower in the mouth.

During the seventh and eighth weeks, the lateral palatine processes elongate and ascend to a horizontal position superior to the tongue. The release of hyaluronic acid in the palatine process mesenchyme helps with this elevation. Gradually, the processes approach each other and fuse in the median plane (see Fig. 10-29D to H). They also fuse with the nasal septum and the posterior part of the primary palate. Elevation of the palatine processes to the horizontal position is believed to be caused by an intrinsic force that is generated by the hydration of hyaluronic acid in the mesenchymal cells within the palatine processes. The medial epithelial seam at the edges of the palatine shelves breaks down, allowing for the fusion of the palatine shelves.

The **nasal septum** develops in a downward growth pattern from internal parts of the merged medial nasal prominences (see Fig. 10-29C, E, and G). The fusion between the nasal septum and the palatine processes begins anteriorly during the ninth week and is completed posteriorly by the 12th week, superior to the primordium of the hard palate (see Fig. 10-29D and F). Bone gradually develops by intramembranous ossification (see Chapter 15) in the primary palate, forming the premaxillary part of the maxilla, which lodges the incisor teeth (see Fig. 10-28B). Concurrently, bone extends from the maxillae and palatine bones into the lateral palatine processes to form the **hard palate** (see Fig. 10-29E and G). The posterior parts of these processes do not become ossified; they extend posteriorly beyond the nasal septum and fuse to form the **soft palate**, including its conical projection, the **uvula** (see Fig. 10-29D, F, and H). The

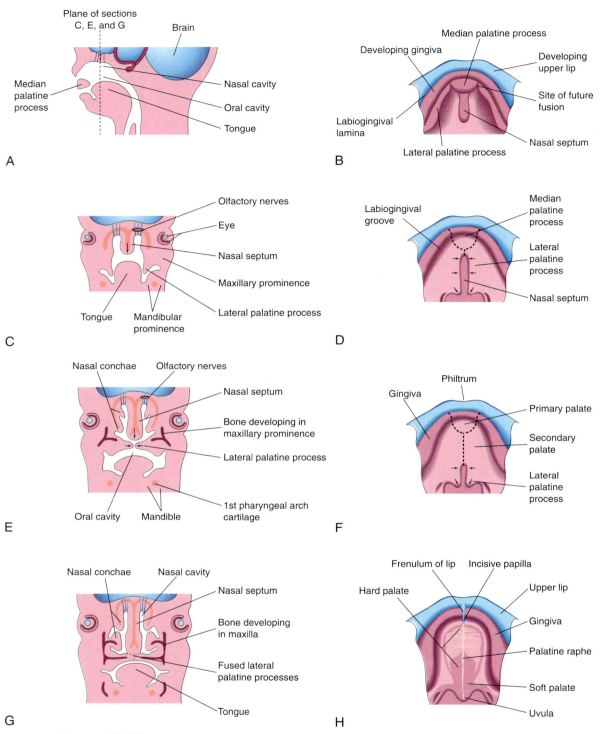

Figure 10–29 **A,** Sagittal section of the embryonic head at the end of the sixth week showing the median palatine process. **B, D, F,** and **H,** Roof of the mouth from the sixth to 12th weeks, illustrating the development of the palate. The *broken lines* in **D** and **F** indicate the sites of fusion of the palatine processes. The *arrows* indicate medial and posterior growth of the lateral palatine processes. **C, E,** and **G,** Frontal sections of the head, illustrating fusion of the lateral palatine processes with each other and with the nasal septum, and separation of the nasal and oral cavities.

median palatine raphe indicates the line of fusion of the lateral palatine processes. A small **nasopalatine canal** persists in the median plane of the palate, between the premaxillary part of the maxilla and the palatine processes of the maxillae. This canal is represented in the adult hard palate by the **incisive fossa** (see Fig. 10-28B). An irregular suture runs from the incisive fossa to the alveolar process of the maxilla, between the lateral incisor and the canine teeth on each side, indicating where the embryonic primary and secondary palates fused.

CLEFT LIP AND CLEFT PALATE

Clefts of the upper lip and palate are common. The defects are usually classified according to developmental criteria, with the incisive fossa and papilla used as reference landmarks (see Fig. 10-28B and Fig. 10-33A). Cleft lip and cleft palate are especially conspicuous because they result in an abnormal facial appearance and defective speech (Fig. 10-30). Two major groups of cleft lip and cleft palate are recognized (Fig. 10-31, Fig. 10-32, and Fig. 10-33):

* **Anterior cleft** defects include cleft lip, with or without cleft of the alveolar part of the maxilla. A complete cleft anomaly is one in which the cleft extends through the lip and the alveolar part of the maxilla to the incisive fossa, separating the anterior and posterior parts of the palate (see Fig. 10-33E and F). Anterior cleft anomalies result from a deficiency of mesenchyme in the maxillary prominences and the median palatine process (see Fig. 10-26D and E).
* **Posterior cleft** defects include clefts of the secondary, or posterior, palate that extend through the soft and hard regions of the palate to the incisive fossa, separating the anterior and posterior parts of the palate (see Fig. 10-33G and H). Posterior cleft defects are caused by defective development of the secondary palate and result from growth distortions in the lateral palatine processes that, in turn, prevent the medial migration and fusion of these processes.

Clefts involving the upper lip, with or without cleft palate, occur in approximately 1 in 1000 births; however, their frequency varies widely, and 60% to 80% of those affected are males. The clefts vary in severity from small notches in the vermilion border of the lip (see Fig. 10-32G) to larger clefts that extend into the floor of the nostril and through the alveolar part of the maxilla (see Fig. 10-31A and Fig. 10-33E). *Cleft lip can be unilateral or bilateral.*

Unilateral cleft lip (see Fig. 10-31A) results from failure of the maxillary prominence on the affected side to unite with the merged medial nasal prominences (see Fig. 10-32A to H), in turn causing a persistent labial groove. The tissues in the floor of the persistent groove break down. As a result, the lip is divided into medial and lateral parts. Sometimes, a bridge of tissue, a *Simonart band*, joins the parts of the incomplete cleft lip.

Bilateral cleft lip (see Figs. 10-31B and 10-33F) results from failure of the mesenchymal masses in the maxillary prominences to meet and unite with the merged medial nasal prominences. When there is a complete bilateral cleft of the lip and the alveolar part of the maxilla, the intermaxillary segment hangs free and projects anteriorly. These defects are especially deforming because of the loss of continuity of the **orbicularis oris muscle**, which closes the mouth and purses the lips.

Median cleft lip is an extremely rare defect. It results from partial or complete failure of the medial nasal prominences to merge and form the intermaxillary segment. Median cleft of the lower lip is also very rare and is caused by failure of the mandibular prominences to merge completely (see Fig. 10-23). The landmark for distinguishing anterior from posterior cleft anomalies is the **incisive fossa** (see Fig. 10-28B). Anterior and posterior cleft defects are embryologically distinct.

Cleft palate, with or without cleft lip, occurs in approximately 1 in 2500 births and is more common in girls than in boys. The cleft may involve only the uvula—cleft uvula—giving it a fish-tail appearance (see Fig. 10-33B), or it may extend through the soft and hard regions of the palate (see Fig. 10-33C and D). In severe cases associated with cleft lip, the cleft in the palate extends through the alveolar part of the maxilla and lips on both sides (see Fig. 10-33G and H).

Unilateral and bilateral clefts in the palate are classified into three groups:

* *Clefts of the anterior palate* result from failure of the lateral palatine processes to meet and fuse with the primary palate (see Fig. 10-33F).
* *Clefts of the posterior palate* result from failure of the lateral palatine processes to meet and fuse with each other and with the nasal septum (see Fig. 10-29E).
* *Clefts of the anterior and posterior parts of the palate* result from failure of the lateral palatine processes to meet and fuse with the primary palate, with each other, and with the nasal septum.

Most clefts of the lip and palate result from multiple factors (*multifactorial inheritance*; see Chapter 19). Some clefts of the lip, palate, or both appear as part of syndromes determined by single mutant genes. Other clefts are features of chromosomal syndromes, especially **trisomy 13** (see Chapter 19, Fig. 19-6). A few cases of cleft lip or cleft palate appear to be caused by teratogenic agents (e.g., anticonvulsant drugs). A sibling of a child with a cleft palate has an elevated risk of having a cleft palate, but no increased risk of cleft lip. A cleft of the lip and the alveolar process of the maxilla that continues through the palate is usually transmitted through a male sex-linked gene.

FACIAL CLEFTS

Various types of facial cleft occur, but they are extremely rare. Severe clefts are usually associated with gross anomalies of the head. *Oblique facial clefts* (orbitofacial fissures) are often bilateral and extend from the upper lip to the medial margin of the orbit. When this occurs, the nasolacrimal ducts are open grooves (persistent nasolacrimal grooves). Oblique facial clefts associated with cleft lip result from failure of the maxillary prominences to merge with the lateral and medial nasal prominences. Lateral, or transverse, facial clefts run from the mouth toward the ear. Bilateral clefts result in a very large mouth—*macrostomia*. In severe cases, the clefts in the cheeks extend almost to the ears.

Figure 10–30   Infant with unilateral cleft lip and cleft palate. Clefts of the lip, with or without a cleft palate, occur in approximately 1 in 1000 births; most affected individuals are males.

Figure 10–31   Birth defects of the lip and palate. **A,** Infant with a left unilateral cleft lip and cleft palate. **B,** Infant with a bilateral cleft lip and cleft palate.

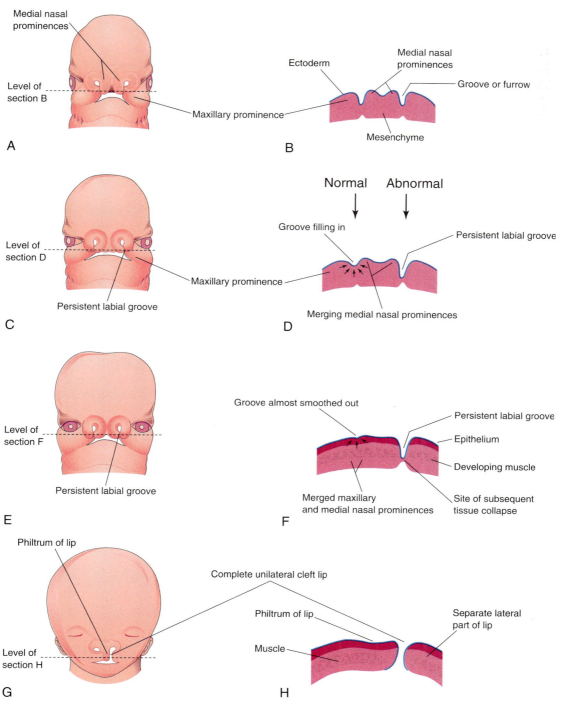

Figure 10–32 Drawings illustrating the embryologic basis for a complete unilateral cleft lip. **A,** 5-week embryo. **B,** Horizontal section through the head illustrating the grooves between the maxillary prominences and the merging medial nasal prominences. **C,** 6-week embryo showing a persistent labial groove on the left side. **D,** Horizontal section through the head showing the groove gradually filling in on the right side after proliferation of the mesenchyme (*arrows*). **E,** 7-week embryo. **F,** Horizontal section through the head showing that the epithelium on the right has almost been pushed out of the groove between the maxillary and medial nasal prominences. **G,** 10-week fetus with a complete unilateral cleft lip. **H,** Horizontal section through the head after stretching of the epithelium and breakdown of the tissues in the floor of the persistent labial groove on the left side, forming complete unilateral cleft lip.

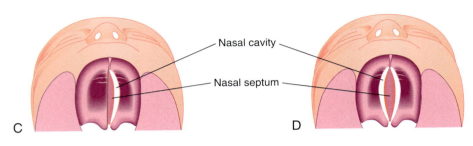

Figure 10–33 Various types of cleft lip and cleft palate. **A,** Normal lip and palate. **B,** Cleft uvula. **C,** Unilateral cleft of the posterior (secondary) palate. **D,** Bilateral cleft of the posterior palate. **E,** Complete unilateral cleft of the lip and alveolar process of the maxilla with a unilateral cleft of the anterior (primary) palate. **F,** Complete bilateral cleft of the lip and the alveolar processes of the maxillae with bilateral cleft of the anterior palate. **G,** Complete bilateral cleft of the lip and the alveolar processes of the maxillae with bilateral cleft of the anterior palate and unilateral cleft of the posterior palate. **H,** Complete bilateral cleft of the lip and the alveolar processes of the maxillae with complete bilateral cleft of the anterior and posterior palate.

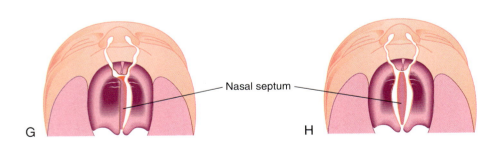

CLINICALLY ORIENTED QUESTIONS

1. Do embryos have cleft lips? Does this common facial defect represent a persistence of such an embryonic condition?

2. Neither Clare nor her husband Jack has a cleft lip or a cleft palate, and no one in either one of their families is known to have or to have had these anomalies. What are their chances of having a child with a cleft lip, with or without a cleft palate?

3. Mary's son has a cleft lip and a cleft palate. Her brother has a similar defect involving his lip and palate. Although Mary does not plan to have any more children, her husband says that Mary is entirely to blame for their son's birth defects. Was the defect likely inherited only from Mary's side of the family?

4. A patient's son has minor anomalies involving his external ears, but he does not have hearing problems or a facial malformation. Would his ear abnormalities be considered pharyngeal (branchial) arch defects?

The answers to these questions are at the back of this book.

Respiratory System

T he **lower respiratory organs** (larynx, trachea, bronchi, and lungs) begin to form during the fourth week of development. The respiratory system starts as a median outgrowth—the **laryngotracheal groove**—that appears in the floor of the caudal end of the primordial pharynx (Fig. 11-1*A* and *B*). The primordium of the **tracheobronchial tree** develops caudal to the fourth pair of pharyngeal pouches. The endodermal lining of the **laryngotracheal groove** gives rise to the pulmonary epithelium and glands of the larynx, trachea, and bronchi. The connective tissue, cartilage, and smooth muscle in these structures develop from the splanchnic mesoderm surrounding the foregut (see Fig. 11-4*A*). *Signaling pathways of* BMP, Wnt, *and* FGF *control patterning of the expression of* Sox2 *and* Nkx2.1 *in the early foregut for the differentiation of the trachea from the esophagus. In the ventral areas,* Nkx2.1 *is activated while* Sox2 *is suppressed.*

By the end of the fourth week, the laryngotracheal groove has evaginated (protruded) to form a pouch-like **laryngotracheal diverticulum** (lung bud), which is located ventral to the caudal part of the foregut (see Fig. 11-1*A* and Fig. 11-2*A*).

As the diverticulum elongates, its distal end enlarges to form a globular **respiratory bud** (see Fig. 11-2*B*). The laryngotracheal diverticulum soon separates from the **primordial pharynx**, but it maintains communication with it through the **primordial laryngeal inlet** (see Fig. 11-2*A* and *C*). As the diverticulum elongates, it is invested with splanchnic mesoderm (see Fig. 11-2*B*). Longitudinal **tracheoesophageal folds** develop in the laryngotracheal diverticulum, approach each other, and fuse to form a partition—the **tracheoesophageal septum** (see Fig. 11-2*D* and *E*).

This septum divides the cranial part of the foregut into a *ventral part*, the **laryngotracheal tube** (primordium of the larynx, trachea, bronchi, and lungs), and a *dorsal part* (primordium of the oropharynx and esophagus) (see Fig. 11-2*F*). The opening of the laryngotracheal tube into the pharynx becomes the **primordial laryngeal inlet** (see Fig. 11-2*F* and Fig.11-3*C*).

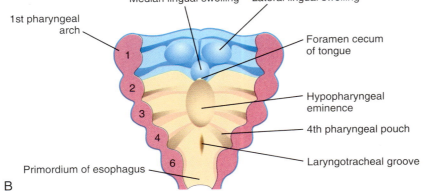

Figure 11–1 **A,** Sagittal section of the cranial half of a 4-week embryo. **B,** Horizontal section of the embryo, illustrating the floor of the primordial pharynx and the location of the laryngotracheal groove.

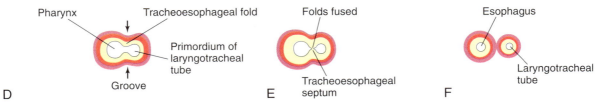

Figure 11–2 Successive stages in the development of the tracheoesophageal septum during the fourth and fifth weeks of development. **A** to **C,** Lateral views of the caudal part of the primordial pharynx, showing the laryngotracheal diverticulum and partitioning of the foregut into the esophagus and the laryngotracheal tube. **D** to **F,** Transverse sections, illustrating the formation of the tracheoesophageal septum and how it separates the foregut into the laryngotracheal tube and esophagus. The *arrows* represent cellular changes resulting from growth.

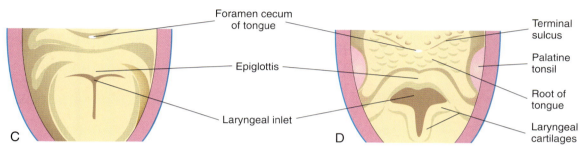

Figure 11–3 Successive stages in the development of the larynx. **A,** 4 weeks. **B,** 5 weeks. **C,** 6 weeks. **D,** 10 weeks. The epithelium lining the larynx is of endodermal origin. The cartilages and muscles of the larynx arise from the mesenchyme in the fourth and sixth pairs of pharyngeal arches. Note that the laryngeal inlet changes in shape from a slit-like opening to a T-shaped inlet as the mesenchyme surrounding the developing larynx proliferates.

DEVELOPMENT OF LARYNX

The epithelial lining of the larynx develops from the endoderm of the cranial end of the laryngotracheal tube. The cartilages of the larynx develop from cell populations in the fourth and sixth pairs of pharyngeal arches (see Chapter 10). The **laryngeal cartilages** develop from mesenchyme that is derived from *neural crest cells*. The mesenchyme at the cranial end of the laryngotracheal tube proliferates rapidly, producing paired **arytenoid swellings** (see Fig. 11-3*B*). These swellings grow toward the tongue, converting the **primordial glottis** into a T-shaped **laryngeal inlet** (see Fig. 11-3*C* and *D*). The laryngeal epithelium proliferates rapidly, resulting in *temporary occlusion of the laryngeal lumen*. Recanalization of the larynx occurs by the 10th week. The laryngeal ventricles form during this recanalization process. These recesses are bound by folds of mucous membrane that evolve into the *vocal folds* (cords) and the *vestibular folds*.

The **epiglottis** develops from the caudal part of the *hypopharyngeal eminence*, a prominence produced by the proliferation of the mesenchyme in the ventral ends of the third and fourth pharyngeal arches (see Chapter 10, Fig. 10-21; and Fig. 11-3*B* to *D*). The rostral part of this eminence forms the posterior third or pharyngeal part of the tongue (see Chapter 10, Fig. 10-21). The **laryngeal muscles** develop from myoblasts in the fourth and sixth pairs of pharyngeal arches and are therefore innervated by the laryngeal branches of the vagus nerves (CN X) that supply these arches (see Table 10-1). Growth of

LARYNGEAL ATRESIA

Laryngeal atresia (obstruction) is a rare birth defect that results in obstruction of the upper fetal airway—**congenital high airway obstruction syndrome**. Distal to the atresia or stenosis (narrowing), the airways become dilated, the lungs are hyperplastic (causing compression of the heart and great vessels), the diaphragm is either flattened or inverted, and **fetal hydrops** (accumulation of fluid in two or more compartments) and/or **ascites** (abdominal fluid) is present. Prenatal ultrasonography permits diagnosis of these anomalies.

the larynx and epiglottis is rapid during the first 3 years after birth, by which time the epiglottis has reached its adult form and position.

DEVELOPMENT OF TRACHEA

The endodermal lining of the laryngotracheal tube distal to the larynx differentiates into the epithelium and the glands of the trachea and the pulmonary epithelium. The cartilage, connective tissue, and muscles of the trachea are derived from the splanchnic mesoderm surrounding the laryngotracheal tube (Fig. 11-4).

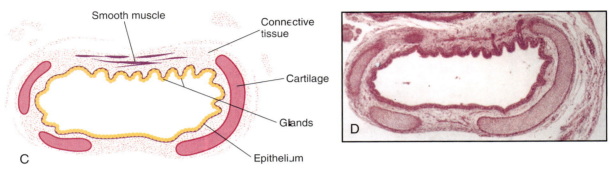

Figure 11–4   Transverse sections through the laryngotracheal tube, illustrating progressive stages in the development of the trachea. **A,** 4 weeks. **B,** 10 weeks. **C,** 11 weeks (drawing of micrograph in **D**). Note that the endoderm of the tube gives rise to the epithelium and the glands of the trachea and that the mesenchyme surrounding the tube forms the connective tissue, muscle, and cartilage (drawing of the micrograph shown in **D**). **D,** Photomicrograph of a transverse section of the developing trachea at 12 weeks. *(From Moore KL, Persaud TVN, Shiota K: Color Atlas of Clinical Embryology, 2nd ed. Philadelphia, Saunders, 2000.)*

TRACHEOESOPHAGEAL FISTULA

A **tracheoesophageal fistula** (**TEF**) is an abnormal passage between the trachea and esophagus (Fig. 11-5 and Fig.11-6*A*). This birth defect occurs at a rate of approximately 1 in 3000 to 1 in 4500 live births and predominantly affects males. In most cases, the fistula is associated with **esophageal atresia**. TEF results from incomplete division of the cranial part of the foregut into respiratory and esophageal parts during the fourth week. Incomplete fusion of the tracheoesophageal folds results in a **defective tracheoesophageal septum** and communication between the trachea and esophagus.

TEF is the most common anomaly of the lower respiratory tract. Four main varieties of TEF may develop (see Fig. 11-5). The usual anomaly is a blind ending of the superior part of the esophagus (**esophageal atresia**) and a joining of the inferior part to the trachea near its bifurcation (see Fig. 11-5*A* and Fig. 11-6*B*). Infants with this type of TEF and esophageal atresia cough and choke when swallowing because of the accumulation of excessive amounts of liquid in the mouth and upper respiratory tract. When the infant attempts to swallow milk, it rapidly fills the esophageal pouch and is regurgitated. Gastric contents may also reflux from the stomach through the fistula into the trachea and lungs, which may result in **pneumonia** or **pneumonitis** (inflammation of the lungs). Other varieties of TEF are shown in Fig. 11-5*B* to *D*. **Polyhydramnios** (see Chapter 8) is often associated with esophageal atresia. Excess amniotic fluid accumulates because fluid cannot pass to the stomach and intestines for absorption and subsequent transfer through the placenta to the maternal blood for disposal.

TRACHEAL STENOSIS AND ATRESIA

Narrowing (stenosis) and obstruction (atresia) of the trachea are uncommon birth defects that are usually associated with one of the varieties of TEF. Stenoses and atresias probably result from unequal partitioning of the foregut into the esophagus and trachea (see Fig. 11-5). In some cases, a web of tissue obstructs airflow (*incomplete tracheal atresia*).

DEVELOPMENT OF BRONCHI AND LUNGS

The **respiratory bud** (lung bud) develops at the caudal end of the laryngotracheal diverticulum during the fourth week (see Fig. 11-2*B*). The bud soon divides into two outpouchings—**primary bronchial buds** (see Fig. 11-2*C*). Later, **secondary and tertiary bronchial buds** form and grow laterally into the *pericardioperitoneal canals* (see Fig. 11-7*A*).

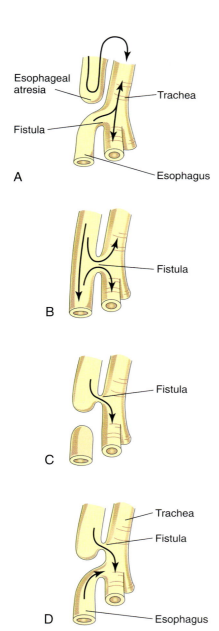

Figure 11–5 The four main varieties of tracheoesophageal fistula (TEF) are shown in order of frequency. Possible directions of the flow of the contents are indicated by *arrows*. **A,** Esophageal atresia is associated with TEF in more than 85% of cases. **B,** Fistula between the trachea and esophagus; this type of birth defect accounts for approximately 4% of cases. **C,** Atresia of the proximal esophagus ending in a tracheoesophageal fistula with the distal esophagus having a blind pouch. Air cannot enter the distal esophagus and stomach. **D,** Atresia of the proximal segment of the esophagus with fistulas between the trachea and both the proximal and distal segments of the esophagus. Air can enter the distal esophagus and stomach. All neonates born with TEF have esophageal dysmotility disorders, and most have reflux (regurgitation of contents of the stomach).

Figure 11–6 **A,** Tracheoesophageal fistula in a 17-week fetus. The upper esophageal segment ends blindly *(arrow)*. (**A,** *From Kalousek DK, Fitch N, Paradice BA: Pathology of the Human Embryo and Previable Fetus. New York, Springer Verlag, 1990.*) **B,** Radiograph of an infant with esophageal atresia. Air in the distal gastrointestinal tract indicates the presence of a tracheoesophageal fistula *(arrow, blind proximal esophageal sac).*

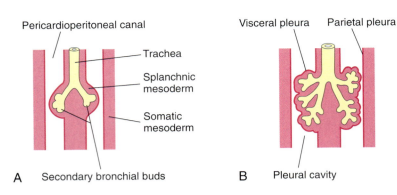

Figure 11–7 Illustrations of the growth of the developing lungs into the splanchnic mesoderm adjacent to the medial walls of the pericardioperitoneal canals (primordial pleural cavities). Development of the layers of the pleura is also shown. **A,** 5 weeks. **B,** 6 weeks.

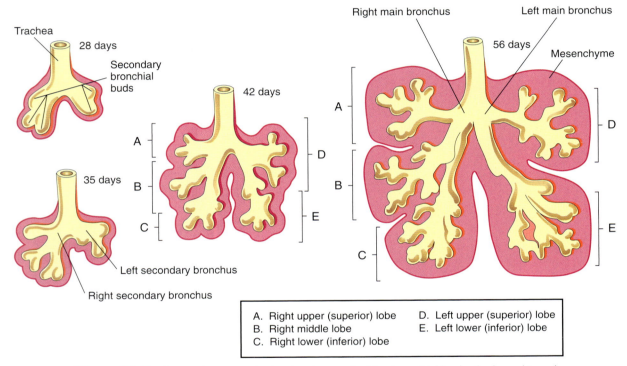

A. Right upper (superior) lobe	D. Left upper (superior) lobe
B. Right middle lobe	E. Left lower (inferior) lobe
C. Right lower (inferior) lobe	

Figure 11–8 Successive stages in the development of the bronchial buds, the bronchi, and the lungs.

Together with the surrounding splanchnic mesoderm, the bronchial buds differentiate into the **bronchi** and their ramifications in the lungs (see Fig. 11-7*B*). Early in the fifth week, the connection of each bronchial bud with the trachea enlarges to form the primordia of **main bronchi** (Fig. 11-8).

The embryonic right main bronchus is slightly larger than the left one and is oriented more vertically. This embryonic relationship persists in adults; consequently, a foreign body is more liable to enter the right main bronchus than the left one.

The main bronchi subdivide into **secondary bronchi that form lobar, segmental, and intrasegmental branches** (see Fig. 11-8). On the right, the superior secondary bronchus supplies the upper (superior) lobe of the lung, whereas the inferior secondary bronchus subdivides into two bronchi, one connecting to the middle lobe of the right lung and the other connecting to the lower (inferior) lobe. On the left, the two secondary bronchi supply the upper and lower lobes of the lung. Each secondary bronchus undergoes progressive branching.

The **segmental bronchi**, 10 in the right lung and 8 or 9 in the left lung, begin to form by the seventh week. As this occurs, the surrounding mesenchyme also divides. Each segmental bronchus, with its surrounding mass of mesenchyme, is the primordium of a **bronchopulmonary segment**. By 24 weeks, approximately 17 orders of branching have occurred and **respiratory bronchioles** have developed (Fig. 11-9*B*). An additional seven orders of airways develop after birth.

As the bronchi develop, cartilaginous plates are formed from the surrounding splanchnic mesenchyme. The bronchial smooth muscle and connective tissue and the pulmonary connective tissue and capillaries are also derived

A   Pseudoglandular period (5–17 weeks)

B   Canalicular period (16–25 weeks)

C   Terminal saccular period (24 weeks–late fetal period)

D   Alveolar period (late fetal period–8 years)

Figure 11–9   Diagram of histologic sections showing progressive stages of lung development. **A** and **B,** Early stages of lung development. In **C** and **D,** note that the alveolocapillary membrane is thin and that some capillaries bulge into the terminal saccules.

from this mesenchyme. As the lungs develop, they acquire a layer of **visceral pleura** from the splanchnic mesoderm (see Fig. 11-7). With expansion, the lungs and pleural cavities grow caudally into the mesenchyme of the body wall and soon lie close to the heart. The thoracic body wall becomes lined by a layer of **parietal pleura** derived from the somatic mesoderm (see Fig. 11-7*B*). The space between the visceral and parietal pleura is the **pleural cavity.**

Maturation of Lungs

Maturation of the lungs is divided into four histologic stages: pseudoglandular, canalicular, terminal saccular, and alveolar.

Pseudoglandular Period (5–17 Weeks)

The developing lungs resemble, on a histologic basis, an exocrine gland during the early part of this period (see Fig. 11-9*A*). By 16 weeks, all of the major elements of the lung have formed, except those involved with gas

exchange. Respiration is not possible; hence, *fetuses born during this period are unable to survive.*

Canalicular Period (16–25 Weeks)

This period overlaps the pseudoglandular period because cranial segments of the lungs mature faster than caudal segments. During the canalicular period, the lumina of the bronchi and the **terminal bronchioles** become larger and the lung tissue becomes highly vascular (see Fig. 11-9*B*). By 24 weeks, each terminal bronchiole has given rise to two or more **respiratory bronchioles,** each of which then divides into three to six tubular passages— **primordial alveolar ducts.**

Respiration is possible toward the end of the canalicular stage because some thin-walled **terminal sacs** (primordial alveoli) have developed at the ends of the respiratory bronchioles and *the lung tissue is well vascularized (rendered vascular by formation of new vessels).* Although a fetus born at 24 to 26 weeks may survive if given intensive care, it often dies because its respiratory and other systems are relatively immature.

Terminal Saccular Period (24 Weeks to Late Fetal Period)

During this period, many more terminal sacs (primordial alveoli) develop, and their *epithelium becomes very thin*. Capillaries begin to bulge into these sacs (see Fig. 11-9C). The intimate contact between epithelial and endothelial cells, establishes the **blood-air barrier**, which permits adequate gas exchange for survival.

By 26 weeks, the terminal sacs are lined mainly by squamous epithelial cells of endodermal origin—**type I pneumocytes**—across which gas exchange occurs. The capillary network proliferates rapidly in the mesenchyme around the developing alveoli, and there is concurrent active development of lymphatic capillaries. Scattered among the squamous epithelial cells are rounded secretory epithelial cells—**type II pneumocytes**, *which secrete pulmonary surfactant*, a complex mixture of phospholipids and proteins.

Surfactant forms as a monomolecular film over the interior walls of the alveolar sacs and counteracts surface tension forces at the air-alveolar interface. This facilitates expansion of the terminal sacs.

The maturation of alveolar type II cells and the production of surfactant vary widely in fetuses of different ages. *Surfactant production begins by 20 to 22 weeks*, but surfactant is present in only small amounts in premature infants. It does not reach adequate levels until the late fetal period. Both increased surfactant production, induced by antenatal corticosteroids, and **postnatal surfactant replacement therapy** have increased the rates of survival of these infants.

Alveolar Period (Late Fetal Period to 8 Years)

Exactly when the terminal saccular period ends and the alveolar period begins depends on the definition of the term *alveolus* (see Fig. 11-9D). At the beginning of the alveolar period, each respiratory bronchiole terminates in a cluster of thin-walled terminal sacs that are separated from one another by loose connective tissue. These terminal sacs represent future **alveolar ducts**. The **alveolocapillary membrane** (pulmonary diffusion barrier, or respiratory membrane) is sufficiently thin to allow gas exchange. The transition from dependence on the placenta for gas exchange to autonomous gas exchange after birth requires the following adaptive changes in the lungs:

- Production of surfactant in the alveolar sacs
- Transformation of the lungs into gas-exchanging organs
- Establishment of parallel pulmonary and systemic circulations

Approximately 95% of **mature alveoli** develop in the postnatal period. Before birth, the primordial alveoli appear as small bulges on the walls of the respiratory bronchioles and alveolar sacs (see Fig. 11-9D). After birth, the primordial alveoli enlarge as the lungs expand; however, most of the increase in the size of the lungs results from a continued increase in the number of respiratory bronchioles and primordial alveoli rather than from an increase in the size of the alveoli. Alveolar development is largely complete by 3 years of age, but new alveoli may be added until approximately 8 years of age. Unlike mature alveoli, *immature alveoli have the potential for forming additional primordial alveoli*.

Approximately 150 million primordial alveoli, one half the number in adults, are present in the lungs of full-term neonates. On chest radiographs, therefore, the lungs of neonates appear denser than adult lungs. Between the third and eighth year, the adult complement of 300 million alveoli is achieved.

Three factors that are essential for normal lung development are:

- Adequate thoracic space for lung growth
- Adequate amniotic fluid volume
- Fetal breathing movements

The mechanism modulating lung morphogenesis and formation of blood vessels in the lungs involves the transcription factors Sox17 and Wnt signaling.

Fetal breathing movements occur before birth, exerting sufficient force to cause aspiration of some amniotic fluid into the lungs. These fetal breathing movements occur approximately 50% of the time and only during rapid eye movement sleep. These movements stimulate lung development, possibly by creating a pressure gradient between the lungs and the amniotic fluid. By birth, the fetus has had the advantage of several months of breathing exercise. Fetal breathing movements increase as the time of delivery approaches.

At birth, the lungs are approximately half-filled with fluid derived from the amniotic cavity, the lungs, and the tracheal glands. Aeration of the lungs at birth occurs not so much by the inflation of empty collapsed organs as by the rapid replacement of intra-alveolar fluid by air. The fluid in the lungs is cleared at birth by three routes:

- Through the mouth and nose by pressure on the thorax during vaginal delivery
- Into the pulmonary capillaries and pulmonary arteries and veins
- Into the lymphatic vessels

OLIGOHYDRAMNIOS AND LUNG DEVELOPMENT

When **oligohydramnios** (insufficient amount of amniotic fluid) is severe and chronic, lung development is retarded. It is thought that reduced hydraulic pressure in the lungs and its consequential effects on lung calcium regulation may result in **pulmonary hypoplasia**, which may be severe.

NEONATAL RESPIRATORY DISTRESS SYNDROME

Respiratory distress syndrome (RDS) affects approximately 2% of live newborns, and those born prematurely are the most susceptible. RDS is also known as *hyaline membrane disease*. *Surfactant deficiency is a major cause of RDS. Prolonged intrauterine asphyxia* may produce irreversible changes in type II alveolar cells, making them incapable of producing surfactant. *Corticosteroids* are potent stimulators of fetal surfactant production and may be given to the mother if early delivery is a risk. Neonates with RDS have rapid, labored breathing shortly after birth. An estimated 30% of all neonatal disease results from RDS or its complications. The lungs are underinflated and the alveoli contain amorphous materials (*hyaline membrane*) from substances in the circulation and the injured pulmonary epithelium. Treatment includes supplementary oxygen and artificial surfactant—more than 90% of neonates with RDS survive.

LUNGS OF NEONATES

Fresh healthy lungs always contain some air; consequently, pulmonary tissue samples float in water. By contrast, a diseased lung that is partially filled with fluid may not float. Of medicolegal significance is the fact that the lungs of a *stillborn* neonate are firm and sink when placed in water because they contain fluid, not air.

LUNG HYPOPLASIA

In infants with a **congenital diaphragmatic hernia** (see Chapter 9), the lungs may not develop normally. This hypoplasia may be caused by changes in growth factors that exist before the abdominal viscera become abnormally positioned. **Lung hypoplasia (underdevelopment)** is characterized by markedly reduced lung volume. Many infants with a congenital diaphragmatic hernia die of pulmonary insufficiency, despite optimal postnatal care, because their lungs are too hypoplastic to support extrauterine life.

CLINICALLY ORIENTED QUESTIONS

1. What stimulates the infant to start breathing at birth? Is "slapping the buttocks" necessary?
2. A neonate reportedly died approximately 72 hours after birth from the effects of respiratory distress syndrome. What is respiratory distress syndrome? By what other name is this condition known? Is its cause genetic or environmental?
3. Can a neonate born 22 weeks after fertilization survive? What can be done to reduce the severity of respiratory distress syndrome?

The answers to these questions are at the back of this book.

Alimentary System

T he **alimentary system** (digestive system) is the digestive tract from the mouth to the anus with all its associative glands and organs. The **primordial gut (earliest stage of development)** forms during the fourth week as the head, caudal eminence (tail), and lateral folds incorporate the dorsal part of the **umbilical vesicle** (yolk sac) (see Chapter 6, Fig. 6-1). The primordial gut is initially closed at its cranial end by the **oropharyngeal membrane** (see Chapter 10, Fig. 10-1*B*), and at its caudal end by the **cloacal membrane** (Fig. 12-1). The endoderm of the primordial gut gives rise to most of the gut, epithelium, and glands. The epithelium at the cranial and caudal ends of the alimentary tract is derived from the ectoderm of the **stomodeum** and **anal pit** (proctodeum), respectively (see Fig. 12-1).

The muscular and connective tissue and other layers of the wall of the **alimentary tract** are derived from the splanchnic mesenchyme surrounding the **primordial gut**. For descriptive purposes, the gut is divided into three parts: foregut, midgut, and hindgut. *The regional differentiation of the primordial gut is established by sonic and Indian hedgehog genes (SHH and IHH) that are expressed in the endoderm and the surrounding mesoderm.* The endodermal signaling provides temporal and positional information for the development of the gut.

FOREGUT

The derivatives of the foregut are the:

- Primordial pharynx and its derivatives
- Lower respiratory system
- Esophagus and stomach
- Duodenum, just distal to the opening of the bile duct
- Liver, biliary apparatus (hepatic ducts, gallbladder, and bile duct), and pancreas

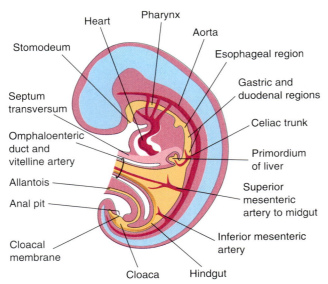

Figure 12–1 Drawing of median section of a 4-week embryo, showing the early alimentary system and its blood supply.

These foregut derivatives, other than the pharynx, lower respiratory tract, and most of the esophagus, are supplied by the **celiac trunk**, the artery of the foregut (see Fig. 12-1 and Fig. 12-2*A*).

Development of Esophagus

10 The esophagus develops from the foregut immediately caudal to the pharynx (see Fig. 12-1). Initially, the esophagus is short, but it elongates rapidly and reaches its final relative length by the seventh week. Its epithelium and glands are derived from the endoderm. The epithelium proliferates and, partly or completely, obliterates the esophageal lumen; however, recanalization normally occurs by the end of the eighth week. The striated muscle of the esophagus is derived from mesenchyme in the fourth and sixth pharyngeal arches (see Chapter 10, Figs. 10-1 and 10-5*B*). The smooth muscle, mainly in the inferior third of the esophagus, develops from the surrounding splanchnic mesenchyme.

ESOPHAGEAL ATRESIA

Blockage (atresia) of the esophageal lumen occurs in approximately 1 in 3000 to 1 in 4500 neonates. Approximately one third of affected infants are born prematurely. **Esophageal atresia** is frequently associated with **tracheoesophageal fistula** (see Chapter 11, Fig. 11-5 and Fig. 11-6). The atresia results from deviation of the *tracheoesophageal septum* in a posterior direction (see Chapter 11, Fig. 11-2 and Fig. 11-6); as a result, separation of the esophagus from the laryngotracheal tube is incomplete. In some cases, the atresia results from *failure of esophageal recanalization* during the eighth week of development. A fetus with esophageal atresia is unable to swallow amniotic fluid, resulting in **polyhydramnios**, the accumulation of excessive amniotic fluid.

ESOPHAGEAL STENOSIS

Narrowing of the lumen of the esophagus (stenosis) can occur anywhere along the esophagus, but it usually occurs in the distal one third, either as a web or as a long segment of esophagus. with a thread-like lumen. The stenosis usually results from incomplete recanalization of the esophagus during the eighth week.

Development of Stomach

During the fourth week, a slight dilation of the tubular foregut indicates the site of the primordial stomach. It first appears as a fusiform enlargement of the caudal part of the foregut that is oriented in the median plane (see Fig. 12-2*B*). The primordial stomach enlarges and broadens ventrodorsally. Its dorsal border grows more quickly than its ventral border. This site of rapid growth demarcates the **greater curvature of the stomach** (see Fig. 12-2*D*).

Rotation of Stomach

As the stomach enlarges, it rotates 90 degrees in a clockwise direction around its longitudinal axis. The effects of rotation on the stomach are (see Fig. 12-2 and Fig. 12-3):

- The ventral border (lesser curvature) moves to the right and the dorsal border (greater curvature) moves to the left (see Fig. 12-2*C* to *F*).
- Before rotation, the cranial and caudal ends of the stomach are in the median plane (see Fig. 12-2*B*).
- During rotation and growth of the stomach, its cranial region moves to the left and slightly inferiorly, and its caudal region moves to the right and superiorly (see Fig. 12-2*C* to *E*).
- After rotation, the stomach assumes its final position, with its long axis almost transverse to the long axis of the body (see Fig. 12-2*E*). This rotation and growth explains why the **left vagus nerve** supplies the anterior wall of the adult stomach, and the **right vagus nerve** innervates its posterior wall.

HYPERTROPHIC PYLORIC STENOSIS

Birth defects of the stomach are uncommon, except for hypertrophic pyloric stenosis, which affects 1 in 150 males and 1 in 750 females. Infants with this birth defect have marked **muscular thickening of the pylorus** *of the stomach, the distal* **sphincteric region** *of the stomach. The muscles in the pyloric region are hypertrophied, which results in* **severe stenosis (narrowing) of the pyloric canal** *and obstruction to the passage of food. As a result, the stomach becomes markedly distended and its contents are expelled with considerable force* **(projectile vomiting)**. *Surgical relief of the obstruction is the usual treatment.*

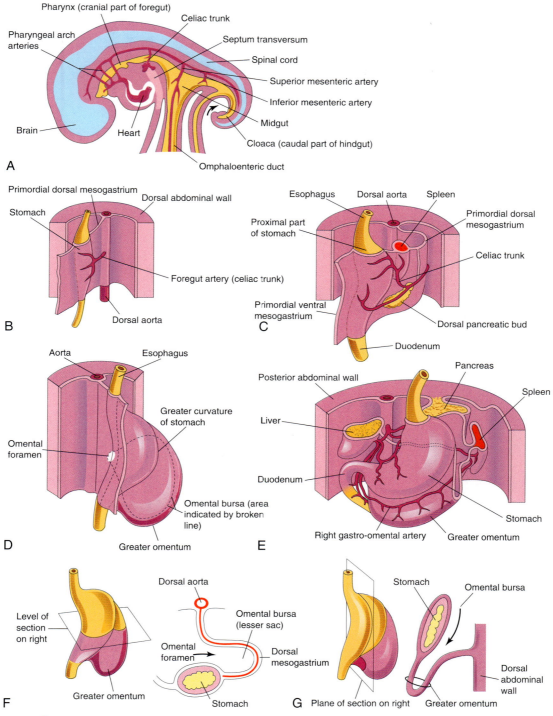

Figure 12–2   Illustrations of the development and rotation of the stomach and formation of the omental bursa and greater omentum. **A,** Median section of the abdomen of a 28-day embryo. **B,** Anterolateral view of the embryo shown in **A. C,** Embryo of approximately 35 days. **D,** Embryo at approximately 40 days. **E,** Embryo of approximately 48 days. **F,** Lateral view of the stomach and greater omentum of an embryo of approximately 52 days. **G,** Sagittal section, showing the omental bursa and greater omentum. The *arrows* in **F** and **G** indicate the site of the omental foramen.

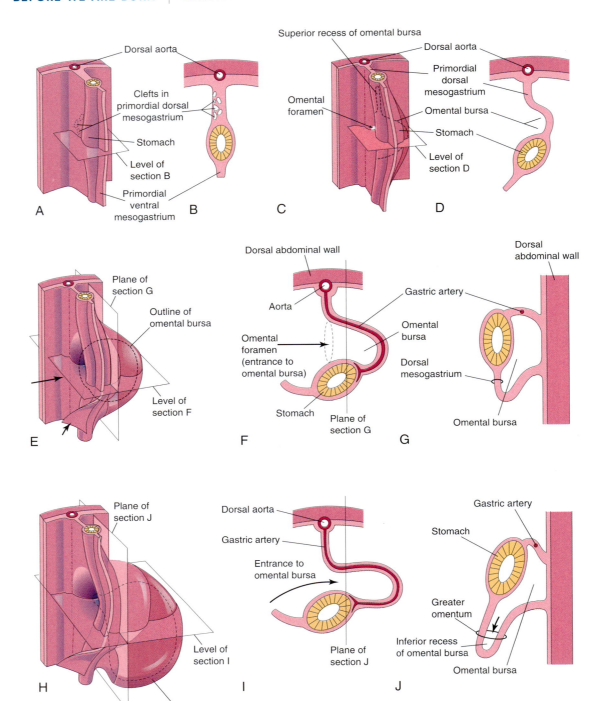

Figure 12–3 Development of stomach and mesenteries and formation of omental bursa. **A,** Embryo of 5 weeks. **B,** Transverse section showing clefts in the dorsal mesogastrium. **C,** Later stage after coalescence of the clefts to form the omental bursa. **D,** Transverse section showing the initial appearance of the omental bursa. **E,** The dorsal mesentery has elongated and the omental bursa has enlarged. **F** and **G,** Transverse and sagittal sections, respectively, showing elongation of the dorsal mesogastrium and expansion of the omental bursa. **H,** Embryo of 6 weeks, showing the greater omentum and expansion of the omental bursa. **I** and **J,** Transverse and sagittal sections, respectively, showing the inferior recess of the omental bursa and omental foramen. The *arrows* in **E, F,** and **I** indicate the site of the omental foramen. In **J,** the *arrow* indicates the recess of the omental bursa.

Mesenteries of Stomach

The stomach is suspended from the **dorsal wall** of the abdominal cavity by the **primordial dorsal mesogastrium** (see Fig. 12-2*B* and *C* and Fig. 12-3*A* to *E*). This mesentery, originally located in the median plane, is carried to the left during rotation of the stomach and formation of the omental bursa. The **primordial ventral mesogastrium** attaches to the stomach, duodenum, liver, and ventral abdominal wall (see Fig. 12-2*C* and Fig. 12-3*A* and *B*).

▶ Omental Bursa

10 Isolated clefts develop in the mesenchyme forming the dorsal mesogastrium (see Fig. 12-3*A* and *B*). The clefts soon coalesce to form a single cavity—the **omental bursa** *(lesser peritoneal sac)*—a large recess of the peritoneal cavity (see Fig. 12-2*F* and *G* and Fig. 12-3*C* and *D*). Rotation of the stomach pulls the dorsal mesogastrium to the left, thereby enlarging the bursa. The pouch-like bursa facilitates movements of the stomach.

The omental bursa lies between the stomach and posterior abdominal wall. As the stomach enlarges, the bursa expands and hangs over the developing intestines (see Fig. 12-3*J*). This part of the bursa is the **greater omentum** (see Fig. 12-3*G* to *J* and Fig. 12-13*A*). The two layers of the greater omentum eventually fuse (see Fig. 12-13*F*). The **omental bursa** communicates with the main part of the peritoneal cavity through a small opening—the **omental foramen** (see Fig. 12-2*D* and *F* and Fig. 12-3*C* and *F*).

▶ Development of Duodenum

10 Early in the fourth week, the duodenum begins to develop from the caudal part of the foregut and the cranial part of the midgut (Fig. 12-4*A*). The developing duodenum elongates, forming a C-shaped loop that projects ventrally (see Fig. 12-4*B* to *D*). As the stomach rotates, the duodenal loop rotates to the right and lies **retroperitoneal** (external to peritoneum). Because of its derivation from the foregut and midgut, the duodenum is supplied by branches of both the celiac and superior mesenteric arteries (see Fig. 12-1). During the fifth and sixth weeks, the lumen of the duodenum is temporarily obliterated because of proliferation of its epithelial cells; normally the lumen is recanalized by the end of the embryonic period (8 weeks).

▶ Development of Liver and Biliary Apparatus

10 The liver, gallbladder, and biliary duct system arise as a ventral outgrowth—**hepatic diverticulum**—from the

DUODENAL STENOSIS

Partial occlusion of the duodenal lumen—**duodenal stenosis**—is usually caused by incomplete recanalization of the duodenum, resulting from defective vacuolization. Most stenoses involve the horizontal (third) and/or ascending (fourth) parts of the duodenum. Because of the stenosis, the stomach's contents (usually containing bile) are often vomited.

DUODENAL ATRESIA

Complete occlusion of the duodenum—**duodenal atresia**—is not common. During early development, the duodenal lumen is completely occluded by epithelial cells. If complete recanalization of the lumen fails to occur, a short segment of the duodenum is occluded (Fig. 12-5*B*). Most atresias involve the descending and horizontal parts of the duodenum and are located distal to the opening of the bile duct. In neonates with duodenal atresia, vomiting begins within a few hours of birth. The vomitus almost always contains bile. **Polyhydramnios** (excess of amniotic fluid) also occurs because duodenal atresia prevents normal absorption of amniotic fluid by the intestines. A diagnosis of duodenal atresia is suggested by the presence of a "double-bubble sign" on plain radiographs or ultrasound scans (see Fig. 12-5*B*). This sign is caused by a distended, gas-filled stomach and the proximal duodenum. Between 20% and 30% of affected infants have Down syndrome and an additional 20% are premature neonates.

caudal part of the foregut early in the fourth week (see Fig. 12-4*A* and Fig. 12-6*A*). *Wnt/β-catenin signaling is involved in the induction of the hepatic diverticulum.*

The diverticulum extends into the **septum transversum** (see Fig. 12-6*B*), a mass of splanchnic mesoderm between the developing heart and midgut. The diverticulum enlarges and divides into two parts as it grows between the layers of the **ventral mesogastrium** (see Fig. 12-4*A*). The larger cranial part of the diverticulum is the **primordium of the liver**; the smaller caudal portion becomes the **gallbladder**. The proliferating endodermal cells give rise to interlacing cords of **hepatocytes** (parenchymal liver cells) and to the epithelial lining of the intrahepatic part of the biliary apparatus. The **hepatic cords** anastomose around endothelium-lined spaces, the primordia of the hepatic sinusoids. The fibrous and hematopoietic tissue and **Kupffer cells** of the liver are derived from mesenchyme in the septum transversum. The liver grows rapidly from the 5th to 10th weeks and fills a large part of the upper abdominal cavity (see Fig. 12-4 and Fig. 12-6*C* and *D*).

Hematopoiesis (formation and development of various types of blood cells) begins in the liver during the sixth week. By the ninth week, the liver accounts for approximately 10% of the total weight of the fetus. **Bile formation** by the hepatic cells begins during the 12th week.

The small caudal part of the hepatic diverticulum becomes the **gallbladder** and the stalk forms the **cystic duct** (see Fig. 12-4*B* and *C*). Initially, the *extrahepatic biliary apparatus* is occluded with epithelial cells. The stalk connecting the hepatic and cystic ducts to the duodenum becomes the **bile duct**; this duct attaches to the ventral aspect of the duodenal loop. As the duodenum grows and rotates, the entrance of the bile duct is carried to the dorsal aspect of the duodenum (see Fig. 12-4*C* and *D*). The bile entering the duodenum through the bile duct after the 13th week gives the meconium (first intestinal discharges of neonate) a dark green color.

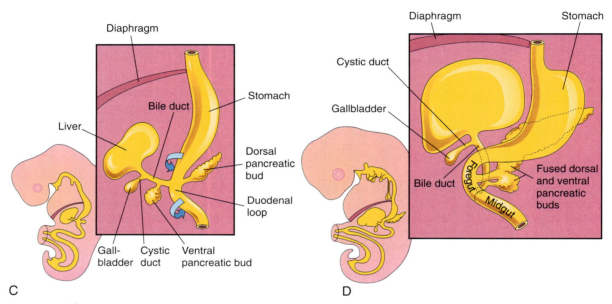

Figure 12–4 Progressive stages in the development of the duodenum, liver, pancreas, and extrahepatic biliary apparatus. **A,** Embryo of 4 weeks. **B** and **C,** Embryo of 5 weeks. **D,** Embryo of 6 weeks. The pancreas develops from the dorsal and ventral pancreatic buds that fuse to form the pancreas. Note that the entrance of the bile duct into the duodenum gradually shifts from its initial position to a posterior one. This explains why the bile duct in adults passes posterior to the duodenum and the head of the pancreas.

BIRTH DEFECTS OF LIVER

Minor variations of liver lobulation are common; however, birth defects are rare. Variations of hepatic ducts, bile duct, and cystic duct are common and clinically significant. **Accessory hepatic ducts** are present in approximately 5% of the population, and awareness of their possible presence is of importance in surgery (e.g., liver transplantation).

EXTRAHEPATIC BILIARY ATRESIA

This is the most serious birth defect involving the **extrahepatic biliary system,** and it occurs in 1 in 5000 to 20,000 live births. These neonates have loss or absence of all or a significant portion of the extrahepatic biliary system. The cause is unclear. **Jaundice** typically occurs between 2 and 6 weeks postpartum, and surgical correction to enhance bile flow, while not curative, can provide temporary palliation. Definitive therapy requires liver transplantation.

Development of Pancreas

Figure 12–5 Ultrasound scans of a fetus of 33 weeks' gestation (31 weeks after fertilization), showing duodenal atresia. **A,** An oblique scan shows the dilated, fluid-filled stomach *(St)* entering the proximal duodenum *(D)*, which is also enlarged because of the atresia (blockage) distal to it. **B,** Transverse ultrasound scan, showing the characteristic "double-bubble" appearance of the stomach and duodenum when there is duodenal atresia.

The pancreas develops between the layers of the mesenteries from dorsal and ventral **pancreatic buds**, which arise from the caudal part of the foregut (Fig. 12-8*A*). Most of the pancreas is derived from the larger **dorsal pancreatic bud**, which appears first.

Formation of the dorsal pancreatic bud depends on signals from the notochord (activin and fibroblast growth factor 2) that block the expression of sonic hedgehog (Shh) in the endoderm. Expression of pancreatic and duodenal homeobox factors (PDX-1 and MafA) is critical for the development of the pancreas.

The smaller **ventral pancreatic bud** develops near the entry of the bile duct into the duodenum (see Fig. 12-8*A* and *B*). As the duodenum rotates to the right and becomes C-shaped, the bud is carried dorsally with the bile duct (see Fig. 12-8*C* to *F*). It soon lies posterior to the dorsal pancreatic bud and later fuses with it (see Fig. 12-8*G*). As the pancreatic buds fuse, their ducts anastomose (link or be linked by anastomosis). The ventral pancreatic bud forms the **uncinate process** and part of the **head of the pancreas**. As the stomach, duodenum, and ventral mesentery rotate, the pancreas comes to lie along the dorsal abdominal wall (retroperitoneal) (see Fig. 12-8*D* and *G*).

The **pancreatic duct** forms from the duct of the ventral bud and the distal part of the duct of the dorsal bud (see Fig. 12-8*G*). In approximately 9% of people, the proximal part of the duct of the dorsal bud persists as an **accessory pancreatic duct** that opens into the *minor duodenal papilla*. The connective tissue sheath and interlobular septa of the pancreas develop from the surrounding splanchnic mesenchyme. **Insulin secretion** begins at approximately 10 weeks. The glucagon- and somatostatin-containing cells develop before differentiation of the insulin-secreting cells occurs. With increasing fetal age, total pancreatic insulin and glucagon content also increases.

DEVELOPMENT OF SPLEEN

The spleen is derived from a mass of mesenchymal cells located between the layers of the dorsal mesogastrium

Ventral Mesentery

The thin, *double-layered ventral* membrane (see Fig. 12-6*C* and *D* and Fig. 12-7) gives rise to:

- The **lesser omentum**, passing from the liver to the lesser curvature of the stomach (**hepatogastric ligament**) and from the liver to the duodenum (**hepatoduodenal ligament**)
- The **falciform ligament**, extending from the liver to the ventral abdominal wall

The **umbilical vein** passes in the free border of the falciform ligament on its way from the umbilical cord to the liver. The ventral mesentery, derived from the mesogastrium, also forms the **visceral peritoneum of the liver.**

ANNULAR PANCREAS

Annular pancreas is an uncommon birth defect, but it warrants attention because it may cause duodenal obstruction (Fig. 12-9*C*). This defect probably results from the growth of a bifid ventral pancreatic bud around the duodenum (see Fig. 12-9*A* to *C*). The parts of the bifid ventral bud then fuse with the dorsal bud, forming a pancreatic ring. The ring-like, annular part of the pancreas consists of a thin, flat band of pancreatic tissue surrounding the descending or second part of the duodenum. An annular pancreas may cause obstruction of the duodenum shortly after birth, but many cases are not diagnosed until adulthood. Females are affected more frequently than males.

Figure 12–6   **A,** Median section of a 4-week embryo. **B,** Transverse section of the embryo showing expansion of the peritoneal cavity *(arrows)*. **C,** Sagittal section of a 5-week embryo. **D,** Transverse section of the embryo after formation of the dorsal and ventral mesenteries.

(Fig. 12-10*A* and *B*). The spleen, a vascular lymphatic organ, begins to develop during the fifth week, but does not acquire its characteristic shape until early in the fetal period. The spleen in a fetus is lobulated, but the lobules normally disappear before birth. The notches in the superior border of the adult spleen are remnants of the grooves that separated the fetal lobules.

ACCESSORY SPLEENS

One or more small splenic masses (about 1 cm in diameter) of fully functional splenic tissue may exist in one of the peritoneal folds, usually near the hilum of the spleen or the tail of the pancreas. These accessory spleens (**polysplenia**) occur in approximately 10% of people.

MIDGUT

The derivatives of the midgut are:

- The small intestine, including the duodenum distal to the opening of the bile duct
- The cecum, appendix, ascending colon, and right half to two thirds of the transverse colon

Each of these derivatives is supplied by the **superior mesenteric artery** (see Fig. 12-1 and Fig. 12-7). The **midgut loop** is suspended from the dorsal abdominal wall by an elongated **mesentery** (peritoneum suspending the intestines). The midgut elongates and forms a ventral, U-shaped loop that projects into the proximal part of the **umbilical cord** (Fig. 12-11*A*). The loop of intestine, a **physiologic umbilical herniation**, occurs at the beginning of the sixth week (see Fig. 12-11*C* and Fig. 12-12). The

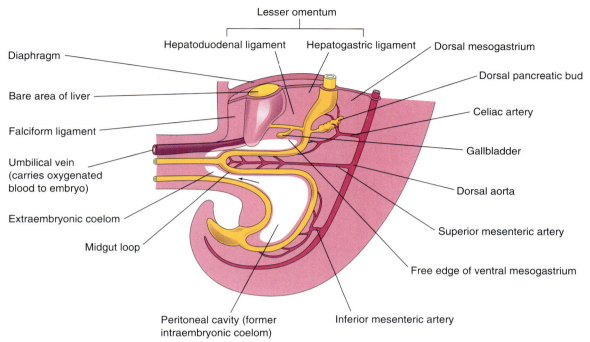

Lesser omentum

Hepatoduodenal ligament | Hepatogastric ligament | Dorsal mesogastrium

Diaphragm

Dorsal pancreatic bud

Bare area of liver

Celiac artery

Falciform ligament

Gallbladder

Umbilical vein (carries oxygenated blood to embryo)

Dorsal aorta

Extraembryonic coelom

Superior mesenteric artery

Midgut loop

Free edge of ventral mesogastrium

Peritoneal cavity (former intraembryonic coelom) | Inferior mesenteric artery

Figure 12–7 Median section of the caudal half of an embryo at the end of the fifth week showing the liver and its associated ligaments. The *arrow* indicates the communication of the peritoneal cavity with the extraembryonic coelom.

loop communicates with the **umbilical vesicle** through the narrow **omphaloenteric duct** until the 10th week (see Fig. 12-11*A* and *C*). The herniation occurs because there is not enough room in the abdominal cavity for the rapidly growing midgut. The shortage of space is caused mainly by the relatively massive liver and kidneys. The cranial limb grows rapidly and forms small **intestinal loops** (see Fig. 12-11*C*). The caudal limb undergoes very little change except for development of the **cecal swelling**, the primordium of the cecum and appendix (see Fig. 12-11*C* to *E*).

Rotation of Midgut Loop

10 While it is in the umbilical cord, the midgut loop rotates 90 degrees counterclockwise around the axis of the **superior mesenteric artery** (see Fig. 12-11*B*). This rotation brings the cranial limb (small intestine) of the midgut loop to the right and the caudal limb (large intestine) to the left. During rotation, the cranial limb elongates and form **intestinal loops** (e.g., primordia of jejunum and ileum).

Retraction of Intestinal Loops

During the 10th week, the intestines return to the abdomen *(reduction of midgut hernia)* (see Fig. 12-11*C* and *D*). The small intestine (formed from the cranial limb) returns first, passing posterior to the superior mesenteric artery, and occupies the central part of the abdomen. As the large intestine returns, it undergoes a further 180-degree counterclockwise rotation (see Fig. 12-11*C₁* and *D₁*). Later, it comes to occupy the right side of the abdomen. The **ascending colon** becomes

recognizable with the elongation of the posterior abdominal wall (see Figs. 12-11*E*).

Fixation of Intestines

Rotation of the stomach and duodenum causes the duodenum and pancreas to fall to the right. The enlarged colon presses the duodenum and pancreas against the posterior abdominal wall. The adjacent layers of peritoneum fuse and subsequently disappear (Fig. 12-13*C* and *F*); consequently, most of the duodenum and head of the pancreas become retroperitoneal (posterior to peritoneum). The mesentery of the ascending colon fuses with the parietal peritoneum on the posterior abdominal wall. The mesentery of the ascending colon becomes retroperitoneal (see Fig. 12-13*B* and *E*). The other derivatives of the midgut loop retain their mesenteries.

Cecum and Appendix

The *primordium of the cecum and appendix*—the cecal 10 swelling (diverticulum)—appears in the sixth week as a swelling on the antimesenteric border of the caudal limb of the midgut loop (see Figs. 12-11*C* to *E* and Fig. 12-14*A*). Initially, the appendix is a small diverticulum (pouch) of the cecum. It subsequently increases rapidly in length so that at birth it is a relatively long tube arising from the distal end of the **cecum** (see Fig. 12-14*D*). After birth, the unequal growth of the walls of the cecum results in the appendix entering its medial side (see Fig. 12-14*E*). *The appendix is subject to considerable variation in position.* As the ascending colon elongates, the appendix may pass posterior to the cecum *(retrocecal appendix)* or colon *(retrocolic appendix)*.

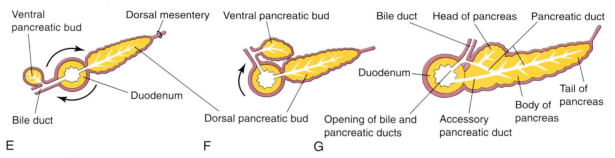

Figure 12–8 **A** to **D**, Successive stages in the development of the pancreas from the fifth to the eighth weeks. **E** to **G**, Transverse sections through the duodenum and developing pancreas. Growth and rotation *(arrows)* of the duodenum bring the ventral pancreatic bud toward the dorsal bud, where the two buds subsequently fuse.

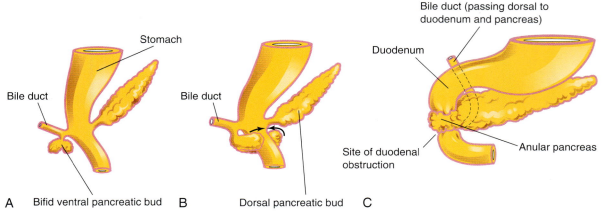

Figure 12–9 **A** and **B,** The probable basis of an annular pancreas. **C,** An annular pancreas encircling the duodenum. This birth defect produces complete obstruction (atresia) or partial obstruction (stenosis) of the duodenum.

CONGENITAL OMPHALOCELE

This birth defect results in persistence of the **herniation of the abdominal contents** into the proximal part of the umbilical cord (Fig. 12-15 and Fig. 12-16). It is caused by failure of the body walls to fuse at the umbilical ring because of defective growth of mesenchyme. Herniation of the intestines occurs in approximately 1 in 5000 births. Herniation of the liver and intestines occurs less frequently (1 in 10,000 births). The size of the hernia depends on its contents. The abdominal cavity is proportionately small when an omphalocele (herniation of viscera) is present because the impetus for it to grow is absent.

GASTROSCHISIS

This birth defect is not common. Gastroschisis results from a defect near the median plane of the abdominal wall (Fig. 12-17). The viscera protrude into the amniotic cavity and are bathed by amniotic fluid. The term *gastroschisis*, which literally means "split stomach," is a misnomer because it is the anterior abdominal wall, not the stomach, that is split. The defect usually occurs on the right side, lateral to the median plane, and is more common in males than females. This birth defect results from incomplete closure of the lateral folds during the fourth week of development (see Chapter 6, Fig. 6-1).

UMBILICAL HERNIA

When the intestines herniate through an imperfectly closed umbilicus, an umbilical hernia forms. This common type of hernia differs from an omphalocele. In umbilical hernias, the protruding mass (usually consisting of part of the greater omentum and small intestine) is covered by subcutaneous tissue and skin. The hernia protrudes during crying, straining, or coughing.

NONROTATION OF MIDGUT

Birth defects of the intestines are relatively common; most of them are defects of gut rotation (e.g., **malrotation of the gut**). Nonrotation of the midgut *(left-sided colon)* is a relatively common defect (Fig. 12-18A and B), resulting in the caudal limb of the midgut loop returning to the abdomen first. The small intestine then lies on the right side of the abdomen and the entire large intestine lies on the left. Although patients are generally asymptomatic, if **volvulus** (twisting) occurs, the superior mesenteric artery may be obstructed, resulting in infarction and gangrene of the associated intestine.

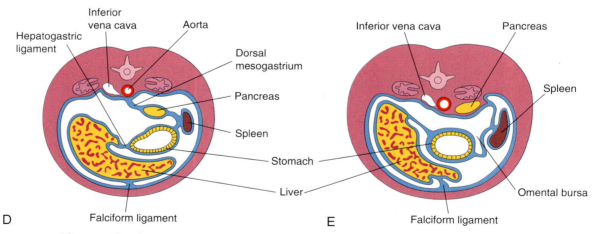

Figure 12–10 **A,** Left side of the stomach and associated structures at the end of the fifth week. Note that the pancreas, spleen, and celiac trunk are between the layers of the dorsal mesogastrium. **B,** Transverse section of the liver, stomach, and spleen at the level shown in **A,** illustrating their relationship to the dorsal and ventral mesenteries. **C,** Transverse section of a fetus showing fusion of the dorsal mesogastrium with the peritoneum on the posterior abdominal wall. **D** and **E,** Similar sections showing movement of the liver to the right and rotation of the stomach. Observe the fusion of the dorsal mesogastrium to the dorsal abdominal wall. As a result, the pancreas becomes retroperitoneal.

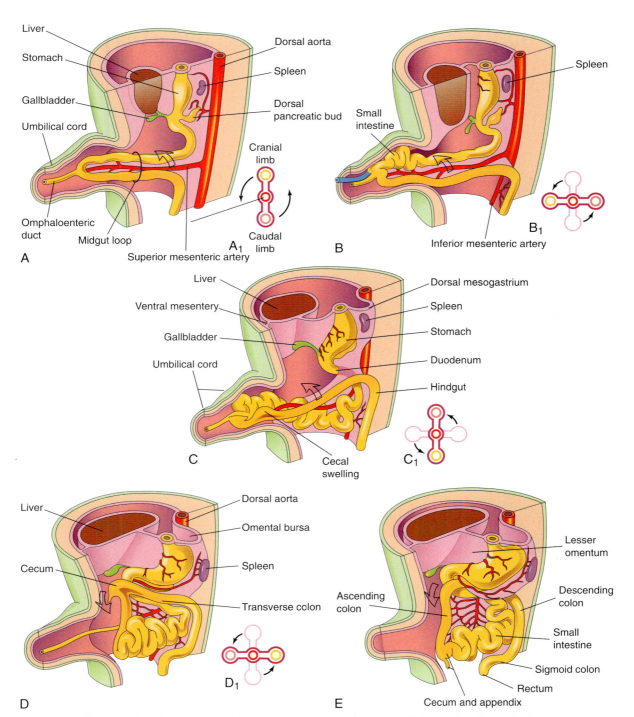

Figure 12–11 Drawings illustrating herniation and rotation of the midgut loop. **A,** At the beginning of the sixth week. **A₁,** Transverse section through the midgut loop, illustrating the initial relationship of the limbs of the midgut loop to the superior mesenteric artery. Note that the midgut loop is in the proximal part of the umbilical cord. **B,** Later stage showing the beginning of midgut rotation. **B₁,** Illustration of the 90-degree counterclockwise rotation that carries the cranial limb of the midgut to the right. **C,** At approximately 10 weeks, showing the intestines returning to the abdomen. **C₁,** Illustration of a further rotation of 90 degrees. **D,** At approximately 11 weeks, showing the location of the viscera (internal organs) after contraction of intestines. **D₁,** Illustrations of a further rotation of 90-degrees rotation of the viscera, for a total of 270 degrees. **E,** Later in the fetal period, showing the cecum rotating to its normal position in the lower right quadrant of the abdomen.

Figure 12–12 **A,** Physiologic hernia in a fetus of approximately 58 days attached to its placenta. Note the herniated intestine in the proximal part of the umbilical cord *(arrow)*. **B,** Transverse section through the abdomen of a 9-week and 5-day-old fetus demonstrates irregular intestinal (bowel) loops just outside the anterior abdominal wall *(thin arrow)*. At this gestational age, this is the normal appearance of physiologic midgut herniation. Conversely, herniation of abdominal contents beyond 12 weeks of gestation would suggest the presence of a pathologic anterior wall defect such as gastroschisis or an omphalocele. Note also the normal location of the umbilical vesicle (yolk sac) *(asterisk)* at this gestational age, just outside the thin-walled amniotic sac *(arrowhead)*.

MIXED ROTATION AND VOLVULUS

With mixed rotation and volvulus, the cecum lies just inferior to the pylorus of the stomach and is fixed to the posterior abdominal wall by peritoneal bands that pass over the duodenum (see Fig. 12-18*B*). These bands and volvulus usually cause **duodenal obstruction**. This type of malrotation results from failure of the midgut loop to complete the final 90 degrees of rotation (see Fig. 12-11*D*); consequently, the terminal part of the ileum returns to the abdomen first.

REVERSED ROTATION

In very unusual cases, the midgut loop rotates in a clockwise rather than a counterclockwise direction (see Fig. 12-18*C*). As a result, the duodenum lies anterior to the superior mesenteric artery, rather than posterior to it, and the transverse colon lies posterior to the superior mesenteric artery instead of anterior to it. In these infants, the transverse colon may be obstructed by pressure from the superior mesenteric artery.

SUBHEPATIC CECUM AND APPENDIX

If the cecum adheres to the inferior surface of the liver when it returns to the abdomen (see Fig. 12-11*D*), it is drawn superiorly with the liver. As a result, the cecum remains in its fetal position (see Fig. 12-18*D*). Subhepatic cecum and appendix are more common in males than in females. This birth defect is not common, but when it occurs, it may create problems in diagnostic procedures for and surgical removal of the appendix in adults.

INTERNAL HERNIA

In this rare birth defect, the small intestine passes into the mesentery of the midgut loop during the return of the intestines to the abdomen (see Fig. 12-18*E*). As a result, a hernia-like sac forms. This very uncommon condition does not usually produce symptoms, and is often detected at postmortem examination.

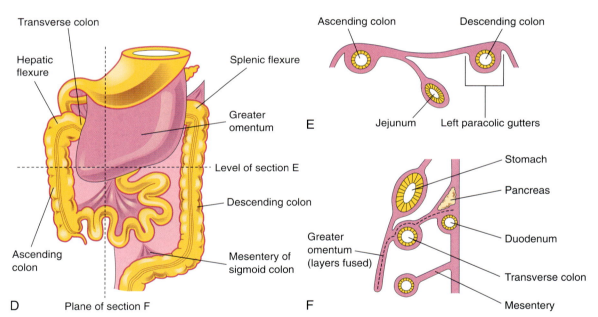

Figure 12–13 Illustration showing the mesenteries and fixation of the intestines. **A,** Ventral view of the intestines before their fixation. **B,** Transverse section at the level shown in **A.** The *arrows* indicate areas of subsequent fusion. **C,** Sagittal section at the plane shown in **A,** illustrating the greater omentum overhanging the transverse colon. The *arrows* indicate areas of subsequent fusion. **D,** Ventral view of the intestines after their fixation. **E,** Transverse section at the level shown in **D** after disappearance of the mesentery of the ascending and descending colon. **F,** Sagittal section at the plane shown in **D,** illustrating fusion of the greater omentum with the mesentery of the transverse colon and fusion of the layers of the greater omentum.

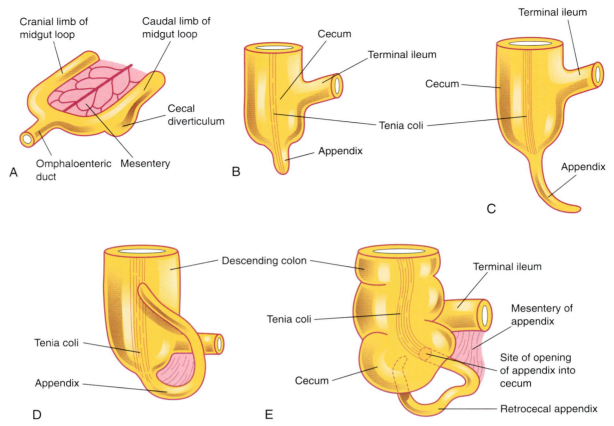

Figure 12–14 Successive stages in the development of the cecum and appendix. **A,** Embryo of 6 weeks. **B,** Embryo of 8 weeks. **C,** Fetus of 12 weeks. **D,** Neonate. Note that the appendix is relatively long and is continuous with the apex of the cecum. **E,** Child. Note that the appendix is now relatively short and its opening is located posterior to the cecum. In approximately 64% of people the appendix is located posterior to the cecum (retrocecal).

MIDGUT VOLVULUS

Midgut volvulus is a birth defect in which the small intestine does not enter the abdominal cavity normally, and the mesenteries do not undergo normal fixation. As a result, **volvulus** (twisting) of the intestines occurs (see Fig. 12-18*F*). Only two parts of the intestine—the duodenum and proximal colon—are attached to the posterior abdominal wall. The small intestine hangs by a narrow stalk that contains the superior mesenteric artery and vein. These vessels are usually twisted in this stalk and become obstructed at or near the **duodenojejunal junction**. The circulation to the twisted intestine is often restricted; if the vessels are completely obstructed, necrosis develops.

STENOSIS AND ATRESIA OF INTESTINE

Partial occlusion *(stenosis)* and complete occlusion *(atresia)* of the intestinal lumen (see Fig. 12-5) account for approximately one third of cases of intestinal obstruction in neonates. The obstructive lesion occurs most often in the ileum (50%) and duodenum (25%). *Stenosis results from failure of recanalization of the intestine.* Most atresias of the ileum are probably caused by infarction of the fetal intestine (bowel) as a result of impairment of its blood supply secondary to volvulus. This impairment most likely occurs during the 10th week as the intestines return to the abdomen.

Figure 12–15 A neonate with a large omphalocele. The defect resulted in herniation of intra-abdominal structures (liver and intestine) into the proximal end of the umbilical cord. The omphalocele is covered by a membrane composed of peritoneum and amnion.

Figure 12–16 Ultrasonogram (sonogram) of the abdomen of a fetus (28 weeks' gestation), showing a large omphalocele (herniation of viscera into the base of the umbilical cord), with much of the liver protruding (herniating) from the abdominal wall. The mass also contains a small, membrane-covered sac *(arrows)*. The umbilical cord was integrally involved in the birth defect.

ILEAL DIVERTICULUM AND OTHER OMPHALOENTERIC DUCT REMNANTS

A congenital **ileal diverticulum**—Meckel diverticulum (Fig. 12-19)—occurs in 2% to 4% of infants, and is three to five times more prevalent in males than in females. It represents a remnant of the proximal portion of the **omphaloenteric duct**. It typically appears as a finger-like pouch approximately 3 to 6 cm long that arises from the *antimesenteric border of the ileum*, 40 to 50 cm from the ileocecal junction. *An ileal diverticulum is of clinical significance because it sometimes becomes inflamed and causes symptoms that mimic appendicitis.* The wall of the diverticulum contains all layers of the ileum and may also contain small patches of gastric and pancreatic tissues. The gastric mucosa often secretes acid, producing ulceration and bleeding (Fig. 12-20A to C). An ileal diverticulum may be connected to the umbilicus by a fibrous cord or an **omphaloenteric fistula** (see Fig. 12-20B and C); other possible remnants of the omphaloenteric duct are shown in Fig. 12-20D to F.

HINDGUT

The derivatives of the hindgut are:

- The left third to half of the transverse colon, the descending colon and sigmoid colon, the rectum, and the superior part of the anal canal
- The epithelium of the urinary bladder and most of the urethra

All hindgut derivatives are supplied by the **inferior mesenteric artery** (see Fig. 12-7). The descending colon becomes retroperitoneal as its mesentery fuses with the peritoneum on the left posterior abdominal wall (see Fig. 12-13B and E). The mesentery of the sigmoid colon is retained (see Fig. 12-13D).

Cloaca

The cloaca is the expanded terminal end of the hindgut 11 before division into the rectum, bladder, and genital primordia. The cloaca is an endoderm-lined chamber that is in contact with the surface ectoderm at the cloacal membrane (Fig. 12-21A and B). This membrane is composed of the endoderm of the cloaca and ectoderm of the anal pit (see Fig. 12-21C and D). The cloaca receives the allantois, which is a finger-like diverticulum (see Fig. 12-21A), ventrally.

Partitioning of Cloaca

The cloaca is divided into dorsal and ventral parts by mesenchyme—the **urorectal septum**—that develops in the angle between the allantois and hindgut (see Fig. 12-21C and D). *Endodermal β-catenin signaling is required for the formation of the urorectal septum.* As the septum grows toward the cloacal membrane, it develops fork-like

Figure 12–17 **A,** Photograph of a neonate with an anterior abdominal wall birth defect—gastroschisis (congenital fissure with protrusion of viscera). The defect was relatively small (2–4 cm long) and involved all layers of the abdominal wall. The defect was located to the right of the umbilicus. **B,** Photograph of the same neonate after the viscera were returned to the abdomen and the defect was surgically closed. **C** and **D,** Sonogram (ultrasonogram) of an 18-week fetus with gastroschisis. Loops of intestine (bowel) can be seen in the amniotic fluid ventral to the fetus on the sagittal scan **(C),** and the axial scan **(D)** of the fetal abdomen.

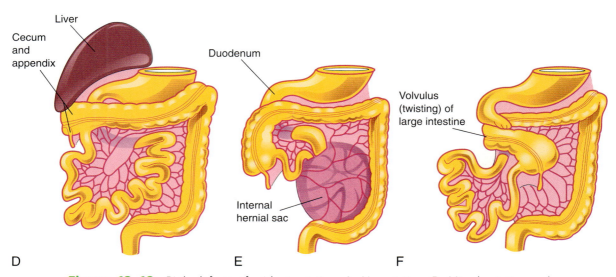

Figure 12–18 Birth defects of midgut rotation. **A,** Nonrotation. **B,** Mixed rotation and volvulus (twisting of intestine). The *arrow* indicates the twisting of the intestine. **C,** Reversed rotation. **D,** Subhepatic (below the liver) cecum and appendix. **E,** Internal hernia. **F,** Midgut volvulus with duodenal obstruction.

extensions that produce infoldings of the lateral walls of the cloaca (see Fig. 12-21B₁). These folds grow toward each other and fuse, forming a partition that divides the cloaca into three parts (see Fig. 12-21D and E)—the **rectum,** the cranial part of the **anal canal,** and the **urogenital sinus.**

The cloaca plays a crucial role in anorectal development. New information indicates that the urorectal septum does not fuse with the cloacal membrane; therefore, an anal membrane does not exist. After the cloacal membrane ruptures by **apoptotic cell death** *(apoptosis),* the **anorectal lumen** is temporarily closed by an **epithelial plug,** which may have been interpreted as the anal membrane (see Fig. 12-21E).

Mesenchymal proliferations produce elevations of the surface ectoderm around the epithelial anal plug. Recanalization of the anorectal canal occurs by apoptotic cell death of the epithelial anal plug, which forms the **anal pit** (see Fig. 12-21) by the eighth week of development.

Anal Canal

The superior two thirds of the adult anal canal are derived from the **hindgut;** the inferior one third develops from the anal pit (Fig. 12-22). The junction of the epithelium derived from the ectoderm of the anal pit and the endoderm of the hindgut is roughly indicated by an irregular **pectinate line,** located at the inferior limit of the **anal valves.** Approximately 2 cm superior to the anus is the **anocutaneous line** ("white line"). This is approximately where the composition of the anal epithelium changes from columnar to stratified squamous cells. At the anus, the epithelium is keratinized (keratin formation) and continuous with the skin around the anus.

Figure 12–19 A typical ileal diverticulum—Meckel diverticulum (cadaveric specimen). Only a small percentage of these diverticula produce symptoms. Ileal diverticula are one of the most common birth defects of the alimentary tract. *(From Moore KL, Persaud TVN, Shiota K: Color Atlas of Clinical Embryology, 2nd ed. Philadelphia, Saunders, 2000.)*

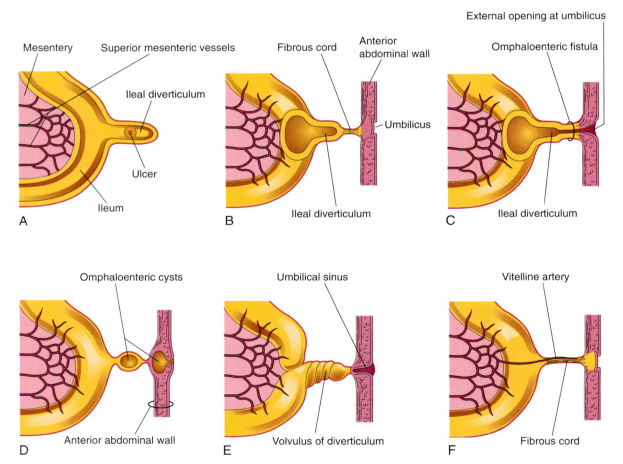

Figure 12–20 Ileal diverticula and remnants of the omphaloenteric duct. **A,** Section of the ileum and a diverticulum with an ulcer. **B,** A diverticulum connected to the umbilicus by a fibrous remnant of the omphaloenteric duct **C,** Omphaloenteric fistula resulting from persistence of the intra-abdominal part of the omphaloenteric duct. **D,** Omphaloenteric cysts at the umbilicus and in a fibrous remnant of the omphaloenteric duct. **E,** Volvulus (twisted) ileal diverticulum and an umbilical sinus resulting from the persistence of the omphaloenteric duct in the umbilicus. **F,** The omphaloenteric duct has persisted as a fibrous cord connecting the ileum with the umbilicus. A persistent vitelline artery extends along the fibrous cord to the umbilicus. This artery carried blood to the umbilical vesicle from the anterior wall of the embryo.

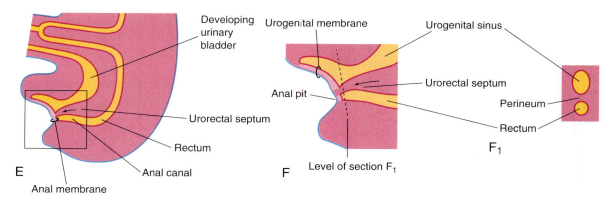

Figure 12–21 Successive stages in the partitioning of the cloaca into the rectum and urogenital sinus by the urorectal septum. **A, C,** and **E,** Views from the left side at 4, 6, and 7 weeks, respectively. **B, D,** and **F,** Enlargements of the cloacal region. **B₁, D₁,** and **F₁,** Transverse sections of the cloaca at the levels shown in **B, D,** and **F,** respectively. Note that the postanal portion (shown in **B**) degenerates and disappears as the rectum forms. The *arrows* in **A** to **E** indicate the growth of the urorectal septum.

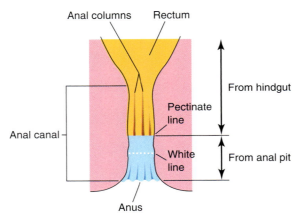

Figure 12–22   The rectum and anal canal, showing their developmental origins. Note that the superior two thirds of the anal canal are derived from the hindgut, whereas the inferior one third of the anal canal is derived from the anal pit. Because of their different embryologic origins, the superior and inferior parts of the anal canal are supplied by different arteries and nerves and have different venous and lymphatic drainages.

Because of its hindgut origin, the superior two thirds of the anal canal are supplied mainly by the *superior rectal artery*, the continuation of the *inferior mesenteric artery* (hindgut artery). Its nerves are from the autonomic nervous system. Because of its origin from the anal pit, the inferior one third of the anal canal is supplied mainly by the *inferior rectal arteries*, branches of the internal pudendal artery. The inferior part of the anal canal is innervated by the inferior rectal nerve and is sensitive to pain, temperature, touch, and pressure.

The differences in blood supply, nerve supply, and venous and lymphatic drainage of the anal canal are important clinically, such as when considering the metastasis (spread) of cancer cells. The characteristics

CONGENITAL MEGACOLON

In infants with **congenital megacolon**, or **Hirschsprung disease** (Fig. 12-23), a part of the colon is dilated because of the *absence of autonomic ganglion cells* in the **myenteric plexus** distal to the dilated segment of colon. The enlarged colon—**megacolon**—has the normal number of ganglion cells. The dilation results from *failure of peristalsis in the aganglionic segment*, which prevents movement of the intestinal contents, resulting in dilation.

Males are affected more than females (4 to 1). **Megacolon** results from failure of neural crest cells to migrate into the wall of the colon during the fifth to seventh weeks of development. Of the genes involved in the pathogenesis of Hirschsprung disease, the *RET (oncogene product) proto-oncogene* accounts for most cases. Megacolon is the most common cause of neonatal obstruction of the colon and accounts for 33% of all neonatal obstructions; this disease affects 1 in 5000 neonates.

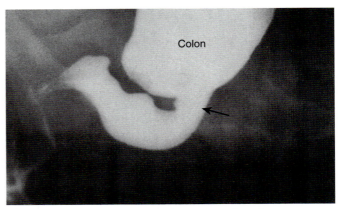

Figure 12–23   Radiograph of the colon, after a barium enema, in a 1-month-old infant with megacolon (Hirschsprung disease). The distal aganglionic segment is narrow, with a dilated proximal colon full of fecal material. Note the transition zone *(arrow)*.

Figure 12–24   Female neonate with membranous anal atresia (imperforate anus—lacking a normal opening). In most cases of this atresia, a thin layer of tissue separates the anal canal from the exterior. Some form of imperforate anus occurs approximately once in every 5000 neonates; it is more common in males.

ANORECTAL BIRTH DEFECTS

Imperforate anus occurs in approximately 1 in 5000 neonates, and it is more common in males than females (Fig. 12-24 and Fig. 12-25C). *Most anorectal defects result from abnormal development of the urorectal septum*, resulting in incomplete separation of the cloaca into urogenital and anorectal parts (see Fig. 12-25A). Lesions are classified as low or high, depending on whether the rectum ends superior or inferior to the puborectalis muscle, which maintains fetal continence and relaxes to allow defecation.

of **carcinomas** (cancer arising in the epithelial tissue of skin) involving the two parts differ. Tumors in the superior part are painless and arise from the columnar epithelium, whereas those in the inferior part are painful and arise from the squamous epithelium.

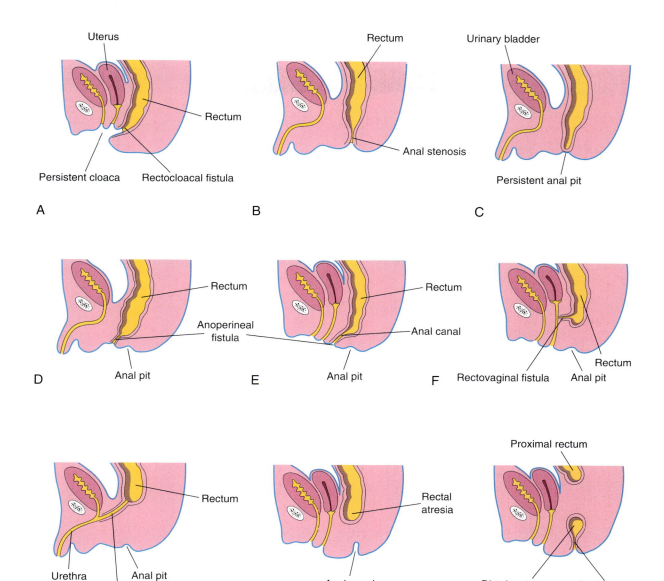

Figure 12–25 Various types of anorectal birth defects. **A,** Persistent cloaca. Note the common outlet of the intestinal, urinary, and reproductive tracts. **B,** Anal stenosis. **C,** An atresia (imperforate anus). **D** and **E,** Anal agenesis with a perineal fistula. **F,** Anorectal agenesis with a rectovaginal fistula. **G,** Anorectal agenesis with a rectourethral fistula. **H** and **I,** Rectal atresia.

LOW RECTAL BIRTH DEFECTS

ANAL AGENESIS, WITH OR WITHOUT A FISTULA

The anal canal may end blindly or there may be an **ectopic anus** or an **anoperineal fistula (abnormal passage)** that opens into the perineum (see Fig. 12-25D and E). The abnormal canal may, however, open into the vagina in females or the urethra in males (see Fig. 12-25F and G). Most low anorectal defects are associated with an external fistula. **Anal agenesis with a fistula** results from incomplete separation of the cloaca by the urorectal septum. *These anomalies have been associated with disruption of β-catenin signaling.*

ANAL STENOSIS

In anal stenosis, the anus is in a normal position but the anus and anal canal are narrow (see Fig. 12-25B). This defect is probably caused by a slight dorsal deviation of the **urorectal septum** as it grows caudally (see Fig. 12-21D).

MEMBRANOUS ATRESIA OF ANUS

In this birth defect, the anus is in the normal position, but a thin layer of tissue separates the anal canal from the exterior (see Fig. 12-24 and Fig. 12-25C). The remnant of the epithelial plug is thin enough to bulge on straining and appears blue from the presence of **meconium (feces of neonate) superior to it.** This defect results from failure of the epithelial plug to perforate at the end of the eighth week.

HIGH ANORECTALBIRTH DEFECTS

ANORECTAL AGENESIS WITH OR WITHOUT A FISTULA

In high defects of the anorectal region, the rectum ends superior to the puborectalis muscle when there is anorectal agenesis. *This is the most common type of anorectal defect* and it accounts for approximately two thirds of anorectal defects. Although the rectum ends blindly, there is usually a fistula to the bladder (**rectovesical fistula**) or urethra (**rectourethral fistula**) in males, or to the vagina (**rectovaginal fistula**) or the vestibule of the vagina (**rectovestibular fistula**) in females (see Fig. 12-25F and G). Anorectal agenesis with a fistula is the result of incomplete separation of the cloaca from the urogenital sinus by the urorectal septum (see Fig. 12-21C to E).

RECTAL ATRESIA

In this atresia, the anal canal and rectum are present but are separated (see Fig. 12-25H and I). Sometimes the two segments of intestine are connected by a fibrous cord, the remnant of the atretic portion of the rectum. The cause of rectal atresia may be abnormal recanalization of the colon or, more likely, a defective blood supply.

⬤ CLINICALLY ORIENTED QUESTIONS

1. About 2 weeks after birth, a neonate began to vomit shortly after feeding. Each time, the vomitus was propelled approximately 2 feet. The physician told the mother that her infant has an obstructing benign growth that causes a narrow outlet from the stomach. Is there an embryologic basis for this defect?

2. Do infants with Down syndrome have an increased incidence of duodenal atresia? Can the condition be corrected?

3. A man claimed that his appendix was on his left side. Is this possible and, if so, how could this happen?

4. A patient reported that she had two appendices and separate operations to remove them. Do people ever have two appendices?

5. What is Hirschsprung disease? Some sources state that it is a congenital condition resulting from large intestine obstruction. Is this correct? If so, what is its embryologic basis?

6. A nurse observed what appeared to be feces being expelled from a baby's umbilicus. How could this happen? If so, what conditions would likely be present?

The answers to these questions are at the back of this book.

CHAPTER

13

Urogenital System

T he **urogenital system** is divided functionally into the **urinary system** and **genital system**. The urogenital system includes all the organs involved in reproduction and forming and voiding urine. Embryologically, the systems are closely associated, especially during their early stages of development.

The **urogenital system** develops from the **intermediate mesenchyme** (embryonic connective tissue in the **mesoderm**) derived from the dorsal body wall of the embryo (Fig. 13-1*A* and *B*). During folding of the embryo in the horizontal plane (see Chapter 6), the mesenchyme is carried ventrally and loses its connection with the somites (see Fig. 13-1*C* and *D*). A longitudinal elevation of the mesenchyme—the **urogenital ridge**—forms on each side of the dorsal aorta (see Fig. 13-1*D*). The part of the urogenital ridge giving rise to the urinary system is the **nephrogenic cord** (see Fig. 13-1*C and D*); the part that gives rise to the genital system is the **gonadal ridge** (see Fig. 13-18*C*).

▶ DEVELOPMENT OF URINARY SYSTEM

The urinary system begins to develop before the genital system and consists of the kidneys, ureters, urinary bladder, and urethra.

Development of Kidneys and Ureters

Three sets of successive kidneys develop in human embryos. The first set—the *pronephroi*—is rudimentary and nonfunctional. The second set—the *mesonephroi*—is well developed and functions briefly during the early period. The third set—the *metanephroi*—forms the permanent kidneys.

Figure 13–1 **A,** Dorsal view of an embryo during the third week (approximately 18 days). **B,** Transverse section of the embryo showing the position of the intermediate mesenchyme before lateral folding occurs. **C,** Transverse section of the embryo after the commencement of folding, showing the nephrogenic cords. **D,** Transverse section of the embryo, showing the lateral folds meeting each other ventrally.

Pronephroi

The bilateral, transitory pronephroi appear early in the fourth week. They are represented by a few cell clusters in the neck region (Fig. 13-2A). The pronephric ducts run caudally and open into the *cloaca* (see Fig. 13-2B). The pronephroi soon degenerate; however, most parts of the **pronephric ducts** persist and are used by the second set of kidneys.

Mesonephroi

These large, elongated excretory organs appear late in the fourth week, caudal to the pronephroi (see Fig. 13-2). The mesonephric kidneys consist of approximately 40 **glomeruli** with **mesonephric tubules** (Fig. 13-3C to F). The tubules open into the **mesonephric ducts**, originally the pronephric ducts. The mesonephric ducts open into the cloaca (see Chapter 12, Fig. 12-21A). The mesonephroi create urine between weeks 6 to 10, until the permanent kidneys begin to function (see Fig. 13-3). The mesonephroi degenerate toward the end of the first

trimester (3 months); however, their tubules become the **efferent ductules of the testes.** The mesonephric ducts have several adult derivatives in males (Table 13-1).

Metanephroi

The metanephroi—**primordia of the permanent kidneys**—begin to develop early in the fifth week (Fig. 13-4) and become functional approximately 4 weeks later. **Urine formation** continues throughout fetal life. The urine is excreted into the amniotic cavity and forms a portion of the amniotic fluid.

The permanent kidneys develop from two sources (see Fig. 13-4A):

- The ureteric bud (metanephric diverticulum)
- The metanephrogenic blastema (metanephric mass of mesenchyme)

The **ureteric bud** is a diverticulum (outgrowth) from the mesonephric duct near its entrance into the cloaca.

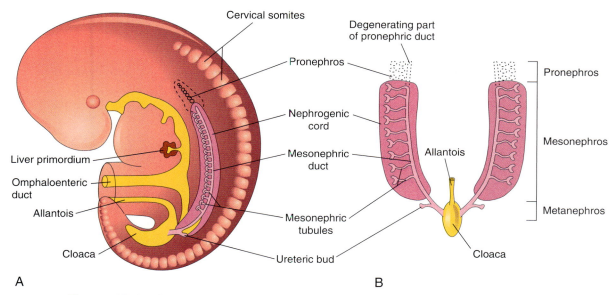

Figure 13–2 Illustrations of the three sets of nephric systems in an embryo during the fifth week. **A,** Lateral view. **B,** Ventral view. The mesonephric tubules are pulled laterally; their normal position is shown in **A.**

Table 13–1   Adult Derivatives and Vestigial Remains of Embryonic Urogenital Structures*

MALE	EMBRYONIC STRUCTURE	FEMALE
Testis	**Indifferent gonad**	*Ovary*
Seminiferous tubules	**Cortex**	*Ovarian follicles*
Rete testis	**Medulla**	Rete ovarii
Gubernaculum	**Gubernaculum**	*Ovarian ligament*
		Round ligament of uterus
Efferent ductules of testis	**Mesonephric tubules**	Epoophoron
Paradidymis		Paroophoron
Appendix of epididymis	**Mesonephric duct**	Appendix vesiculosa
Duct of epididymis		Duct of epoophoron
Ductus deferens		Longitudinal duct, Gartner duct
Ureter, pelvis, calices, and collecting tubules		*Ureter, pelvis, calices, and collecting tubules*
Ejaculatory duct and seminal gland		
Appendix of testis	**Paramesonephric duct**	Hydatid (of Morgagni)
		Uterine tube
		Uterus
Urinary bladder	**Urogenital sinus**	*Urinary bladder*
Urethra (except navicular fossa)		*Urethra*
Prostatic utricle		*Vagina*
Prostate		*Urethral and paraurethral glands*
Bulbourethral glands		*Greater vestibular glands*
Seminal colliculus	**Sinus tubercle**	Hymen
Penis	**Primordial phallus**	*Clitoris*
Glans penis		*Glans clitoris*
Corpora cavernosa of penis		*Corpora cavernosa of clitoris*
Corpus spongiosum of penis		*Bulb of vestibule*
Ventral aspect of penis	**Urogenital folds**	*Labia minora*
Scrotum	**Labioscrotal swellings**	*Labia majora*

*Functional derivatives are shown in italics.

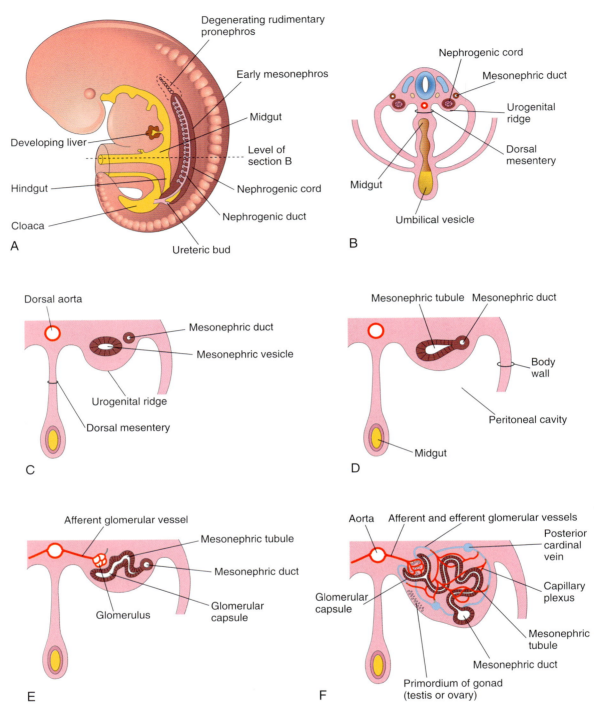

Figure 13–3 **A,** Lateral view of a 5-week embryo showing the extent of the early mesonephros and ureteric bud, the primordium of the metanephros (primordium of the permanent kidney). **B,** Transverse section of the embryo showing the nephrogenic cords from which the mesonephric tubules develop. **C** to **F,** Successive stages in the development of mesonephric tubules between the 5th and 11th weeks. The expanded medial end of the mesonephric tubule is invaginated by blood vessels to form a glomerular capsule.

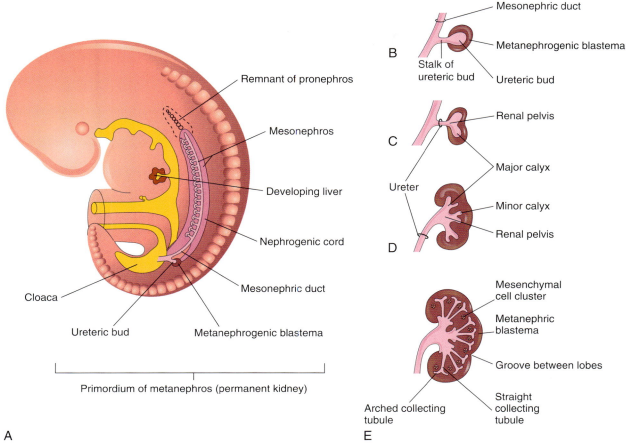

Figure 13–4 Development of the permanent kidney. **A,** Lateral view of a 5-week embryo showing the ureteric bud, the primordium of the metanephros. **B** to **E,** Successive stages in the development of the ureteric bud (fifth to eighth weeks). Observe the development of the kidney: ureter, renal pelvis, calices, and collecting tubules.

The ureteric bud is the primordium of the ureter, renal pelvis, calices (subdivisions of the renal pelvis), and collecting tubules (see Fig. 13-4B to E). The elongating bud penetrates the **metanephrogenic blastema**—a mass of cells derived from the **nephrogenic cord**—that forms the nephrons (see Fig. 13-4A). The **stalk of the ureteric bud** becomes the **ureter**, and the cranial part of the diverticulum undergoes repetitive branching. The branches differentiate into the **collecting tubules of the metanephros** (see Figs. 13-4C to E and Fig. 13-5).

The **straight collecting tubules** undergo repeated branching, forming successive generations of collecting tubules. The first four generations of tubules enlarge and coalesce to form the **major calices** (see Fig. 13-4C to E); the second four generations coalesce to form the **minor calices**. The end of each **arched collecting tubule** induces clusters of mesenchymal cells in the metanephrogenic blastema to form small **metanephric vesicles** (see Fig. 13-5A). These vesicles elongate and become the *metanephric tubules* (see Fig. 13-5B and C). The proximal ends of these tubules are invaginated by **glomeruli**. The renal corpuscle (glomerulus and its capsule) and its proximal convoluted tubule, the **nephron loop** (Henle loop),

and the distal convoluted tubule constitute a **nephron** (Fig. 13-5D). Each distal convoluted tubule contacts an arched collecting tubule. The collecting tubules become confluent, forming a **uriniferous tubule**.

Branching of the metanephric diverticulum depends on an inductive signal from the metanephric mesoderm—differentiation of the nephrons depends on induction by the collecting tubules. The **molecular aspects** of the reciprocal interactions between the metanephric mesenchyme and collecting tubules are shown in Figure 13-6.

The **fetal kidneys are subdivided into lobes**. The lobulation usually disappears during infancy as the nephrons increase in size. Nephron formation is complete by approximately week 36—each kidney **contains approximately 2 million nephrons**. Functional maturation of the kidneys occurs after occurs after birth.

Positional Changes of Kidneys

The developing metanephric kidneys lie close to each other in the pelvis (Fig. 13-7A). As the abdomen and pelvis grow, the kidneys gradually relocate to the abdomen and move farther apart (see Fig. 13-7B and C). They

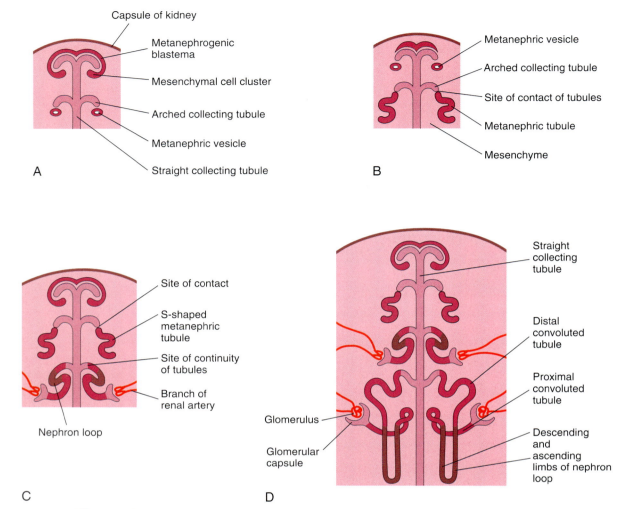

Figure 13–5 Development of nephrons. **A,** Nephrogenesis commences around the beginning of the eighth week. **B** and **C,** Note that the metanephric tubules, the primordia of the nephrons, become connect with the collecting tubules to form uriniferous tubules. **D,** Observe that nephrons are derived from the metanephric blastema and the collecting tubules are derived from the ureteric bud.

attain their adult position on either side of the vertebral column by the ninth week (see Fig. 13-7D). This "ascent" results mainly from the relative growth of the embryo's body caudal to the kidneys. As the kidneys change their positions, they also rotate medially almost 90 degrees. By the ninth week, the kidneys come in contact with the **suprarenal glands** as the former attain their adult position (see Fig. 13-7D).

Changes in Blood Supply of Kidneys

Initially, the **renal arteries** are branches of the **common iliac arteries** (see Fig. 13-7A and B). Later, the kidneys receive their blood supply from the distal end of the **aorta** (see Fig. 13-7C). The kidneys receive their most cranial arterial branches, which become the **renal arteries**, from the **abdominal aorta**. Normally, the caudal primordial branches undergo involution and disappear (see Fig. 13-7C and D).

ACCESSORY RENAL ARTERIES

The common variations in the blood supply to the kidneys reflect the manner in which the blood supply continually changes during embryonic and early fetal life (see Fig. 13-7). Approximately 25% of adult kidneys have two to four renal arteries. **Accessory (supernumerary) renal arteries** usually arise from the aorta, superior or inferior to the main renal artery (Fig. 13-8A and B). An accessory artery to the inferior pole (polar renal artery) may cross anterior to the ureter and obstruct it, causing **hydronephrosis**—distention of the pelvis and calices with urine (see Fig. 13-8B). *Accessory renal arteries are end arteries;* consequently, if an accessory artery is damaged or ligated, the part of the kidney supplied by it will become **ischemic**. Accessory arteries are approximately twice as common as accessory veins.

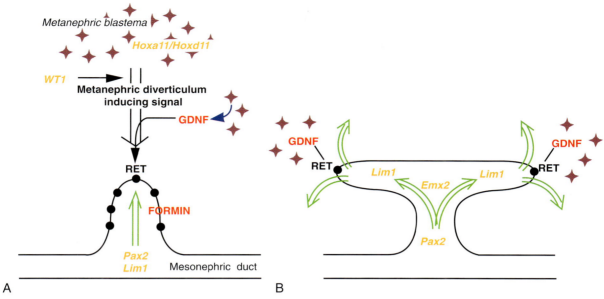

Figure 13–6 Molecular control of kidney development. **A,** The ureteric bud requires inductive signals derived from the metanephric blastema under control of transcription factors (*yellow text*), such as WT1, and signaling molecules (*red text*), including glial-derived neurotropic factor (GDNF) and its epithelial receptor, RET. The normal ureteric bud response to these inductive signals is under the control of transcription factors such as Pax2, Pax8, Lim1, and the *FORMIN* gene. **B,** Branching of the ureteric bud is initiated and maintained by interaction with the mesenchyme under the regulation of transcription factors such as Emx2 and specified expression of GDNF and RET at the tips of the invading ureteric bud. *(From Piscione TD, Rosenblum ND: The malformed kidney: disruption of the glomerular and tubular development. Clin Genet 56:342, 1999.)*

Figure 13–7 **A** to **D,** Diagrammatic ventral views of the abdominopelvic region of embryos and fetuses (sixth to ninth weeks), showing medial rotation and relocation of the kidneys from the pelvis to the abdomen. **C** and **D,** Note that, as the kidneys relocate (ascend), they are supplied by arteries at successively higher levels and that the hila of the kidneys (where the vessels and nerves enter) are directed anteromedially.

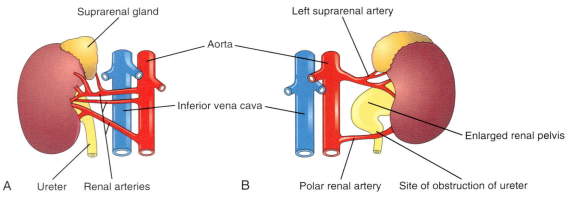

Figure 13–8   Common variations of the renal arteries. **A** and **B,** Multiple renal arteries. The polar renal artery shown in **B** has obstructed the ureter and produced an enlarged renal pelvis.

CONGENITAL ANOMALIES OF KIDNEYS AND URETERS

Unilateral renal agenesis (absence of kidney) occurs in approximately 1 in 1000 neonates (Fig. 13-9A). Males are affected more often than females, and the left kidney is usually the one that is absent. The other kidney usually undergoes **compensatory hypertrophy** and performs the function of the missing kidney.

   Bilateral renal agenesis *is associated with oligohydramnios* (small amount of amniotic fluid) because little or no urine is excreted into the amniotic cavity. This condition occurs in approximately 1 in 3000 births and is incompatible with postnatal life. This defect is three times more common in males. These infants also have **pulmonary hypoplasia (incomplete development of the lungs)**. Failure of the ureteric bud to penetrate the metanephric blastema results in absence of renal development because no nephrons are induced by the collecting tubules to develop from the blastema.

MALROTATION OF KIDNEYS

If the kidney does not rotate, the hilum faces anteriorly—embryonic position—(see Fig. 13-9C). If the hilum faces posteriorly, rotation has progressed too far; if it faces laterally, medial rotation has occurred. Abnormal rotation of the kidneys is often associated with ectopic kidneys.

ECTOPIC KIDNEYS

One or both kidneys may be in an abnormal position (see Fig. 13-9B and E). Most ectopic kidneys are located in the pelvis, but some lie in the inferior part of the abdomen. Pelvic kidneys and other forms of ectopia result from failure of the kidneys to ascend.

FUSION ANOMALIES

CROSSED FUSED ECTOPIA

Sometimes a kidney crosses to the other side, resulting in crossed renal ectopia, with or without fusion. An unusual kidney defect is **unilateral fused kidneys** (see Fig. 13-9D). In such cases, the developing kidneys fuse while they are in the pelvis, and one kidney moves to its normal position, carrying the other one with it.

HORSESHOE KIDNEY

In 0.2% of the population, the poles of the kidneys are fused (usually the inferior poles) (Fig. 13-10). The large U-shaped (horseshoe) kidney is usually located in the pelvic region, anterior to the inferior lumbar vertebrae. Normal ascent of the fused kidneys is prevented by the root of the **inferior mesenteric artery**. The function of these kidneys is preserved and each has a normal ureter and blood supply. A horseshoe kidney may produce no symptoms but is prone to increased occurrence of renal stones and infection. Approximately 15% of persons with Turner syndrome have horseshoe kidneys (see Chapter 19, Fig. 19-3).

DUPLICATIONS OF URINARY TRACT

Duplications of the abdominal part of the ureter and renal pelvis are common, but a kidney in excess of the normal number (**supernumerary kidney**) is rare (see Fig. 13-9C and F). These duplicates often result from division of a ureteric bud. Partial division results in a divided kidney with a bifid ureter (see Fig. 13-9B). Complete division results in a double kidney with a bifid ureter or with separate ureters (see Fig. 13-9C). A supernumerary kidney with its own ureter probably results from the formation of two ureteric buds (see Fig. 13-9F).

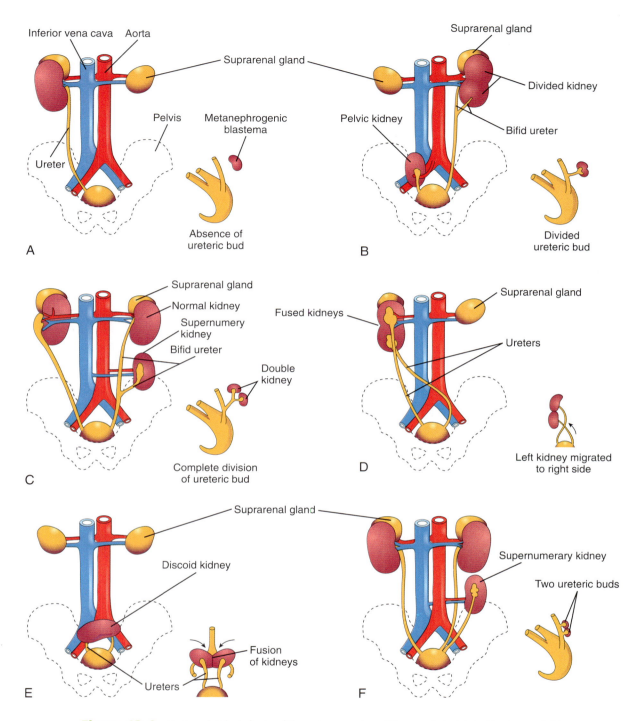

Figure 13–9 Various birth defects of the urinary system. The small sketch to the lower right of each drawing illustrates the probable embryologic basis of the defect. **A,** Unilateral renal agenesis. **B,** Right side, pelvic kidney; left side, divided kidney with a bifid ureter. **C,** Right side, malrotation of the kidney; the hilum is facing laterally. Left side, bifid ureter and the normal and a supernumerary kidney. **D,** Crossed renal ectopia. The left kidney crossed to right and fused with the right kidney. **E,** Pelvic kidney or discoid kidney, resulting from fusion of the kidneys while they were in the pelvis. **F,** Supernumerary left kidney resulting from the development of two ureteric buds.

Figure 13–10 Horseshoe kidney in the lower abdomen of a 13-week female fetus. This anomaly resulted from fusion of the inferior poles of the kidneys while they were in the pelvis.

▶ Development of Urinary Bladder

11 For descriptive purposes, the urogenital sinus is divided into three parts (Fig. 13-11C):

- A *vesical part* that forms most of the bladder and is continuous with the allantois
- A *pelvic part* that becomes the urethra in the neck of the bladder, the prostatic part of the urethra in males, and the entire urethra in females
- A *phallic part* that grows toward the genital tubercle—the primordium of the penis or the clitoris

The bladder develops mainly from the vesical part of the **urogenital sinus** (see Fig. 13-11C), but the **trigone** (triangular area at the base of the bladder between the openings of the ureters) is derived from the caudal ends of the mesonephric ducts (see Fig. 13-11A and B). Initially, the bladder is continuous with the **allantois** (see Fig. 13-11C). This fetal membrane soon constricts and becomes a thick, fibrous cord, the **urachus** (see Fig. 13-11G and H). In adults, the urachus is represented by the **median umbilical ligament**. As the bladder enlarges, distal parts of the mesonephric ducts are incorporated into its dorsal wall (see Fig. 13-11B to H). These ducts contribute to the formation of the connective tissue in the *trigone of the bladder*. The epithelium of the entire bladder is derived from the endoderm of the urogenital sinus. The other layers of the bladder wall develop from the adjacent splanchnic mesenchyme. As the mesonephric ducts are absorbed, the ureters open separately into the urinary bladder (see Fig. 13-11C to H). In males, the orifices of the mesonephric ducts move close together and enter the *prostatic part of the urethra* (see Fig. 13-22C) as the caudal ends of these ducts become the *ejaculatory ducts* (see Fig. 13-22A). In females, the distal ends of the mesonephric ducts degenerate.

ECTOPIC URETER

An ectopic ureter does not enter the urinary bladder. In males, an ectopic ureter may open into the neck of the bladder or the prostatic part of the urethra. It may also enter the ductus deferens, prostatic utricle, or seminal gland (see Fig. 13-22). In females, an ectopic ureter may enter the neck of the bladder, urethra, vagina, or vestibule of vagina. An ectopic ureter results when the ureter is carried caudally with the mesonephric duct, and is incorporated into the caudal portion of the vesical part of the urogenital sinus. **Incontinence** may result and urine may leak from the urethra in males and the urethra and/or vagina in females.

URACHAL ANOMALIES

A remnant of the urachal lumen may persist, typically in the inferior part of the **urachus**. In approximately 50% of cases, the lumen is continuous with the cavity of the bladder. Remnants of the epithelial lining of the urachus may give rise to **urachal cysts** (Fig. 13-12A). The patent inferior end of the urachus may dilate to form a **urachal sinus** that opens into the bladder. The lumen in the superior part of the urachus may also remain patent and form a urachal sinus that opens at the umbilicus (see Fig. 13-12B). Very rarely, the entire urachus remains patent and forms a **urachal fistula** that allows urine to escape from its umbilical orifice (see Fig. 13-12C).

EXSTROPHY OF BLADDER

Exstrophy of the bladder (deficiency of the anterior wall of the bladder and anterior abdominal wall) is a severe birth defect than occurs in approximately 1 in every 10,000 to 40,000 births, predominantly affecting males (Fig. 13-13). *Exposure and protrusion of the mucosal surface of the posterior wall of the bladder characterize this birth defect.* The trigone of the bladder and ureteric orifices are exposed, and urine dribbles intermittently from the everted bladder.

Epispadias is a birth defect in which the urethra opens on the dorsum of the penis. Epispadias and wide separation of the pubic bones are associated with complete exstrophy of the bladder. In some cases, the penis is divided into two parts and the scrotum is bifid (split). **Exstrophy of the bladder** is believed to be caused by failure of the mesenchymal cells to migrate between the ectoderm and endoderm of the abdominal wall (**cloacal membrane**) during the fourth week (Fig. 13-14B and C). As a result, no muscle or connective tissue forms in the abdominal wall over the urinary bladder. **Rupture of the cloacal membrane** results in wide communication between the exterior and the mucous membrane of the bladder. Rupture of the membrane before division of the cloaca by the urorectal septum leads to **exstrophy of the cloaca**, resulting in exposure of both the bladder and hindgut.

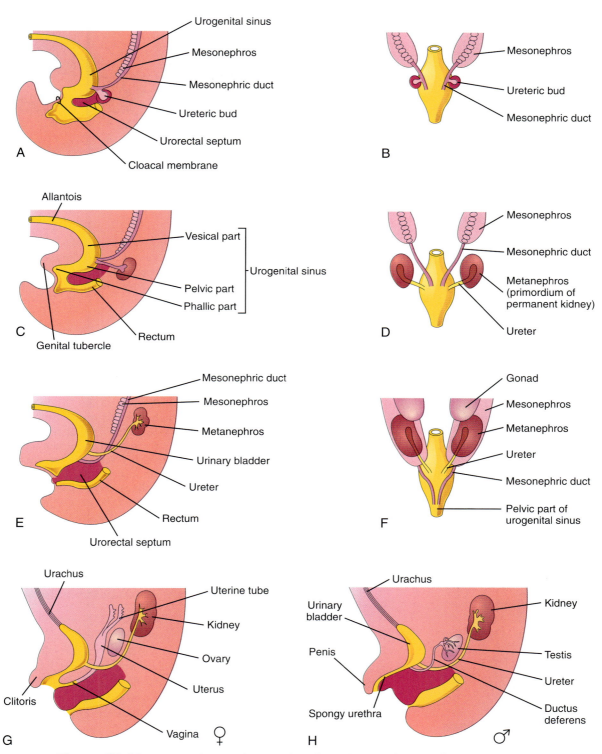

Figure 13–11 **A,** Lateral view of a 5-week embryo showing division of the cloaca by the urorectal septum into the urogenital sinus and rectum. **B, D,** and **F,** Dorsal views showing the development of the kidneys and bladder, and changes in the location of kidneys. **C, E, G,** and **H,** Lateral views. The stages shown in **G** and **H** are reached by the 12th week.

Figure 13–12 Urachal anomalies. **A,** Urachal cysts; the common site for them is in the superior end of the urachus, just inferior to the umbilicus. **B,** Two types of urachal sinus are shown: one that opens into the bladder and another that opens at the umbilicus. **C,** A urachal fistula connects the bladder and umbilicus.

Development of Urethra

The epithelium of most of the male urethra and the entire female urethra is derived from the endoderm of the **urogenital sinus** (see Fig. 13-11A and B and Fig. 13-15). The distal part of the urethra in the **glans penis** is derived from a solid cord of ectodermal cells that grows from the tip of the glans and joins the rest of the spongy urethra (see Chapter 2, Fig. 2-1B and Fig. 13-15A to C). Consequently, the epithelium of the terminal part of the urethra is derived from the surface ectoderm. The connective tissue and smooth muscle of the urethra in both sexes are derived from splanchnic mesenchyme.

Figure 13–13 A male neonate with exstrophy of the bladder. Because of defective closure of the inferior part of the anterior abdominal wall and anterior wall of the bladder, the urinary bladder appears as an everted, bulging mass inferior to the umbilicus.

DEVELOPMENT OF SUPRARENAL GLANDS

The **cortex and medulla** of the suprarenal glands (adrenal glands) have different origins (Fig. 13-16). The **cortex** develops from mesenchyme and the **medulla** from **neural crest cells** (see Fig. 13-16A and B). During the sixth week, the cortex begins an aggregation of mesenchymal cells on each side of the embryo between the root of the dorsal mesentery and the developing gonad (see Fig. 13-18C). Differentiation of the characteristic suprarenal cortical zones begins during the late fetal period (see Fig. 13-16C to E). The *zona glomerulosa* and the *zona fasciculata* are present at birth, but the *zona reticularis* is not recognizable until the end of the third year (see Fig. 13-16H).

CONGENITAL ADRENAL HYPERPLASIA

Congenital adrenal hyperplasia (CAH) represents a group of *autosomal recessive disorders* in which an abnormal increase in the cells of the suprarenal cortex results in **excessive androgen production** during the fetal period. In females, this usually causes masculinization of the external genitalia (Fig. 13-17). Affected male infants have normal external genitalia and the disorder may go undetected in early infancy. Later in childhood in both sexes, androgen excess leads to rapid growth and accelerated skeletal maturation.

CAH is most often caused by a genetically determined mutation in the cytochrome-P450c 21-steroid, 21-hydroxylase gene, which results in a deficiency of suprarenal cortical enzymes. These are necessary for the biosynthesis of various steroid hormones. The reduced hormone output results in increased release of adrenocorticotropic hormone by the anterior pituitary, which causes CAH and overproduction of androgens by the hyperplastic suprarenal glands.

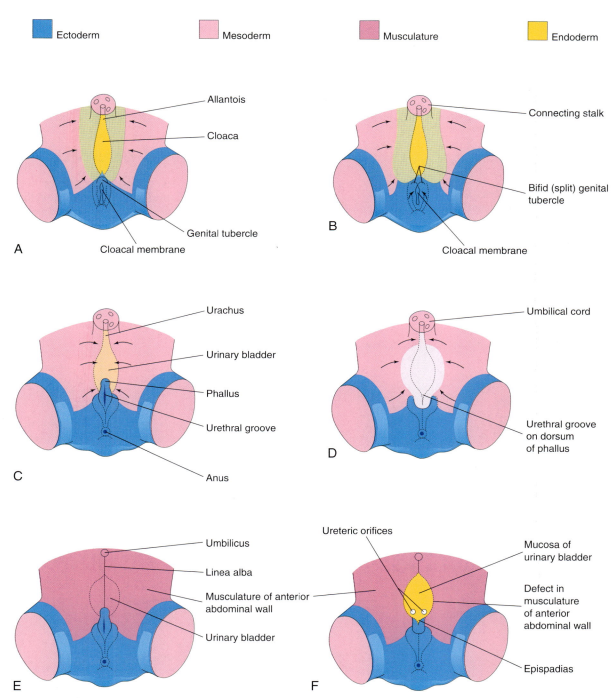

Figure 13–14 **A, C,** and **E,** Normal stages in the development of the infraumbilical abdominal wall and the penis during the fourth to eighth weeks. **B, D,** and **F,** Probable stages in the development of epispadias and exstrophy of the bladder with epispadias. **B** and **D,** note that the mesoderm fails to extend into the anterior abdominal wall anterior to the urinary bladder. Also note that the genital tubercle is located in a more caudal position than usual, and that the urethral groove has formed on the dorsal surface of the penis. **F,** The surface ectoderm and anterior wall of the bladder have ruptured, resulting in exposure of the posterior wall of the bladder. Note that the musculature of the anterior abdominal wall is present on each side of the defect. *(Modified from Patten BM, Barry A: The genesis of exstrophy of the bladder and epispadias. Am J Anat 90:35, 1952.)*

A

B

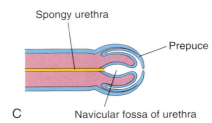

C

Figure 13–15 Schematic longitudinal sections of the developing penis, illustrating development of the prepuce (foreskin) and the distal part of the spongy urethra. **A,** At 11 weeks. **B,** At 12 weeks. **C,** At 14 weeks. The epithelium of the spongy urethra has a dual origin; most of it is derived from endoderm of the phallic part of the urogenital sinus; the distal part of the urethra lining the navicular fossa is derived from surface ectoderm.

Relative to body weight, the **suprarenal glands** of the fetus are 10 to 20 times larger than the adult glands and are large compared with the kidneys because of the extensive size of the fetal suprarenal cortex. The medulla remains small until after birth (see Fig. 13-16*F*). The suprarenal glands rapidly become smaller as the cortex regresses during the first year of infancy (see Fig. 13-16*G*).

DEVELOPMENT OF GENITAL SYSTEM

The early genital systems in the two sexes are similar; therefore, the initial period of genital development is referred to as the *indifferent stage of sexual development.*

Development of Gonads

The gonads (testes and ovaries) are the organs that produce cells (sperms and oocytes). The gonads are derived from three sources (Fig. 13-18):

- Mesothelium (mesodermal epithelium) lining the posterior abdominal wall
- Underlying mesenchyme (embryonic connective tissue)
- Primordial germ cells (earliest undifferentiated sex cells)

Indifferent Gonads

Gonadal development begins during the fifth week when a thickened area of mesothelium develops on the medial side of the **mesonephros** (see Fig. 13-18*A* to *C*). Proliferation of this epithelium and underlying mesenchyme produces a bulge on the medial side of the mesonephros—the **gonadal ridge** (see Fig. 13-18*A* and *C*). Finger-like epithelial cords—**gonadal cords**—soon grow into the underlying mesenchyme (see Fig. 13-18*D*). The **indifferent gonads** now consist of an external cortex and an internal medulla.

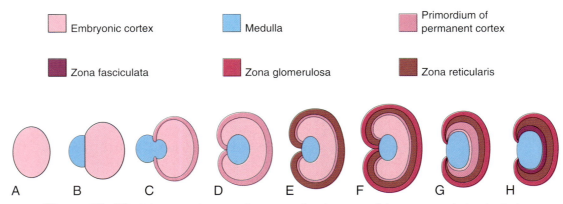

Figure 13–16 Schematic drawings illustrating development of the suprarenal glands. **A,** At 6 weeks, showing the mesodermal primordium of the embryonic cortex. **B,** At 7 weeks, showing the addition of neural crest cells. **C,** At 8 weeks, showing the fetal cortex and early permanent cortex beginning to encapsulate the medulla. **D** and **E,** Later stages of encapsulation of the medulla by the cortex. **F,** Gland of a neonate showing the fetal cortex and two zones of the permanent cortex. **G,** At 1 year, the fetal cortex has almost disappeared. **H,** At 4 years, showing the adult pattern of cortical zones. Observe that the fetal cortex has disappeared and that the gland is smaller than it was at birth **(F).**

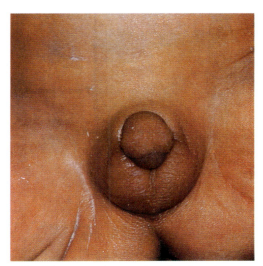

Figure 13–17 External genitalia of a female neonate with congenital adrenal hyperplasia. The virilization was caused by excessive androgens produced by the suprarenal glands during the fetal period. Note the enlarged clitoris and fusion of the labia majora to form a scrotum.

In embryos with an **XX sex chromosome complex**, the cortex of the indifferent gonad differentiates into an ovary, and the medulla regresses. In embryos with an **XY sex chromosome complex**, the medulla differentiates into a testis and the cortex regresses (see Fig. 13-18D).

Primordial Germ Cells

The **primordial germ cells** originate in the wall of the umbilical vesicle (from the epiblast) and migrate along the dorsal mesentery of the hindgut to the gonadal ridges (see Fig. 13-18D). *Early chemotactic signaling by stem cell factor (SCF) and later nerve tract guidance appears to help the cells migrate to the gonadal ridges.* During the sixth week, the primordial germ cells enter the underlying mesenchyme and are incorporated into the **gonadal cords** (see Fig. 13-18D). They eventually differentiate into oocytes or sperms.

Sex Determination

Chromosomal and genetic sex, established at fertilization, depends on whether an X-bearing or a Y-bearing sperm fertilizes the X-bearing oocyte. The type of gonads that develop is normally determined by the **sex chromosome complex** of the embryo (XX or XY). Before the seventh week, the gonads of the two sexes are identical in appearance and are called **indifferent gonads** (Fig. 13-19). Development of a male phenotype (characteristics) requires a functional Y chromosome. Two X chromosomes are required for the development of the female phenotype.

Development of Testes

A coordinated sequence of genes induces the development of testes. The *SRY* gene (**sex determining region on the Y**) for a testis-determining factor (TDF) gene on the short arm of the Y chromosome acts as the switch that directs the development of the indifferent gonad into a testis.

ABNORMAL SEX CHROMOSOME COMPLEXES

In embryos with abnormal sex chromosome complexes, such as XXX or XXY, the number of X chromosomes appears to be unimportant in sex determination. If a normal Y chromosome is present, the embryo develops as a male. If no Y chromosome is present or if the testis-determining region of the Y chromosome has been lost, female development occurs. The loss of an X chromosome does not appear to interfere with the migration of primordial germ cells to the gonadal ridges because some germ cells have been observed in the fetal gonads of 45,XO females with **Turner syndrome** (see Chapter 19, Fig. 19-3). Two X chromosomes are needed, however, to bring about complete ovarian development.

TDF induces the gonadal cords to condense and extend into the medulla of the indifferent gonad, where they branch and anastomose to form the **rete testis** (see Fig. 13-19). The connection of the prominent gonadal cords—the **seminiferous cords**—with the surface epithelium is lost when the **tunica albuginea** develops. This dense tunica, a thick fibrous capsule, is a characteristic feature of testicular development. Gradually, the testis separates from the degenerating mesonephros and becomes suspended by its own mesentery, the **mesorchium**. The seminiferous cords develop into the seminiferous tubules, tubuli recti (straight tubules), and rete testis.

The **seminiferous tubules** are separated by mesenchyme, giving rise to the **interstitial cells** (Leydig cells). By the eighth week, these cells secrete the **androgenic hormone** *testosterone,* which induces masculine differentiation of the mesonephric ducts and external genitalia. Testosterone production is stimulated by **human chorionic gonadotropin**, which reaches peak amounts during the 8th to 12th week. The fetal testes also produce a glycoprotein—**anti-müllerian hormone (AMH)** or müllerian-inhibiting substance (MIS). AMH is produced by the **sustentacular cells (Sertoli cells)**, which continues until puberty, after which the levels of the hormone decrease. *Expression of the transcription factor SOX9 is essential in the differentiation of Sertoli cells in the testes. AMH suppresses the development of the paramesonephric ducts,* which form the uterus and uterine tubes. The seminiferous tubules remain until puberty (i.e., without lumina), when lumina begin to develop. In addition to sustentacular cells, the walls of the **seminiferous tubules** are composed of (see Fig. 13-19)

- Spermatogonia, the primordial sperm cells derived from the primordial germ cells
- Sertoli cells, which constitute most of the seminiferous epithelium in the fetal testis (see Fig. 13-19)

The **rete testis** becomes continuous with 15 to 20 mesonephric tubules, which become **efferent ductules**. These ductules are connected with the mesonephric duct,

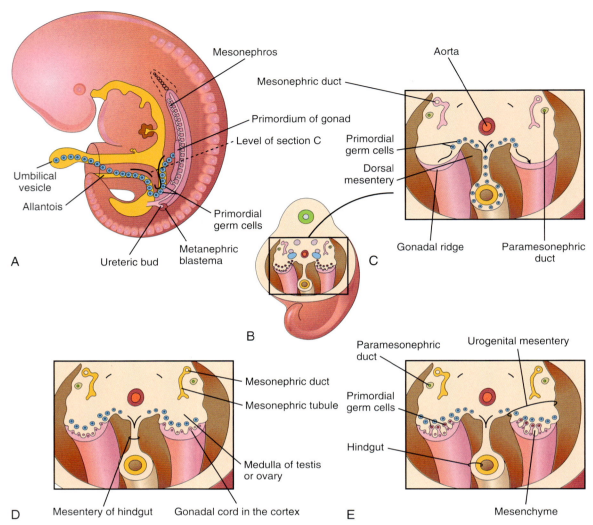

Figure 13–18 **A,** Sketch of a 5-week embryo illustrating the migration of primordial germ cells from the umbilical vesicle into the embryo. **B,** Three-dimensional sketch of the caudal region of the 5-week embryo, showing the location and extent of the gonadal ridges. **C,** Transverse section showing the gonadal ridges and the migration of primordial germ cells into the developing gonads. **D,** Transverse section of a 6-week embryo showing the gonadal cords. **E,** Similar section at a later stage showing the indifferent gonads and paramesonephric ducts.

which becomes the **ductus epididymis** (see Fig. 13-19 and Fig. 13-20*A*).

Development of Ovaries

Ovarian development occurs approximately 3 weeks later (by week 10) than testicular development. The X chromosomes have genes that contribute to ovarian development; autosomal genes also appear to play a role in **ovarian organogenesis.** The ovary is not identifiable by histologic examination until approximately the 10th week. **Gonadal cords** extend into the medulla of the ovary and form a rudimentary *rete ovarii* (see Fig. 13-18*D* and Fig. 13-19). This network of canals and gonadal cords normally degenerate and disappear. **Cortical cords** extend from the surface epithelium of the developing ovary into the underlying mesenchyme during the early

fetal period. As the cortical cords increase in size, **primordial germ cells** are incorporated into them. At approximately 16 weeks, these cords begin to break up into isolated cell clusters—**primordial follicles**—each of which consists of an **oogonium** (derived from a primordial germ cell). The follicles are surrounded by a layer of follicular cells derived from the surface epithelium (see Fig. 13-19). Active mitosis produces many oogonia during fetal life.

No oogonia form postnatally. Although many oogonia degenerate before birth, 2 million or so enlarge to become **primary oocytes** (see Chapter 2, Fig. 2-5) before birth. After birth, the surface epithelium of the ovary flattens to a single layer of cells that is continuous with the mesothelium of the peritoneum. The surface epithelium becomes separated from the follicles in the cortex by a thin fibrous capsule, the **tunica albuginea.** As the ovary

Development of Testes

Development of Ovaries

Section of seminiferous tubule   Section of ovarian cortex

Figure 13–19   Schematic illustrations showing differentiation of the indifferent gonads in a 5-week embryo *(top)* into ovaries or testes. The **left side** of the drawing shows the development of testes resulting from the effects of the testis-determining factor (TDF) located on the Y chromosome. Note that the gonadal cords become seminiferous cords, the primordia of the seminiferous tubules. The parts of the gonadal cords that enter the medulla of the testis form the rete testis. In the section of the testis at the *bottom left,* observe that there are two kinds of cells: spermatogonia, derived from the primordial germ cells; and sustentacular or Sertoli cells, derived from mesenchyme. The **right side** shows the development of ovaries in the absence of TDF. Cortical cords have extended from the surface epithelium of the gonad, and primordial germ cells have entered them. They are the primordia of the oogonia. Follicular cells are derived from the surface epithelium of the gonad and primordial germ cells have entered them. They are the primordia of the oogonia. Follicular cells are derived from the surface epithelium of the ovaries. The *arrows* indicate the changes that occur as the gonads (testes and ovaries) develop.

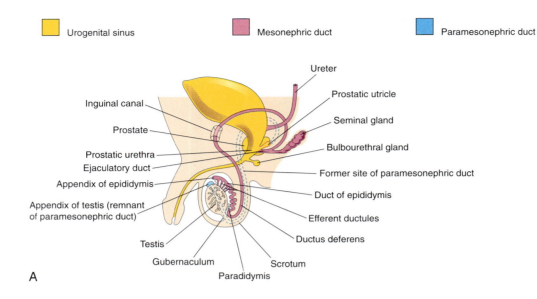

Urogenital sinus   Mesonephric duct   Paramesonephric duct

Figure 13–20 Schematic drawings illustrating development of the male and female reproductive systems from the genital ducts and urogenital sinus. Vestigial structures are also shown. **A,** Reproductive system in a male neonate. **B,** Female reproductive system in a 12-week fetus. **C,** Reproductive system in a female neonate.

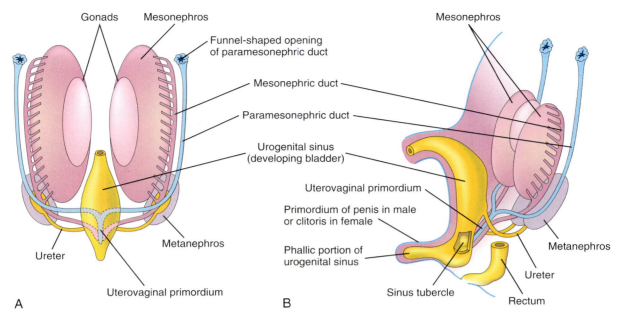

Figure 13–21 A, Sketch of a ventral view of the posterior abdominal wall of a 7-week embryo, showing the two pairs of genital ducts present during the indifferent stage of sexual development. **B,** Lateral view of a 9-week fetus showing the sinus tubercle on the posterior wall of the urogenital sinus. It becomes the hymen in females (see Fig. 13-20C) and the seminal colliculus in males.

separates from the regressing mesonephros, it is suspended by its mesentery, the **mesovarium** (see Fig. 13-19).

Development of Genital Ducts

Both male and female embryos have two pairs of genital ducts: **mesonephric ducts** (wolffian ducts) and **paramesonephric ducts**—müllerian ducts (Fig. 13-21A). The mesonephric ducts play an essential role in the development of the male reproductive system (see Fig. 13-20A), and the paramesonephric ducts play an essential role in the development of the female reproductive system (see Table 13-1 and Fig. 13-20B and C). During conversion of the mesonephric and paramesonephric ducts into adult structures, some parts of the ducts remain as **vestigial structures** (see Fig. 13-20A, B, and C). These vestiges are rarely seen unless pathologic changes develop in them (e.g., Gartner duct cysts, see Fig. 13-20C).

Development of Male Genital Ducts and Glands

The fetal testes produce testosterone beginning in the eighth week and peaking at approximately week 12 and **AMH** at 6 to 7 weeks. **Testosterone** stimulates the mesonephric ducts to form male genital ducts, whereas AMH causes the paramesonephric ducts to disappear by epithelial-mesenchymal transformation. As the mesonephros degenerates, some mesonephric tubules persist and are transformed into **efferent ductules** (see Fig. 13-20A). These ductules open into the mesonephric duct, which has been transformed into the **duct of epididymis** in this region. Distal to the epididymis, the mesonephric duct acquires a thick investment of smooth muscle and becomes the **ductus deferens** (see Fig. 13-20A).

Seminal Glands. Lateral outgrowths from the caudal end of each mesonephric duct become **seminal glands** (vesicles). The secretions of this pair of glands nourish the sperms. The part of the mesonephric duct between the duct of this gland and the urethra becomes the **ejaculatory duct** (see Fig. 13-20A).

Prostate. Multiple endodermal outgrowths arise from the prostatic part of the urethra and grow into the surrounding mesenchyme (Fig. 13-22). The glandular epithelium of the prostate differentiates from these endodermal cells, and the associated mesenchyme differentiates into the dense stroma and smooth muscle of the prostate. Secretions from the prostate contribute to the semen.

Bulbourethral Glands. The bulbourethral glands are pea-sized structures that develop from paired outgrowths derived from the spongy part of the urethra (see Fig. 13-20A). The smooth muscle fibers and the stroma differentiate from the adjacent mesenchyme. Secretions from these glands also contribute to the semen.

Development of Female Genital Ducts and Glands

The **mesonephric ducts** of female embryos regress because of the absence of testosterone. The **paramesonephric ducts** develop because of the absence of AMH. Female sexual development does not depend on the presence of ovaries or hormones until puberty. The **paramesonephric ducts** form most of the female genital tract. The **uterine tubes** develop from the unfused cranial parts of the paramesonephric ducts (see Fig. 13-20B and C). The caudal, fused portions of these ducts form the **uterovaginal primordium**, which gives rise to the **uterus** and the superior portion of the **vagina** (see Fig. 13-21).

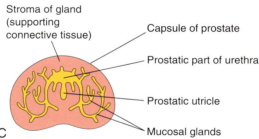

Figure 13–22 **A,** Dorsal view of the developing prostate in an 11-week fetus. **B,** Sketch of a median section of the developing urethra and prostate showing numerous endodermal outgrowths from the prostatic urethra. The vestigial prostatic utricle is also shown. **C,** Section of the prostate (16 weeks) at the level shown in **B.**

Expression of Hox genes in the paramesonephric ducts regulates the development of the female genital ducts. The endometrial stroma and myometrium are derived from splanchnic mesenchyme. Fusion of the paramesonephric ducts also forms a peritoneal fold that becomes the **broad ligament,** and forms two peritoneal compartments—the **rectouterine pouch** and **vesicouterine pouch** (Fig. 13-23B to D).

Development of Vagina. The vaginal epithelium is derived from the endoderm of the **urogenital sinus.** The fibromuscular wall of the vagina develops from the surrounding mesenchyme. Contact of the *uterovaginal primordium* with the urogenital sinus, forming the **sinus tubercle** (see Fig. 13-21B), induces the formation of paired endodermal outgrowths—**sinovaginal bulbs** (see Fig. 13-23A). They extend from the urogenital sinus to

the caudal end of the uterovaginal primordium. The sinovaginal bulbs fuse to form a **vaginal plate** (see Fig. 13-20B). The central cells of this plate break down, forming the **lumen of the vagina.** The peripheral cells of the plate form the vaginal epithelium or lining (see Fig. 13-20C). Until late in fetal life, the lumen of the vagina is separated from the cavity of the urogenital sinus by a membrane—the **hymen** (see Fig. 13-20C and Fig. 13-24H). The hymen is formed by invagination of the posterior wall of the urogenital sinus. The hymen usually ruptures during the perinatal period (first 28 days after birth), and remains as a thin mucous membrane just within the vaginal orifice.

Female Auxiliary Genital Glands. Outgrowths from the urethra into the surrounding mesenchyme form the bilateral mucus-secreting urethral glands and **paraurethral glands** (see Fig. 13-20B). Outgrowths from the urogenital sinus form the **greater vestibular glands** in the lower one third of the **labia majora** (see Fig. 13-24F). These tubuloalveolar glands also secrete mucus and are homologous to the bulbourethral glands in males (see Table 13-1).

Development of External Genitalia

Up to the seventh week, the external genitalia are sexually undifferentiated (see Fig. 13-24A and B). Distinguishing sexual characteristics begin to appear during the 9th week, but the external genitalia are not fully differentiated until the 12th week. Early in the fourth week, the proliferating mesenchyme produces a **genital tubercle** (see Fig. 13-24A)—**primordium of penis or clitoris**—in both sexes at the cranial end of the cloacal membrane. *Fgf8 is involved in the signaling pathways in the early development of the external genitalia.*

Labioscrotal swellings and **urogenital folds** soon develop on each side of the cloacal membrane. The genital tubercle soon elongates to form a **primordial phallus**—**penis or clitoris** (see Fig. 13-24B). The **urogenital membrane** lies in the floor of a median cleft, the **urethral groove,** which is bound by the urogenital folds (see Fig. 13-24C and D). In female fetuses, the urethra and vagina open into a common cavity, the **vestibule of the vagina** (see Fig. 13-24B and H).

DETERMINATION OF FETAL SEX

Assessment of fetal sex by **transabdominal ultrasound** is important for decision making, especially in pregnancies at risk of serious X-linked birth defects. Assessment is based on the direct visualization of the external genitalia. By the 12th week of gestation, the primordial phallus has differentiated to form the penis (see Fig. 13-24G). Several studies indicate that sex assignment is highly accurate in most cases (99%–100%) after 13 weeks of gestation providing the external genitalia are not malformed. The accuracy of diagnosis increases with gestational age, and it depends on the experience of the sonographer, equipment, the position of the fetus, and the amount of amniotic fluid.

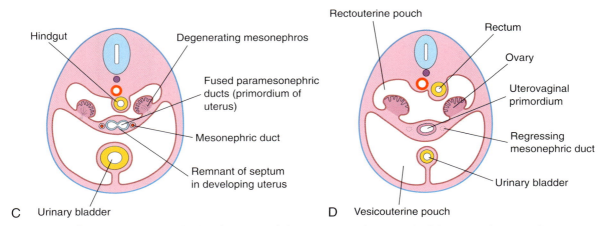

Figure 13–23 Early development of the ovaries and uterus. **A,** Schematic drawing of a sagittal section of the caudal region of an 8-week female embryo. **B,** Transverse section showing the paramesonephric ducts approaching each other. **C,** Similar section at a more caudal level illustrating fusion of the paramesonephric ducts. A remnant of the septum that separates the paramesonephric ducts is shown. **D,** Similar section showing the uterovaginal primordium, broad ligament, and pouches in the pelvic cavity. Note that the mesonephric ducts have regressed.

Development of Male External Genitalia

Masculinization of the indifferent external genitalia is induced by dihydrotestosterone that is produced peripherally by 5α-reductase conversion of testosterone from the testicular Leydig cells (see Fig. 13-24C, E, and G). As the **primordial phallus** enlarges and elongates to become the penis, the **urogenital folds** form the lateral walls of the **urethral groove** on the ventral surface of the penis. This groove is lined by a proliferation of endodermal cells, the **urethral plate** (see Fig. 13-24C), which extends from the phallic portion of the urogenital sinus. The **urethral folds** fuse with each other along the ventral surface of the penis to form the **spongy urethra** (see Fig. 13-24E_1 to E_3). The surface ectoderm fuses in the median plane of the penis, forming the **penile raphe** and enclosing the spongy urethra within the penis. At the tip of the **glans penis,** an ectodermal ingrowth forms a cellular ectodermal cord, which extends toward the root of the penis to meet the spongy urethra (see Fig. 13-15A). This cord canalizes and joins the previously formed spongy urethra (see Fig. 13-15B). This juncture completes the terminal part of the urethra and moves the **external urethral orifice** to the tip of the glans penis (see Fig. 13-15C and Fig. 13-24G). During the 12th week, a circular ingrowth of ectoderm occurs at the periphery of the glans penis (see Fig. 13-15B). When this ingrowth breaks down, it forms the **prepuce** (foreskin) (see Fig. 13-24G). The **corpora cavernosa** and **corpus spongiosum** develop from mesenchyme in the phallus. The **labioscrotal swellings** grow toward each other and fuse to form the **scrotum** (see Fig. 13-24E). The line of fusion of these folds is clearly visible as the **scrotal raphe** (see Fig. 13-24G).

Development of Female External Genitalia

Growth of the primordial phallus in the female fetus gradually decreases as it becomes the **clitoris** (see

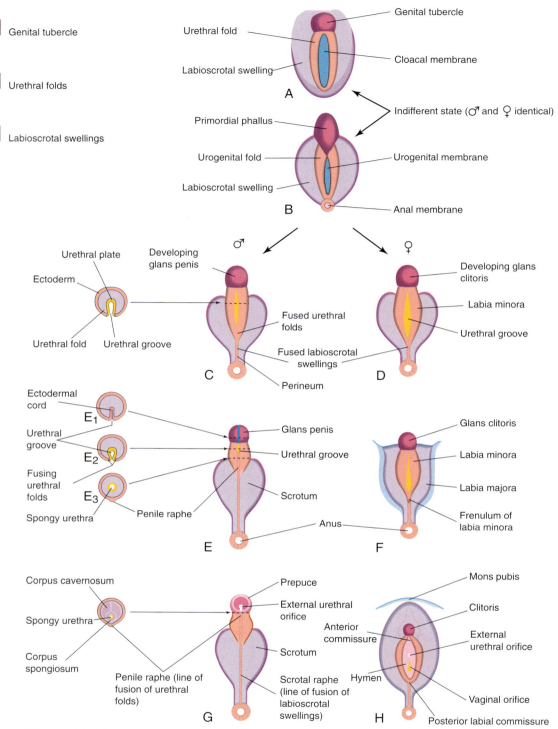

Figure 13–24 Development of the external genitalia. **A** and **B,** Diagrams illustrating appearance of the genitalia during the indifferent stage (fourth to seventh weeks). **C, E,** and **G,** Stages in the development of the male external genitalia at 9, 11, and 12 weeks, respectively. To the *left* are schematic transverse sections of the developing penis illustrating formation of the spongy urethra and scrotum. **D, F,** and **H,** Stages in the development of the female external genitalia at 9, 11, and 12 weeks, respectively. The mons pubis is a pad of fatty tissue over the symphysis pubis.

Fig. 13-24*D*, *F*, and *H*). The clitoris is still relatively large at 18 weeks (see Fig. 13-24*D*). The clitoris develops in a similar way to the penis, except that the urogenital folds do not fuse, except posteriorly, where they join to form the **frenulum of labia minora**. The unfused parts of the urogenital folds form the **labia minora**. The labioscrotal folds fuse posteriorly to form the **posterior labial commissure** and anteriorly to form the **anterior labial commissure** and the **mons pubis**. Most parts of the **labioscrotal folds** remain unfused and form two large folds of skin, the **labia majora** (see Fig. 13-24*H*).

INTERSEX DISORDERS

Advances in molecular genetics have led to a better understanding of **abnormal sexual development** and ambiguous genitalia. Because of psychosocial stigma and in order to provide better clinical management for neonates with atypical chromosomal constitution or gonads, a new nomenclature has been introduced to describe these conditions, which are now called **disorders of sex development (DSD)**. The new classification avoids using the term "hermaphrodite" and instead uses the term "intersex." (See Lee PA, Houk CP, Ahmed SF, Hughes IA: Consensus statement on management of intersex disorders. Pediatrics 118:e488, 2006.)

OVOTESTICULAR DSD (TRUE GONADAL INTERSEX)

Persons with the extremely rare intersexual condition of ovotesticular DSD usually have a 46,XX sex chromosome constitution. **Ovotesticular DSD** results from an error in sex determination; these persons have both testicular and ovarian tissue. The phenotype may be male or female, but the external genitalia are always ambiguous.

46,XX DSD (46,XX INTERSEX)

Females with 46,XX DSD have been exposed to **excessive androgens in utero**, the principal effect of which is **virilization (masculinization) of the external genitalia** (Fig. 13-25). Persons with this intersex have *chromatin-positive nuclei* and a 46,XX chromosome constitution. The common cause of 46,XX DSD is **congenital adrenal hyperplasia**. There is no ovarian abnormality, but the excessive production of androgens by the fetal suprarenal glands causes **masculinization of the external genitalia**, varying from enlargement of the clitoris to almost masculine genitalia. Commonly, **clitoral hypertrophy**, partial fusion of the labia majora, and a persistent urogenital sinus are noted.

Figure 13–25 External genitalia of a 6-year-old girl showing an enlarged clitoris and a scrotum-like structure formed by fusion of the labia majora. The *arrow* indicates the opening into the urogenital sinus (see Fig. 13-11*C*). This extreme masculinization is the result of congenital adrenal hyperplasia.

46,XY DSD (46,XY INTERSEX)

Males with 46,XY DSD have sex *chromatin-negative nuclei* and a 46,XY chromosome constitution. The external and internal genitalia are variable, owing to differing degrees of development. These changes are caused by *inadequate production of testosterone and AMH* by the fetal testes. Testicular development ranges from rudimentary to normal.

ANDROGEN INSENSITIVITY SYNDROME

Androgen insensitivity syndrome—previously called **testicular feminization syndrome**—occurs in 1 in 20,000 neonates. Individuals with this form of 46,XY DSD appear as female, despite the presence of testes and a 46,XY chromosome constitution. The external genitalia are female, but the vagina usually ends in a blind pouch and the uterus and uterine tubes are absent or rudimentary. At puberty, there is normal development of breasts and female characteristics, but menstruation does not occur and pubic hair is scanty or absent. In some cases, the external genitalia are abnormal (e.g., enlarged clitoris and a scrotum-like structure; see Fig. 13-25). The failure of masculinization results from a resistance to the action of testosterone at the cellular level in the genital tubercle and the labioscrotal and urogenital folds.

HYPOSPADIAS

There are four types of hypospadias: glanular (most common type), penile, penoscrotal, and perineal hypospadias. **Hypospadias is the most frequent anomaly** involving the penis and is found in 1 in 125 male infants. In **glanular hypospadias**, the external urethral orifice is on the ventral surface of the glans penis. In **penile hypospadias**, the external urethral orifice is on the ventral surface of the body of the penis. The glanular and penile types of hypospadias are the common types (Fig. 13-26). In **penoscrotal hypospadias**, the urethral orifice is at the junction of the penis and scrotum. In **perineal hypospadias**, the external urethral orifice is located between the unfused halves of the scrotum. **Hypospadias results from inadequate production of androgens by the fetal testes.** It is believed that environmental factors may disrupt testosterone-related gene expression.

EPISPADIAS

In 1 of every 30,000 male neonates, the urethra opens on the dorsal surface of the penis. Although epispadias may occur as a separate entity, it is *often associated with exstrophy of the bladder* (see Fig. 13-13). Epispadias may result from inadequate ectodermal-mesenchymal interactions during development of the genital tubercle. As a consequence, the genital tubercle develops more dorsally than in normal embryos. Consequently, when the urogenital membrane ruptures, the urogenital sinus opens on the dorsal surface of the penis. Urine is expelled at the root of the malformed penis.

Figure 13–26   Glanular hypospadias in a male infant. There is a shallow pit in the glans penis at the usual site of the urethral orifice.

BIRTH DEFECTS OF FEMALE GENITAL TRACT

Various types of uterine duplication and vaginal defects result from developmental arrest of the uterovaginal primordium during the eighth week of development (Fig. 13-27B to G). The main developmental defects are:

* Incomplete fusion of the paramesonephric ducts
* Incomplete development of one or both paramesonephric ducts
* Failure of parts of one or both paramesonephric ducts to develop
* Incomplete canalization of the vaginal plate that forms the vagina

In some cases, the uterus is divided internally by a septum (see Fig. 13-27F). If the duplication involves only the superior part of the body of the uterus, the condition is a **bicornuate uterus** (see Fig. 13-27D and E). If growth of one paramesonephric duct is retarded and the duct does not fuse with the other one, a **bicornuate uterus with a rudimentary horn** develops (see Fig. 13-27E). The horn may not communicate with the cavity of the uterus. A **unicornuate uterus** develops when one paramesonephric duct does not develop; this results in a uterus with one uterine tube (see Fig. 13-27G). In many of these cases, the individuals are fertile, but may have an increased incidence of premature delivery. A **double uterus** (uterus didelphys) results from failure of fusion of the inferior parts of the paramesonephric ducts. It may be associated with a double or a single vagina (see Fig. 13-27B and C).

Agenesis of the vagina results from **failure of the sinovaginal bulbs to develop** and form the vaginal plate (see Fig. 13-20B). When the vagina is absent, the uterus is usually also absent, because the developing uterus (uterovaginal primordium) induces the formation of sinovaginal bulbs, which fuse to form the **vaginal plate** (see Fig. 13-24C). Failure of canalization of the vaginal plate results in blockage of the vagina. Failure of the inferior end of the vaginal plate to perforate results in an **imperforate hymen** (see Fig. 13-20C).

DEVELOPMENT OF INGUINAL CANALS

The inguinal canals form pathways for the testes to descend from the dorsal abdominal wall through the anterior abdominal wall into the scrotum. *Inguinal canals develop in both sexes* because of the morphologically indifferent stage of sexual development. As the mesonephros degenerates, a ligament—the **gubernaculum**—develops on each side of the abdomen from the inferior pole of the gonad (Fig. 13-28A). The gubernaculum passes obliquely through the developing anterior abdominal wall at the site of the future inguinal canal (see Fig. 13-28B to D). The gubernaculum attaches caudally to the internal surface of the **labioscrotal swellings (future halves of scrotum or labia majora).**

The **processus vaginalis,** an evagination of peritoneum, develops ventral to the gubernaculum and herniates through the abdominal wall along the path formed by the

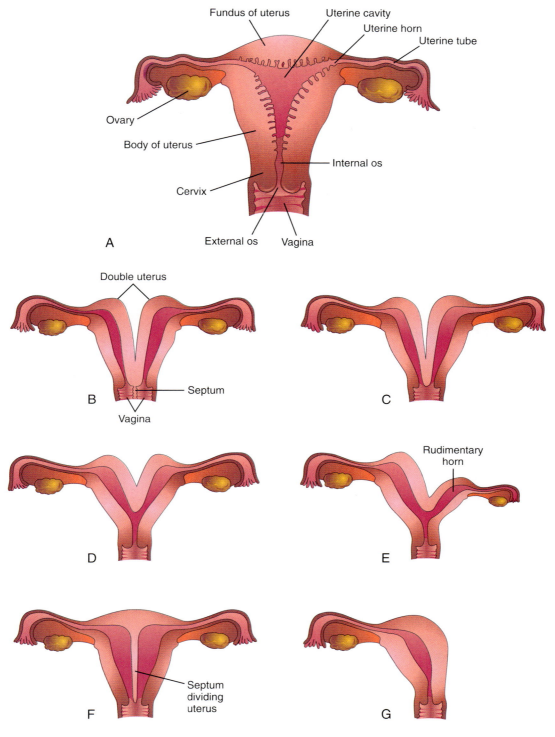

Figure 13–27 Various types of congenital uterine birth defects. **A,** Normal uterus and vagina. **B,** Double uterus (uterus didelphys) and double vagina. Note the septum dividing the vagina. **C,** Double uterus with a single vagina. **D,** Bicornuate uterus (two uterine horns). **E,** Bicornuate uterus with a rudimentary left horn. **F,** Septate uterus. Note the septum dividing the uterus. **G,** Unicornuate uterus. Note that only half of the uterus exists.

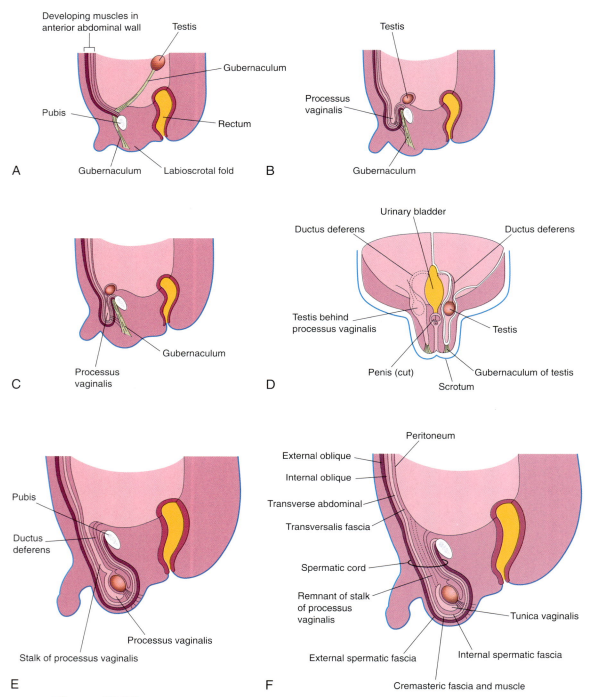

Figure 13–28   Formation of the inguinal canals and descent of the testes. **A,** Sagittal section of a 7-week embryo showing the testis before its descent from the dorsal abdominal wall. **B** and **C,** Similar sections at approximately 28 weeks showing the processus vaginalis and testis beginning to pass through the inguinal canal. Note that the processus vaginalis carries fascial layers of the abdominal wall before it. **D,** Frontal section of a fetus approximately 3 days later illustrating descent of the testis posterior to the processus vaginalis. The processus has been cut away on the *left side* to show the testis and ductus deferens. **E,** Sagittal section of a male infant neonate showing the processus vaginalis communicating with the peritoneal cavity by a narrow stalk. **F,** Similar section of a 1-month-old neonate after obliteration of the stalk of the processus vaginalis. Note that the extended fascial layers of the abdominal wall now form the coverings of the spermatic cord.

gubernaculum (see Fig. 13-28*B* to *E*). The processus vaginalis carries along extensions of the layers of the abdominal wall before it, which form the walls of the inguinal canal. These layers also form the coverings of the spermatic cord and testis (see Fig. 13-28*E* and *F*). The opening in the transversalis fascia produced by the vaginal process becomes the **deep inguinal ring,** and the opening created in the external oblique aponeurosis forms the **superficial inguinal ring.**

RELOCATION OF TESTES AND OVARIES

Descent of Testes

By 26 weeks, the testes have descended retroperitoneally from the posterior abdominal wall to the deep inguinal rings (see Fig. 13-28*B* and *C*). This change in position occurs as the fetal pelvis enlarges and the trunk of the embryo elongates. Transabdominal relocation of the testes is largely a relative movement that results from growth of the cranial part of the abdomen away from the future pelvic region.

Testicular descent through the inguinal canals and into the scrotum is controlled by androgens (e.g., testosterone) produced by the fetal testes. The **gubernaculum** (fibrous cord) guides the testes during their descent. The relocation of the testes through the inguinal canals and into the scrotum usually begins during the 26th week and it may take 2 to 3 days. By 32 weeks, both testes are in the scrotum in most cases. More than 97% of full-term neonates have both testes in the scrotum. During the first 3 months after birth, most undescended testes descend into the scrotum. When the testes descend, they carry the ductus deferens and vessels with them. As the testis and **ductus deferens** descend, they are ensheathed by the fascial extensions of the abdominal wall (see Fig. 13-28*F*):

- The extension of the transversalis fascia becomes the **internal spermatic fascia.**
- The extensions of the internal oblique muscle and fascia become the **cremasteric muscle** and **fascia.**

CRYPTORCHIDISM

Cryptorchidism (hidden or undescended testes) is the most common birth defect in neonates and occurs in about 30% of premature males and in approximately 3% to 4% of full-term males. Cryptorchidism may be unilateral or bilateral. In most cases, the testes descend into the scrotum by the end of the first year. If both testes remain within or just outside the abdominal cavity, they do not mature and sterility is common. If uncorrected, there is a significantly higher risk for the development of **germ cell tumors,** especially in cases of *abdominal cryptorchidism.* **Cryptorchid testes** may be in the abdominal cavity or anywhere along the usual path of descent of the testis, but they are usually in the inguinal canal (Fig. 13-29*A*). The cause of most cases of cryptorchidism is unknown, but a deficiency of androgen production by the fetal testes is an important factor.

- The extension of the transversalis fascia becomes the **external spermatic fascia.**

Within the scrotum, the testis projects into the distal end of the **processus vaginalis.** During the perinatal period (first 4 weeks), the connecting stalk of the process normally obliterates, forming a serous membrane—the **tunica vaginalis**—that covers the front and sides of the testis (see Fig. 13-28*F*).

Descent of Ovaries

The ovaries also descend from the lumbar region of the posterior abdominal wall and relocate to the pelvis; however, *they do not pass from the pelvis and enter the inguinal canals.* The **gubernaculum** (fibrous cord) is attached to the uterus near the attachment of the uterine tube. The cranial part of the gubernaculum becomes the **ovarian ligament** and the caudal part forms the **round ligament** of the uterus (see Fig. 13-20*C*). The round ligaments pass through the inguinal canals and terminate in the labia majora. The relatively small processus vaginalis in the female is usually obliterated and it disappears long before birth. A patent processus in a fetus is known as **a vaginal process of peritoneum** (canal of Nuck).

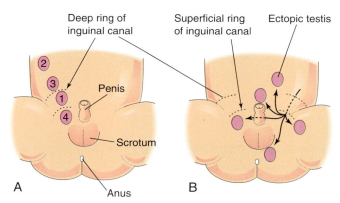

Figure 13–29 Possible sites of cryptorchid and ectopic testes. **A,** Positions of cryptorchid testes, numbered 1 to 4 in order of increasing frequency. **B,** Usual locations of ectopic testes.

ECTOPIC TESTES

After traversing the inguinal canal, the testis may deviate from its usual path of descent and lodge in various abnormal locations (see Fig. 13-29*B*):

- Interstitial (external to the aponeurosis of the external oblique muscle)
- In the proximal part of the medial thigh
- Dorsal to the penis
- On the opposite side (**crossed ectopia**)

All types of ectopic testis are rare, but **interstitial ectopia** occurs most frequently. Ectopic testis occurs when a part of the gubernaculum passes to an abnormal location and the testis follows it.

Figure 13–30 Diagrams of sagittal sections illustrating conditions resulting from failure of closure of the processus vaginalis. **A,** Incomplete congenital inguinal hernia into the scrotum resulting from persistence of the proximal part of the processus vaginalis. **B,** Complete congenital inguinal hernia entering the unobliterated processus in the scrotum. Cryptorchidism, a commonly associated birth defect, is also shown. **C,** Large hydrocele that arose from an unobliterated portion of the processus vaginalis. **D,** Hydrocele of the testis and spermatic cord resulting from peritoneal fluid passing into an unclosed processus vaginalis.

CONGENITAL INGUINAL HERNIA

If the communication between the tunica vaginalis and peritoneal cavity does not close, a **persistent processus vaginalis** occurs. A loop of intestine may herniate through it into the scrotum or labia majora (Fig. 13-30A and B). Embryonic remnants resembling the ductus deferens or epididymis are often found in inguinal hernial sacs. Congenital inguinal hernia is much more common in males, especially when there are undescended testes. The hernias are also common with ectopic testes and in **androgen insensitivity syndrome** (see Fig. 13-25).

HYDROCELE

Occasionally the abdominal end of the processus vaginalis remains open but is too small to permit herniation of intestine (see Fig. 13-30D). Peritoneal fluid passes into the patent processus vaginalis and forms a **scrotal hydrocele.** If only the middle part of the processus vaginalis remains open, fluid may accumulate and give rise to a **hydrocele of the spermatic cord** (see Fig. 13-30C).

CLINICALLY ORIENTED QUESTIONS

1. Does a horseshoe kidney usually function normally? What problems may occur with this anomaly and how can they be corrected?

2. A man was told by a doctor that he has two kidneys on one side and none on the other. How did this birth defect probably happen? Are there likely to be any problems associated with this condition?

3. Are individuals with ovotesticular DSD ever fertile?

4. When a baby is born with ambiguous external genitalia, how long does it take to assign the appropriate sex? What does the physician tell the parents? How is the appropriate sex determined?

5. What is a common type of disorder that produces ambiguous external genitalia? Will masculinizing, or androgenic, hormones given during the fetal period of development cause ambiguity of the external genitalia in female fetuses?

The answers to these questions are at the back of this book.

Cardiovascular System

T *he cardiovascular system is the first major system to function in the embryo.* The primordial heart and vascular system appear in the middle of the third week (Fig. 14-1). *The heart begins to beat at 22 to 23 days* (Fig. 14-2). This precocious development is necessary because the rapidly growing embryo can no longer satisfy its nutritional and oxygen requirements by diffusion alone. The cardiovascular system is derived from:

- *Splanchnic mesoderm*, which forms the primordium of the heart (see Fig. 14-1*A* and *B*)
- *Paraxial and lateral mesoderm* near the otic placodes—plate-like thickenings—(see Fig. 17-9*A* and *B*)

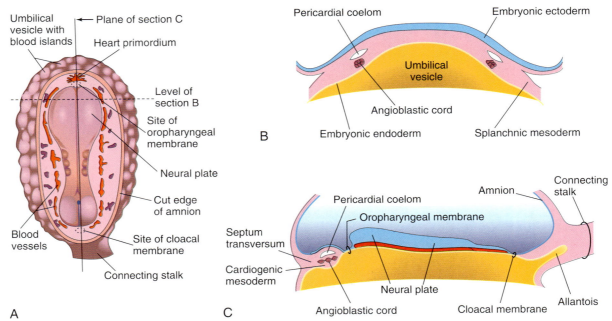

Figure 14–1 Early development of the heart. **A,** Drawing of a dorsal view of an embryo (approximately 18 days). **B,** Transverse section of the embryo showing angioblastic cords in the cardiogenic mesoderm and their relationship to the pericardial coelom. **C,** Longitudinal section through the embryo illustrating the relationship of the angioblastic cords to the oropharyngeal membrane, pericardial coelom, and septum transversum.

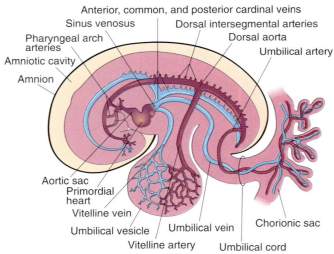

Figure 14–2 Drawing of the embryonic cardiovascular system (at approximately 26 days) showing vessels on the left side only. The umbilical vein carries well-oxygenated blood and nutrients from the chorionic sac to the embryo. The umbilical arteries carry poorly oxygenated blood and waste products from the embryo to the chorionic sac (outermost embryonic membrane; see Chapter 8, Fig. 8-1A and B).

EARLY DEVELOPMENT OF HEART AND BLOOD VESSELS

Multipotential cardiac progenitor cells from several sources contribute to the formation of the heart. These include distinct mesodermal populations—a primary, or first, heart field (FHF) and a secondary heart field (SHF)—as well as neural crest cells. Mesodermal cells from the primitive streak migrate to form bilateral paired strands (FHF), and from the pharyngeal mesoderm, the SHF, located medial to the FHF. These strands canalize to form two thin heart **tubes** that soon fuse to form a single **heart tube** late in the third week as a result of embryo folding (see Fig. 14-5). An inductive influence from the anterior endoderm stimulates early formation of the heart. Cardiac morphogenesis (development) is controlled by a cascade of *regulatory genes and transcription factors*.

Development of Veins Associated with Embryonic Heart

Three paired veins drain into the tubular heart of a 4-week embryo (see Fig. 14-2):

- *Vitelline veins* return poorly oxygenated blood from the umbilical vesicle.
- *Umbilical veins* carry well-oxygenated blood from the chorionic sac
- *Common cardinal veins* return poorly oxygenated blood from the body of the embryo to the heart.

The **vitelline veins** enter the venous end of the heart—the **sinus venosus** of the primordial heart (see Fig. 14-2, Fig. 14-3, and Fig. 14-4A and B). As the liver primordium grows into the septum transversum, the **hepatic cords** anastomose around preexisting endothelium-lined spaces. These spaces, the primordia of the hepatic sinusoids, later become linked to the vitelline veins. The **hepatic**

Figure 14–3 Illustrations of the primordial veins of the trunk of an embryo (ventral views). Initially, three systems of veins are present: the umbilical veins from the chorionic sac, the vitelline veins from the umbilical vesicle, and the cardinal veins from the body of the embryo. Next, the subcardinal veins appear, and finally the supracardinal veins develop. **A,** At 6 weeks. **B,** At 7 weeks. **C,** At 8 weeks. **D,** Drawing illustrating the transformations that produce the adult venous pattern. *IVC*, inferior vena cava. *(Modified from Arey LB: Developmental Anatomy, 7th ed. Philadelphia, Saunders, 1974.)*

Figure 14–4   Dorsal views of the developing heart. **A,** During the fourth week (approximately 24 days), showing the primordial atrium, sinous venosus, and veins draining into them. **B,** At 7 weeks, showing the enlarged right sinus horn and venous circulation through the liver. The organs are not drawn to scale. **C,** At 8 weeks, indicating the adult derivatives of the cardinal veins shown in **A** and **B.** *Arrows* indicate the flow of blood.

veins form from the remains of the right vitelline vein in the region of the developing liver. The **portal vein** develops from a network of vitelline veins around the duodenum (see Fig. 14-4*B*). The transformation of the umbilical veins may be summarized as follows (see Fig. 14-4*B*):

- The right umbilical vein and the cranial part of the left umbilical vein between the liver and the sinus venosus degenerate.
- The persistent caudal part of the left umbilical vein becomes the umbilical vein, which carries well-oxygenated blood from the placenta to the embryo.
- A large venous shunt—the ductus venosus—develops within the liver and connects the umbilical vein with the inferior vena cava (IVC).

The **cardinal veins** (see Fig. 14-2 and Fig. 14-3*A*) constitute the main venous drainage system of the embryo. The anterior and posterior cardinal veins drain the cranial and caudal parts of the embryo, respectively (see Fig. 14-3*A*). These join the **common cardinal veins**, which enter the **sinus venosus** (see Fig. 14-4*A*). During the eighth week, the **anterior cardinal veins** are connected by an oblique anastomosis (see Fig. 14-4*B*) that shunts blood from the left to the right anterior cardinal vein. This anastomotic shunt becomes the **left brachiocephalic vein** when the caudal part of the left anterior cardinal vein degenerates (see Figs. 14-3*D* and 14-4*C*). The **superior vena cava** (SVC) forms from the right anterior cardinal vein and the right common cardinal vein. The only adult derivatives of the **posterior cardinal veins** are the root of the **azygos vein** and the **common iliac veins** (see Figs. 14-3*D* and 14-4*C*). The subcardinal and supracardinal veins gradually replace and supplement the posterior cardinal veins.

The **subcardinal veins** appear first (see Fig. 14-3*A*) and form the stem of the left renal vein, the suprarenal veins, the gonadal veins (testicular and ovarian), and a segment of the inferior vena cava (see Fig. 14-3*D*). The **supracardinal veins** become disrupted in the region of the kidneys (see Fig. 14-3*C*). Cranial to this, they become united by an anastomosis that forms the **azygos** and the **hemiazygos veins** (see Fig. 14-3*D* and Fig. 14-4*C*). Caudal to the kidneys, the left supracardinal vein degenerates but the right supracardinal vein becomes the inferior part of the IVC (see Fig. 14-3*D*). The **inferior vena cava** forms as blood returning from the caudal part of the embryo is shifted from the left to the right side of the body.

ANOMALIES OF VENAE CAVAE

The most common anomaly of the venae cavae is a persistent left SVC. The most common anomaly of the IVC is interruption of its abdominal course; as a result, blood drains from the lower limbs, abdomen, and pelvis to the heart through the azygos system of veins (see Fig. 14-3).

Pharyngeal Arch Arteries and Other Branches of the Dorsal Aorta

As the *pharyngeal arches* form during the fourth and fifth weeks, they are supplied by **pharyngeal arch arteries** arising from the **aortic sac** and terminating in the **dorsal aortae** (see Fig. 14-2). Neural crest cells delaminate from the neural tube and contribute to the formation of the outflow tract of the heart and pharyngeal arches. Initially, the paired dorsal aortae run through the entire length of the embryo. Later, the caudal portions of the paired dorsal aortae fuse to form a single lower thoracic/abdominal aorta. Of the remaining paired dorsal aortae, the right regresses and the left becomes the primordial aorta.

Intersegmental Arteries

Thirty or so branches of the dorsal aorta, the **intersegmental arteries**, pass between and carry blood to the somites (cell masses) and their derivatives (see Fig. 14-2). The intersegmental arteries in the neck join to form the **vertebral arteries**. Most of the original connections of the intersegmental arteries to the dorsal aorta disappear.

In the thorax, the intersegmental arteries persist as **intercostal arteries**. Most of the intersegmental arteries in the abdomen become **lumbar arteries**; however, the fifth pair of lumbar intersegmental arteries remains as the **common iliac arteries**. In the sacral region, the intersegmental arteries form the **lateral sacral arteries**.

Fate of Vitelline and Umbilical Arteries

The unpaired ventral branches of the dorsal aorta supply the umbilical vesicle, allantois, and chorion (see Fig. 14-2). The **vitelline arteries** supply the umbilical vesicle and, later, the primordial gut, which forms from the incorporated part of the umbilical vesicle. Only three vitelline arteries remain: the *celiac arterial trunk* to the foregut, the *superior mesenteric artery* to the midgut, and the *inferior mesenteric artery* to the hindgut.

The paired **umbilical arteries** pass through the connecting stalk (primordial umbilical cord) and join the vessels in the chorion (membrane enclosing the embryo). The umbilical arteries carry poorly oxygenated fetal blood to the placenta (see Fig. 14-2). The proximal parts of these arteries become the **internal iliac arteries** and **superior vesical arteries**, whereas the distal parts are obliterated after birth and become **medial umbilical ligaments**.

LATER DEVELOPMENT OF HEART

The external layer of the embryonic heart tube—the **primordial myocardium** (cardiac precursor of the primary heart field)—is formed from the splanchnic mesoderm surrounding the **pericardial cavity** (Fig. 14-5 and Fig. 14-6*B* and C). At this stage, the developing heart is composed of a thin tube, separated from a thick primordial myocardium by gelatinous-matrix connective tissue—**cardiac jelly** (see Fig. 14-6*C* and *D*).

The **endothelial tube** becomes the internal endothelial lining of the heart—**endocardium**—and the primordial

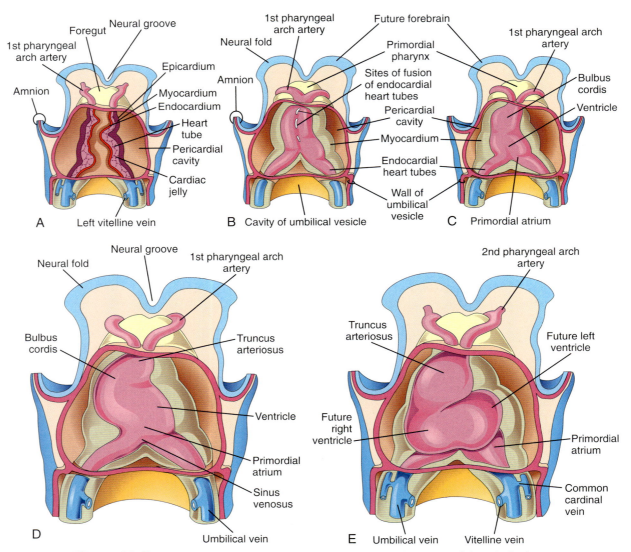

Figure 14–5 Drawings showing fusion of the heart tubes and looping of the tubular heart.
A to C, Ventral views of the developing heart and pericardial region (22–35 days). The ventral
pericardial wall has been removed to show the developing myocardium and fusion of the two
heart tubes to form a tubular heart. The endothelium of the heart tube forms the endocardium
of the heart. **D** and **E**, As the straight tubular heart elongates, it bends and undergoes looping,
which forms a D-loop that produces an S-shaped heart.

myocardium becomes the muscular wall of the heart, the **myocardium**. The **epicardium** is derived from the SHF and from mesothelial cells that arise from the external surface of the sinus venosus and spread over the myocardium (see Fig. 14-6F).

As folding of the head region occurs, the heart and pericardial cavity appear ventral to the foregut and caudal to the **oropharyngeal membrane** (Fig. 14-7A to C). Concurrently, the tubular heart elongates and develops alternate dilations and constrictions (see Fig. 14-5C to E): the **bulbus cordis** (composed of the **truncus arteriosus, conus arteriosus,** and **conus cordis**), ventricle, atrium, and sinus venosus. The growth of the heart tube results from the addition of cells (cardiomyocytes) that differentiate from the mesoderm at the dorsal wall of the pericardium.

The tubular **truncus arteriosus** is continuous cranially with the aortic sac (Fig. 14-8A), from which the pharyngeal arch arteries arise. Progenitor cells from the SHF contribute to the formation of the arterial and venous ends of the developing heart. The **sinus venosus** receives the umbilical, vitelline, and common cardinal veins from the chorion, umbilical vesicle, and embryo, respectively (see Fig. 14-4A). The arterial and venous ends of the heart are fixed in place by the pharyngeal arches and septum transversum, respectively. Because the **bulbus cordis** and ventricle grow faster than the other regions, the heart bends on itself, forming a U-shaped **bulboventricular loop** (see Fig. 14-6E). *Complex signaling pathways involving BMP, Notch, Wnt, and Shh are essential regulators in the remodeling of the heart tube.*

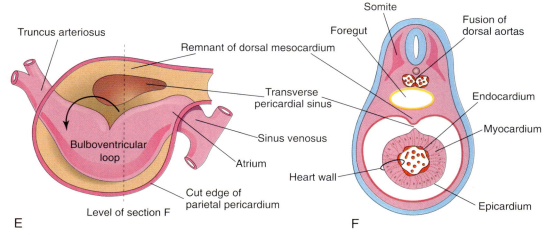

Figure 14–6 **A,** Dorsal view of an embryo (approximately 20 days). **B,** Schematic transverse section of the heart region of the embryo illustrated in **A,** showing the two endocardial heart tubes and lateral folds of the body. **C,** Transverse section of a slightly older embryo, showing the formation of the pericardial cavity and fusion of the heart tubes. **D,** Similar section (approximately 22 days) showing the tubular heart suspended by the dorsal mesocardium. **E,** Schematic drawing of the heart (approximately 28 days) showing degeneration of the central part of the dorsal mesocardium and formation of the transverse pericardial sinus. The *arrow* shows bending of the primordial heart. The tubular heart now has a D-loop. **F,** Transverse section of the embryo at the level seen in **E,** showing the layers of the heart wall.

A

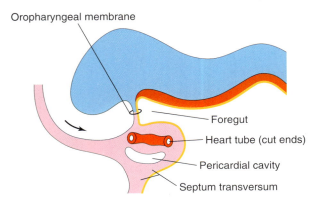

B

Figure 14–7 Illustrations of longitudinal sections through the cranial half of embryos during the fourth week, showing the effect of the head fold *(arrows)* on the position of the heart and other structures. **A** and **B,** As the head fold develops, the heart tube and pericardial cavity move ventral to the foregut and caudal to the oropharyngeal membrane. **C,** Note that the positions of the pericardial cavity and septum transversum have reversed with respect to each other. The septum transversum now lies posterior to the pericardial cavity, where it will form the central tendon of the diaphragm.

C

Nodal (belonging to the transforming growth factor-β superfamily) is involved in looping of the heart tube. As the primordial heart bends, the atrium and sinus venosus appear dorsal to the truncus arteriosus, bulbus cordis, and ventricle (see Fig. 14-8A and B). By this stage, the sinus venosus has developed lateral expansions, the right and left **horns of the sinus venosus.**

As the heart develops, it gradually invaginates the **peri-cardial cavity** (see Figs. 14-6C and D and Fig. 14-7C). The heart is initially suspended from the dorsal wall by a **mesentery** (double layer of peritoneum), the **dorsal mesocardium.** However, the central part of this mesentery degenerates, forming a communication—the **trans-verse pericardial sinus**—between the right and left

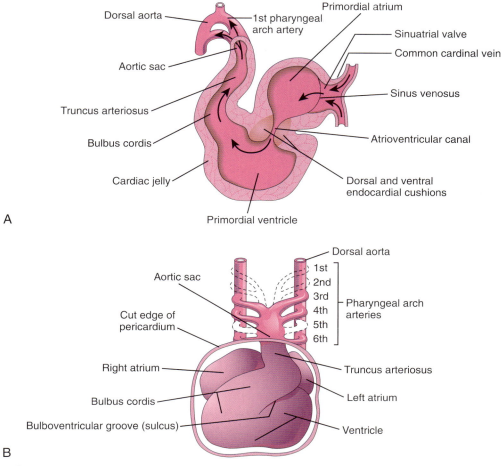

Figure 14–8 **A,** Sagittal section of the primordial heart at approximately 24 days, showing blood flowing through it *(arrows)*. **B,** Ventral view of the heart and pharyngeal arch arteries at approximately 35 days. The ventral wall of the pericardial sac has been removed to show the heart in the pericardial cavity.

sides of the pericardial cavity (see Fig. 14-6*E* and *F*). At this stage, the heart is attached only at its cranial and caudal ends.

Circulation through Primordial Heart

Blood enters the sinus venosus (see Fig. 14-8*A* and Fig. 14-4*A*) from the:

- Embryo through the common cardinal veins
- Developing placenta through the umbilical veins
- Umbilical vesicle through the vitelline veins

Blood from the **sinus venosus** enters the **primordial atrium**; its flow is controlled by **sinuatrial (SA) valves** (see Fig. 14-8*A*). The blood then passes through the **atrioventricular (AV) canal** into the **primordial ventricle**. When the ventricle contracts, blood is pumped through the **bulbus cordis** and **truncus arteriosus** into the **aortic sac**, from which it is distributed to the pharyngeal arch arteries (see Fig. 14-8*B*). The blood then passes into the dorsal

aortae for distribution to the embryo, umbilical vesicle, and placenta (see Fig. 14-2).

Partitioning of Primordial Heart

Partitioning of the AV canal, primordial atrium, ventricle, and outflow tract begins at the middle of the fourth week and is essentially completed by the end of the eighth week.

Toward the end of the fourth week, **atrioventricular endocardial cushions** form on the dorsal and ventral walls of the AV canal (see Fig. 14-8*A*). These cushions approach each other and fuse, dividing the AV canal into right and left AV canals (Fig. 14-9*B*). These canals partially separate the primordial atrium from the ventricle, and the cushions function as AV valves. The endocardial cushions develop from a specialized extracellular **matrix** (intracellular substance of a tissue) related to the myocardium as well as neural crest cells. *Its formation is associated with the expression of transforming growth factor-β₂ and bone morphogenetic proteins 2A and 4.*

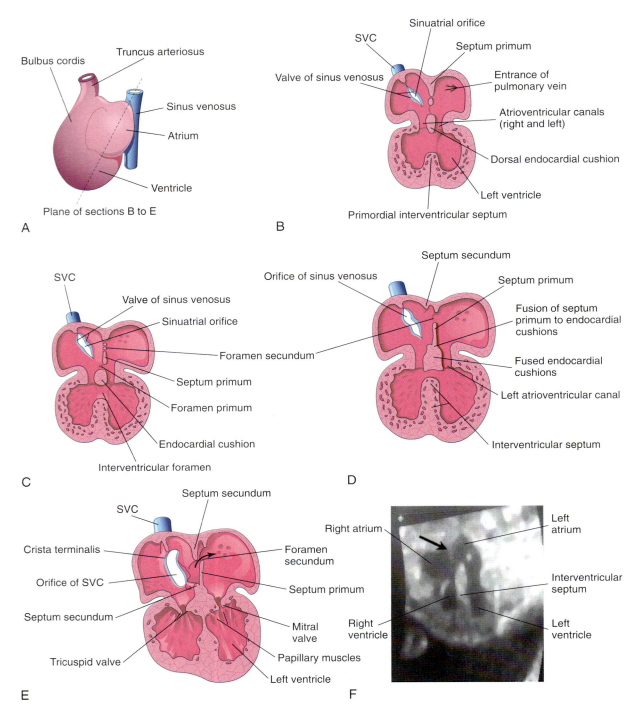

Figure 14–9   Drawings of the heart showing partitioning of the atrioventricular (AV) canal, primordial atrium, and ventricle. **A,** Sketch showing the plane of sections **B** to **E. B,** Frontal section of the heart during the fourth week (approximately 28 days) showing the early appearance of the septum primum, interventricular septum, and dorsal endocardial cushion. **C,** Frontal section of the heart (approximately 32 days) showing perforations in the dorsal part of the septum primum. **D,** Frontal section of the heart (approximately 35 days), showing the foramen secundum. **E,** At approximately 8 weeks, the heart is partitioned into four chambers. The *arrow* indicates the flow of well-oxygenated blood from the right to the left atrium. **F,** Sonogram of a second-trimester fetus showing the four chambers of the heart. Note the septum secundum *(arrow). SVC,* Superior vena cava.

Partitioning of Primordial Atrium

The primordial atrium is divided into right and left atria by the formation and subsequent modification and fusion of two septa, the septum primum and septum secundum (see Fig. 14-9A to E and Fig. 14-10). The **septum primum** grows toward the fusing endocardial cushions from the roof of the primordial atrium, partially dividing the atrium into right and left halves. As this curtain-like muscular septum develops, a large opening—the **foramen primum**—forms between its free edge and the **endocardial cushions** (see Fig. 14-9C and Fig. 14-10A to C). This foramen allows shunting of oxygenated blood from the right to the left atrium. The foramen becomes progressively smaller and disappears as the mesenchymal cap of the septum primum fuses with the fused endocardial cushions to form the **primordial AV septum** (see Fig. 14-10D and D_1). *Molecular biology studies have revealed that a distinct population of extracardiac progenitor cells, from the SHF, migrate through the dorsal mesocardium to complete the atrial septum. Shh signaling plays a critical role in this process.*

Before the foramen primum disappears, perforations produced by **apoptosis (programmed cell death)** appear in the central part of the septum primum. As the septum fuses with the endocardial cushions, obliterating the foramen primum (see Fig. 14-9D and Fig. 14-10D), the perforations coalesce to form another opening in the septum primum—the **foramen secundum** (see Fig. 14-10C). This foramen ensures continued shunting of oxygenated blood from the right to the left atrium.

The **septum secundum** grows from the muscular ventrocranial wall of the atrium, immediately adjacent to the right of the **septum primum** (see Fig. 14-10D_1). As this thick septum grows during the fifth and sixth weeks, it gradually overlaps the **foramen secundum** in the septum primum (see Fig. 14-10E and F). The septum secundum forms an incomplete partition between the atria: the opening in the foramen secundum—**oval foramen** (foramen ovale). The cranial part of the septum primum gradually disappears (see Fig. 14-10G_1). The remaining part of the septum, attached to the endocardial cushions, forms the **valve of the oval foramen**.

Before birth, the oval foramen allows most of the oxygenated blood entering the right atrium from the IVC to pass into the left atrium (see Fig. 14-10H_1). It also prevents the passage of blood in the opposite direction because the septum primum closes against the relatively rigid septum secundum (see Fig. 14-10G_1).

After birth, the oval foramen functionally closes due to higher pressure in the left atrium than in the right atrium. At approximately 3 months, the valve of the oval foramen fuses with the septum secundum, forming the **oval fossa** (fossa ovalis). As a result, the interatrial septum becomes a complete partition between the atria (see Fig. 14-10G).

Changes in Sinus Venosus

Initially, the sinus venosus opens into the center of the posterior wall of the primordial atrium. By the end of the fourth week, the right sinual horn becomes larger than the left sinual horn (Fig. 14-11A and B). As this occurs, the **sinuatrial orifice** moves to the right and opens in the part of the primordial atrium that will become the adult right atrium (see Fig. 14-11C). As the right sinual horn enlarges, it receives all the blood from the head and neck through the SVC, and from the placenta and caudal regions of the body through the IVC.

The **left horn of the sinus venosus** becomes the **coronary sinus**, and the **right horn of the sinus venosus** is incorporated into the wall of the right atrium (see Fig. 14-11B and C) and becomes the smooth part of the internal wall of the right atrium—the **sinus venarum** (see Fig. 14-11B and C). The remainder of the anterior internal surface of the wall of the right atrium, as well as that of the **right auricle**, has a rough, trabeculated appearance (see Fig. 14-11C). These latter two parts are derived from the primordial atrium. The smooth part and rough part are demarcated internally in the right atrium by a vertical ridge—**crista terminalis**, or terminal crest (see Fig. 14-11C)—and externally by a shallow groove—the **sulcus terminalis**, or terminal groove (see Fig. 14-11B).

The crista terminalis represents the cranial part of the **right sinuatrial valve** (see Fig. 14-11C); the caudal part of this valve forms the valves of the IVC and coronary sinus. The **left sinuatrial valve** fuses with the septum secundum and is incorporated with it into the interatrial septum.

Primordial Pulmonary Vein and Formation of Left Atrium

Most of the wall of the left atrium is smooth because it is formed by the incorporation of the **primordial pulmonary vein** (Fig. 14-12A). This vein develops as an outgrowth of the dorsal atrial wall, just to the left of the septum primum. As the atrium expands, the primordial pulmonary vein and its main branches are gradually incorporated into the wall of the left atrium (see Fig. 14-12B). As a result, four pulmonary veins are formed (see Fig. 14-12C and D). The small left auricle is derived from the primordial atrium; its internal surface has a rough, trabeculated appearance (see Fig. 14-12D).

Partitioning of Primordial Ventricle

Division of the primordial ventricle into two ventricles is first indicated by a median ridge—the **muscular interventricular (IV) septum**—in the floor of the ventricle near its apex (see Fig. 14-9B). This fold has a concave superior free edge (Fig. 14-13A). Initially, most of its increase in height results from dilation of the ventricles on each side of the muscular IV septum (see Fig. 14-13B). Myocytes (muscle cells) from both the right and left primordial ventricles contribute to the formation of the *muscular part of the IV septum.*

Until the seventh week, there is a crescent-shaped opening (**IV foramen**) between the free edge of the IV septum and the fused **endocardial cushions**. The IV foramen permits communication between the right and left ventricles (see Fig. 14-13B and Fig. 14-14B). The IV foramen usually closes by the end of the seventh week as the **bulbar ridges** fuse with the endocardial cushion (see Fig. 14-14C to E).

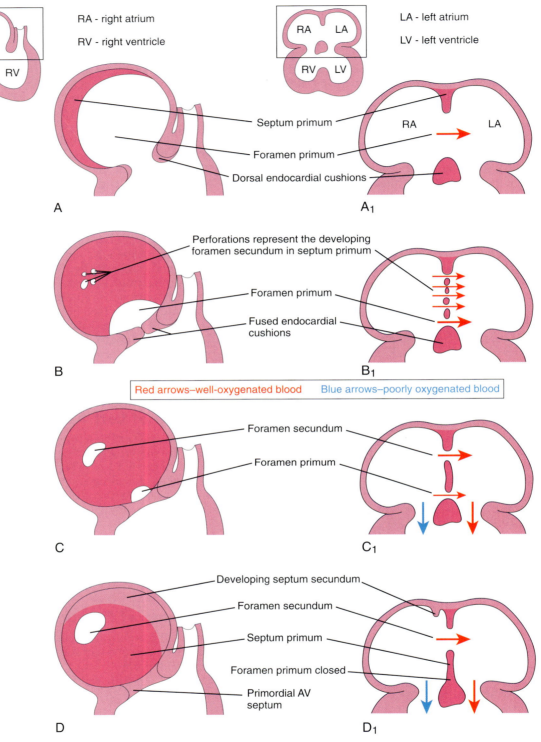

Figure 14–10 Diagrams illustrating progressive stages in partitioning of the primordial atrium. **A** to **H,** The developing interatrial septum, as viewed from the right side. **A₁** to **H₁,** Coronal sections of the developing interatrial septum. As the septum secundum grows, note that it overlaps the opening in the septum primum, the foramen secundum. Observe the valve of the oval foramen in **G₁** and **H₁.** When the pressures are equal or higher in the left atrium, the valve closes the oval foramen **(G₁).**

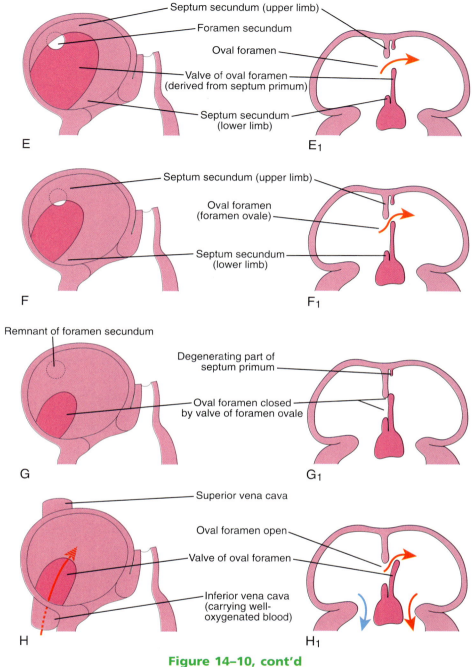

Figure 14–10, cont'd

Closure of the IV foramen and formation of the membranous part of the IV septum result from the fusion of tissues from three sources: the right bulbar ridge, the left bulbar ridge, and the endocardial cushion. The **membranous part of the IV septum** is derived from an extension of tissue from the right side of the endocardial cushion to the muscular part of the IV septum (Fig. 14-15A and B). Closure of the IV foramen and formation of the membranous part of the IV septum result in communication of the pulmonary trunk with the right ventricle and the aorta

communicates with the left ventricle (see Fig. 14-14E). Cavitation of the ventricular walls forms a sponge-like mass of muscular bundles—**trabeculae carneae**. Other bundles become the **papillary muscles** and **tendinous cords** *(chordae tendineae)*. The tendinous cords run from the papillary muscles to the AV valves (see Fig. 14-15B).

Partitioning of Bulbus Cordis and Truncus Arteriosus

During the fifth week, active proliferation of mesenchymal cells in the walls of the **bulbus cordis** results in the

6
13

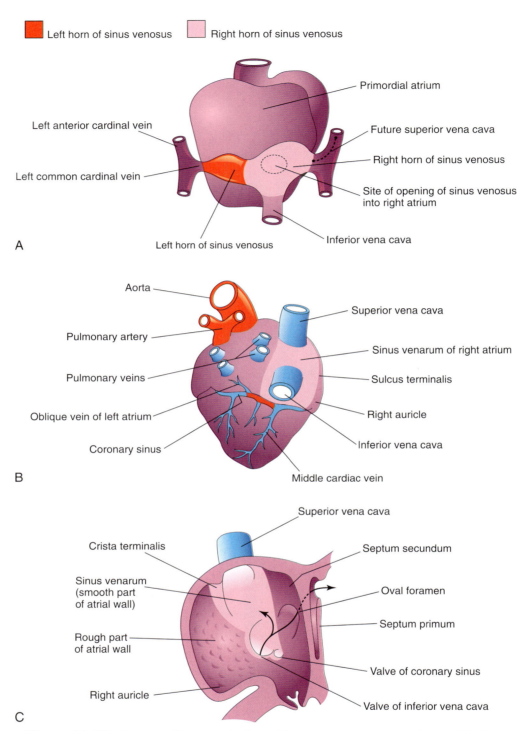

■ Left horn of sinus venosus ☐ Right horn of sinus venosus

A

Primordial atrium

Left anterior cardinal vein

Future superior vena cava

Right horn of sinus venosus

Left common cardinal vein

Site of opening of sinus venosus into right atrium

Inferior vena cava

Left horn of sinus venosus

B

Aorta

Superior vena cava

Pulmonary artery

Sinus venarum of right atrium

Pulmonary veins

Sulcus terminalis

Oblique vein of left atrium

Right auricle

Coronary sinus

Inferior vena cava

Middle cardiac vein

C

Superior vena cava

Crista terminalis

Septum secundum

Sinus venarum (smooth part of atrial wall)

Oval foramen

Septum primum

Rough part of atrial wall

Valve of coronary sinus

Right auricle

Valve of inferior vena cava

Figure 14–11 Diagrams illustrating the fate of the sinus venosus. **A,** Dorsal view of the heart (approximately 26 days) showing the primordial atrium and sinus venosus. **B,** Dorsal view at 8 weeks after incorporation of the right horn of the sinus venosus into the right atrium. The left horn has become the coronary sinus. **C,** Internal view of the fetal right atrium showing: (1) the smooth part of the wall of the right atrium (sinus venarum), derived from the right horn of the sinus venosus; and (2) the crista terminalis and valves of the inferior vena cava and coronary sinus, derived from the right sinuatrial valve. The primordial right atrium becomes the right auricle, a conical muscular pouch. *Arrows* indicate the flow of blood.

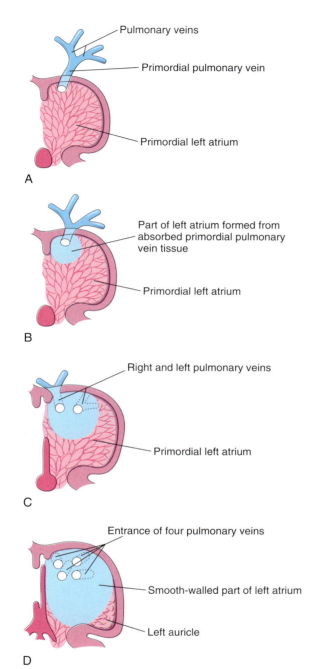

A

B

C

D

Figure 14–12 Diagrammatic sketches illustrating absorption of the pulmonary vein into the left atrium. **A,** At 5 weeks, showing the primordial pulmonary vein opening into the primordial left atrium. **B,** Later stage showing partial absorption of the primordial pulmonary vein. **C,** At 6 weeks, showing the openings of two pulmonary veins into the left atrium resulting from absorption of the primordial pulmonary vein. **D,** At 8 weeks, showing four pulmonary veins with separate atrial orifices. The primordial left atrium becomes the left auricle, a tubular pouch of the atrium. Most of the left atrium is formed by absorption of the primordial pulmonary vein and its branches.

formation of **bulbar ridges** (see Fig. 14-14C and D and Fig. 14-16B and C). Similar ridges form in the truncus arteriosus; these ridges are continuous with the bulbar ridges. The **bulbar** and **truncal ridges** are derived mainly from the neural crest mesenchyme. *Bone morphogenetic protein and other signaling systems in the SHF, such as Wnt and fibroblast growth factor, have been implicated in the induction and migration of neural crest cells through the primordial pharynx and the pharyngeal arches.*

Concurrently, the bulbar and truncal ridges undergo 180-degree spiraling. The spiral orientation of the bulbar and truncal ridges, possibly caused in part by the streaming of blood from the ventricles, results in the formation of a spiral **aorticopulmonary septum** when the ridges fuse (see Fig. 14-16D to G). This septum divides the bulbus cordis and the truncus arteriosus into two arterial channels, the **aorta** and the **pulmonary trunk**. Because of the spiraling of the aorticopulmonary septum, the pulmonary trunk twists around the ascending aorta (see Fig. 14-16H).

The **bulbus cordis** is incorporated into the walls of the definitive ventricles in several ways (see Fig. 14-14A and B):

- In the right ventricle, the bulbus cordis is represented by the **conus arteriosus** (infundibulum), which gives origin to the pulmonary trunk.
- In the left ventricle, the bulbus cordis forms the walls of the **aortic vestibule**, the part of the ventricular cavity just inferior to the aortic valve.

Development of Cardiac Valves

The semilunar valves develop from three swellings of subendocardial tissue around the orifices of the aorta and pulmonary trunk (Fig. 14-17B to F). Cardiac precursors, from neural crest cells, also contribute to this formation. These swellings are hollowed out and reshaped to form three thin-walled cusps. The **atrioventricular valves** (tricuspid and mitral valves) develop similarly from localized proliferations of tissue around the AV canals.

Conducting System of Heart

Initially, the muscle layers of the atrium and ventricle are continuous. As the chambers form, their myocardium conducts the wave of depolarization faster than the rest of the myocardium. Throughout development, the impulse moves from the venous to the arterial pole of the heart. The *atrium acts as the interim pacemaker of*

FETAL CARDIAC ULTRASONOGRAPHY

Echocardiography and Doppler ultrasonography have made it possible for sonographers to recognize normal and abnormal fetal cardiac anatomy. Most studies are first performed at 18 to 22 weeks' gestation, when the heart is large enough to be examined easily; however, real-time ultrasound images of the fetal heart can be obtained at 16 weeks.

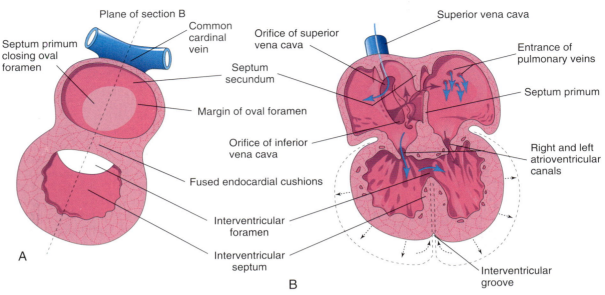

Figure 14–13 Illustrations of partitioning of the primordial heart. **A,** Sagittal section late in the fifth week, showing the cardiac septa and foramina. **B,** Frontal section at a slightly later stage, showing the directions of blood flow through the heart (*blue arrows*) and the expansion of the ventricles (*black arrows*).

the heart, but the sinus venosus soon takes over this function. The **sinuatrial node** develops during the fifth week. This node is located in the right atrium, near the entrance of the SVC (see Fig. 14-15*B*). After incorporation of the sinus venosus, cells from its left wall are found in the base of the interatrial septum, near the opening of the coronary sinus. Together with cells from the AV region, they form the **AV node and bundle**, located just superior to the endocardial cushions (see Fig. 14-15*B*). The atrial and ventricular chambers become electrically isolated from each other by fibrous tissue, resulting in only the AV node and bundle being able to conduct the impulses. The fibers arising from the AV bundle pass from the atrium into the ventricle and split into right and left **bundle branches**, which are distributed throughout the ventricular myocardium (see Fig. 14-15*B*). The SA node, AV node, and AV bundle are richly supplied by nerves; however, the conducting system is well developed before these nerves enter the heart. Parasympathetic innervation of the heart occurs by contributions from the neural crest cells.

BIRTH DEFECTS OF HEART AND GREAT VESSELS

Congenital heart defects (CHDs) occur with a frequency of 6 to 8 cases in 1000 live births and are a leading cause of neonatal morbidity. Some CHDs are caused by single-gene or chromosomal mechanisms; others result from exposure to teratogens such as the *rubella virus* (see Chapter 19). Most CHDs appear to be caused by multiple factors, both genetic and environmental (i.e., multifactorial inheritance). Recent technology, such as real-time, three-dimensional *echocardiography*, has permitted the detection of fetal CHDs as early as the 16th week.

DEXTROCARDIA

If the embryonic heart tube bends to the left instead of to the right, the heart is displaced to the right (Fig. 14-18), and there is transposition whereby the heart and its vessels are reversed, left to right, as in a mirror image. **Dextrocardia** is the most frequent positional defect of the heart. In **dextrocardia with situs inversus** (transposition of abdominal viscera), the incidence of accompanying cardiac defects is low. In **isolated dextrocardia**, the abnormal position of the heart is not accompanied by displacement of other viscera. This defect is usually complicated by severe cardiac defects (e.g., single ventricle and transposition of the great vessels).

ECTOPIA CORDIS

In ectopia cordis (Fig. 14-19), an extremely rare condition, the heart is in an abnormal location. In the **thoracic form of ectopia cordis**, the heart is partly or completely exposed on the surface of the thorax. Death occurs in most cases during the early neonatal period, usually from infection, cardiac failure, or **hypoxemia** (subnormal oxygenation of arterial blood). The most common thoracic form of ectopia cordis results from faulty development of the sternum and pericardium secondary to incomplete fusion of the lateral folds in the formation of the thoracic wall during the fourth week. If no severe cardiac defects are present, surgical therapy usually consists of covering the heart with skin.

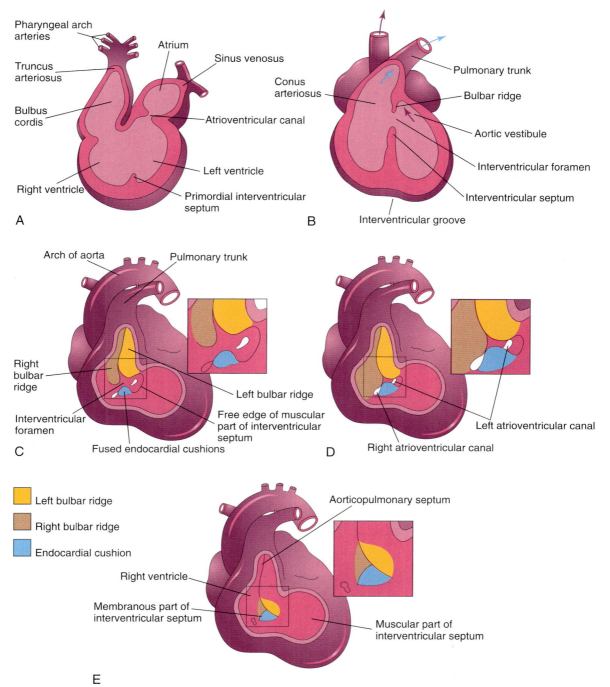

Figure 14–14 Sketches illustrating incorporation of the bulbus cordis into the ventricles and partitioning of the bulbus cordis and truncus arteriosus into the aorta and pulmonary trunk. **A,** Sagittal section at 5 weeks showing the bulbus cordis as one of the chambers of the primordial heart. **B,** Schematic coronal section at 6 weeks, after the bulbus cordis has been incorporated into the ventricles to become the conus arteriosus of the right ventricle, which gives origin to the pulmonary trunk and aortic vestibule of the left ventricle. The *arrows* indicate blood flow. **C** to **E,** Schematic drawings illustrating closure of the interventricular (IV) foramen and formation of the membranous part of the IV septum. The walls of the truncus arteriosus, bulbus cordis, and right ventricle have been removed. **C,** At 5 weeks, showing the bulbar ridges and fused endocardial cushions. **D,** At 6 weeks, showing how the proliferation of subendocardial tissue diminishes the IV foramen. **E,** At 7 weeks, showing the fused bulbar ridges, the membranous part of the IV septum formed by extensions of tissue from the right side of the endocardial cushions, and closure of the IV foramen.

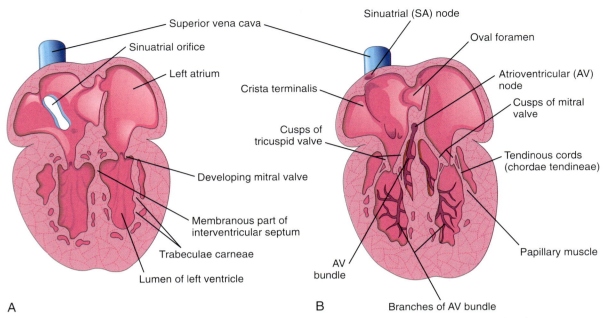

Figure 14–15   Schematic sections of the heart illustrating successive stages in the development of the atrioventricular valves, tendinous cords *(chordae tendineae)*, and papillary muscles. **A,** At 7 weeks. **B,** At 20 weeks, showing the conducting system of the heart.

ATRIAL SEPTAL DEFECTS

Atrial septal defects (ASDs) occur more frequently in females than in males. The most common form of ASD is a **patent oval foramen** (Fig. 14-20A and Fig. 14-21A to D). A small, isolated patent foramen is of no hemodynamic significance. However, if other defects are present (e.g., pulmonary atresia), blood is shunted through the oval foramen into the left atrium, producing **cyanosis**.

A **probe-patent oval foramen** is present in up to 25% of people. In this circumstance, a probe can be passed from one atrium to the other through the superior part of the floor of the oval fossa (see Fig. 14-20B). This defect is not clinically significant, but a probe-patent oval foramen may be forced open because of other cardiac defects. A probe-patent oval foramen results from incomplete adhesion between the flap-like valve of the oval foramen and the septum secundum after birth.

There are four clinically significant types of ASD (see Fig. 14-21), of which the first two are relatively common:

* Ostium secundum defect
* Endocardial cushion defect with a foramen primum defect
* Sinus venosus defect
* Common atrium

Ostium secundum ASDs (see Fig. 14-21A to D) occur in the area of the oval fossa and include defects of the septum primum and septum secundum. Females with ASDs outnumber males 3 to 1. This ASD is one of the most common, yet least severe, types of CHD. The patent oval foramen usually results from abnormal resorption of the septum primum during the formation of the foramen secundum. If resorption occurs in abnormal locations, the septum primum is fenestrated or net-like (see Fig. 14-21A). If excessive resorption of the septum primum occurs, the resulting short septum primum does not close the oval foramen (see Fig. 14-21B). If an abnormally large oval foramen develops as a result of defective development of the septum secundum, a normal septum primum does not close the abnormal oval foramen at birth (see Fig. 14-21D). Large ostium secundum ASDs may also occur because of a combination of excessive resorption of the septum primum and a large oval foramen.

Endocardial cushion defects with a foramen primum are less common forms of ASD (see Fig. 14-21E). The septum primum does not fuse with the endocardial cushions, resulting in a patent foramen primum. Usually there is also a cleft in the anterior cusp of the mitral valve.

Sinus venosus ASDs are located in the superior part of the interatrial septum, close to the entry of the SVC (see Fig. 14-21F). These defects result from incomplete absorption of the sinus venosus into the right atrium, abnormal development of the septum secundum, or both. **Common atrium** occurs in patients with all three types of defect: ostium secundum, ostium primum, and sinus venosus.

Figure 14–16 Partitioning of the bulbus cordis and truncus arteriosus. **A,** Ventral aspect of heart at 5 weeks. The *broken lines* and *arrows* indicate the levels of the sections shown in **B. B,** Transverse sections of the truncus arteriosus and bulbus cordis, illustrating the truncal and bulbar ridges. **C,** The ventral wall of the heart and truncus arteriosus has been removed to demonstrate these ridges. **D,** Ventral aspect of the heart after partitioning of the truncus arteriosus. The *broken lines* and *arrows* indicate the levels of the sections shown in **E. E,** Sections through the newly formed aorta (*A*) and pulmonary trunk (*PT*) showing the aorticopulmonary septum. **F,** 6 weeks. The ventral wall of the heart and pulmonary trunk have been removed to show the aorticopulmonary septum. **G,** Diagram illustrating the spiral form of the aorticopulmonary septum. **H,** Drawing showing the great arteries (ascending aorta and pulmonary trunk) twisting around each other as they leave the heart.

Figure 14–17 Development of the semilunar valves of the aorta and pulmonary trunk. **A,** Sketch of a section of the truncus arteriosus and bulbus cordis showing the valve swellings. **B,** Transverse section of the bulbus cordis. **C,** Similar section after fusion of the bulbar ridges. **D,** Formation of the walls and valves of the aorta and pulmonary trunk. **E,** Rotation of the vessels has established the adult positions of the valves in relation to each other. **F** and **G,** Longitudinal sections of the aorticoventricular junction illustrating successive stages in the hollowing (arrows) and thinning of the valve swellings to form the valve cusps. *A,* anterior; *L,* left; *P,* posterior; *R,* right.

VENTRICULAR SEPTAL DEFECTS

Ventricular septal defects (VSDs) are the most common type of CHD, accounting for approximately 25% of cases. VSDs occur more frequently in males than in females. *Most VSDs involve the membranous part of the IV septum* (Fig. 14-22B). Many small VSDs close spontaneously, usually during the first year. Most people with a large VSD have massive left-to-right shunting of blood. *Muscular VSD* is a less common type of defect that may appear anywhere in the muscular part of the IV septum. **Transposition of great arteries** (Fig. 14-23) and a rudimentary outlet chamber are present in most infants with this severe type of CHD.

NORMAL

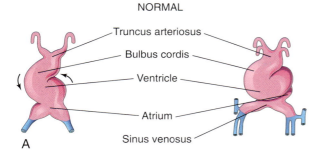

Truncus arteriosus

Bulbus cordis

Ventricle

Atrium

Sinus venosus

A

DEXTROCARDIA

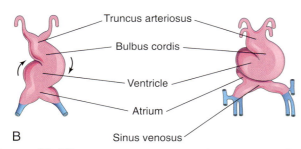

Truncus arteriosus

Bulbus cordis

Ventricle

Atrium

Sinus venosus

B

Figure 14–18 The embryonic heart tube during the fourth week. **A,** Normal looping of the tubular heart to the right *(arrows)*. **B,** Abnormal looping to the left.

Figure 14–19 Magnetic resonance image of a fetus demonstrating exteriorization of the heart (*) from its normal position within the thorax *(t)*. An omphalocele (see Chapter 12) can also be seen *(arrow)*. *(From Leyder M, van Berkel K, Done E, Cannie M, Van Hecke W, Voeselmans A: Ultrasound meets magnetic resonance imaging in the diagnosis of pentalogy of Cantrell with complete ectopy of the heart. Gynecol Obstet [Sunnyvale] 4:200, 2014.)*

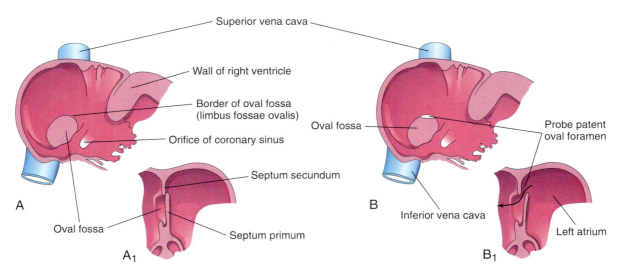

Superior vena cava

Wall of right ventricle

Border of oval fossa (limbus fossae ovalis)

Orifice of coronary sinus

Septum secundum

Oval fossa

A

Oval fossa

Septum primum

A₁

Oval fossa

Probe patent oval foramen

B

Inferior vena cava

Left atrium

B₁

Figure 14–20 **A,** Normal postnatal appearance of the right side of the interatrial septum after adhesion of the septum primum to the septum secundum. **A₁,** Sketch of a section of the interatrial septum illustrating formation of the oval fossa in the right atrium. Note that the floor of the fossa is formed by the septum primum. **B** and **B₁,** Similar views of a probe-patent oval foramen resulting from incomplete adhesion of the septum primum to the septum secundum. Some well-oxygenated blood can enter the right arium via a patent oval foramen; however, if the opening is small it is usually of no hemodynamic significance.

Figure 14–21 Drawings of the right aspect of the interatrial septum. The adjacent sketches of sections of the septa illustrate various types of atrial septal defect *(ASD)*. **A,** Patent oval foramen resulting from resorption of the septum primum in abnormal locations. **B,** Patent oval foramen caused by excessive resorption of the septum primum ("short flap defect"). **C,** Patent oval foramen resulting from an abnormally large oval foramen. **D,** Patent oval foramen resulting from an abnormally large oval foramen and excessive resorption of the septum primum. **E,** Endocardial cushion defect with a primum-type ASD. The adjacent section shows the cleft in the anterior cusp of the mitral valve. **F,** Sinus venosus ASD. The high septal defect resulted from abnormal absorption of the sinus venosus into the right atrium. In **E** and **F,** note that the oval fossa has formed normally. *Arrows* indicate the direction of flow of blood. *LA,* Left atrium; *RA,* right atrium.

Figure 14–22   Illustrations of the main type of persistent truncus arteriosus (PTA). **A,** The common trunk divides into the aorta and a short pulmonary trunk. **B,** Coronal section of the heart shown in **A.** Observe the circulation of blood in this heart *(arrows)* and the ventricular septal defect. *LA,* Left atrium; *RA,* right atrium.

Figure 14–23   Drawing of a heart illustrating transposition of the great arteries (TGA). The ventricular septal defect (VSD) and atrial septal defect (ASD) allow mixing of the arterial and venous blood. TGA is the most common single cause of **cyanotic heart disease** in neonates. This birth defect is often associated with other cardiac defects, as shown (VSD and ASD). The *arrows* indicate the flow of blood. In TGA, when there is an ASD, blood flows from the right atrium to the left atrium.

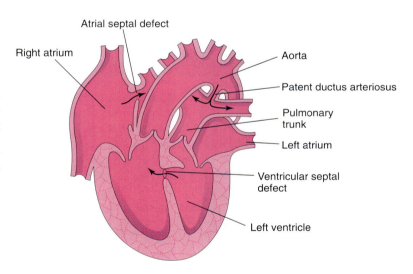

PERSISTENT TRUNCUS ARTERIOSUS

Persistent truncus arteriosus (TA) results from failure of the truncal ridges and aorticopulmonary septum to develop normally, and to divide the TA into the aorta and pulmonary trunk (see Fig. 14-22). The most common type of persistent TA is a **single arterial trunk** that branches to form the pulmonary trunk and ascending aorta (see Fig. 14-22*A* and *B*) supplying the systemic, pulmonary, and coronary circulations. A VSD is always present with a TA defect; the TA straddles the VSD (see Fig. 14-22*B*).

TRANSPOSITION OF GREAT ARTERIES

Transposition of the great arteries (TGA) is the most common cause of **cyanotic heart disease** in neonates (see Fig. 14-23). In typical cases, the aorta lies anterior and to the right of the pulmonary trunk and arises anteriorly from the morphologic right ventricle, whereas the pulmonary trunk arises from the morphologic left ventricle. There is also an ASD, with or without an associated patent ductus arteriosus (PDA) and VSD. This defect is believed to result from **failure of the conus arteriosus to develop normally** during incorporation of the bulbus cordis into the ventricles. Defective neural crest cell migration may also be involved.

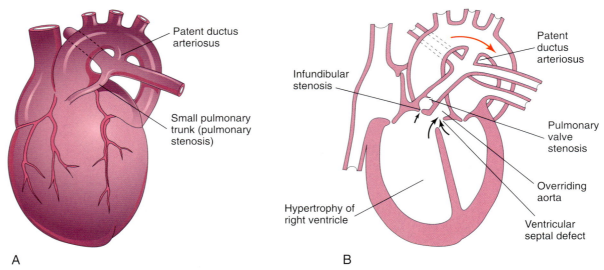

Figure 14–24 Drawings illustrating tetralogy of Fallot. **A,** Drawing of an infant's heart showing a small **(pulmonary stenosis)** and a large aorta resulting from unequal partitioning of the truncus arteriosus. There is also hypertrophy of the right ventricle and a patent ductus arteriosus. **B,** Frontal section of this heart, illustrating the tetralogy of Fallot. Observe the four cardiac defects of this tetralogy: pulmonary valve stenosis, ventricular septal defect, overriding aorta, and hypertrophy of the right ventricle. In this case, infundibular stenosis is also shown. The *arrows* indicate the flow of blood into the great vessels (aorta and pulmonary trunk).

UNEQUAL DIVISION OF TRUNCUS ARTERIOSUS

Unequal division of the truncus arteriosus (see Fig. 14-22 and Fig. 14-24A and B) results when partitioning of the TA superior to the valves is unequal, producing one large great artery and one small one. As a result, the aorticopulmonary septum is not aligned with the IV septum, and a VSD results. The larger vessel (aorta or pulmonary trunk) usually straddles the VSD (see Fig. 14-24A and B).

In **pulmonary valve stenosis,** the cusps of the pulmonary valve are fused to form a dome with a narrow central opening. In **infundibular stenosis,** the conus arteriosus of the right ventricle is underdeveloped. The two types of pulmonary stenosis may be concurrent. Depending on the degree of obstruction to blood flow, there is a variable degree of hypertrophy of the right ventricle (see Fig. 14-24B).

TETRALOGY OF FALLOT

The classic group of four cardiac defects—*tetralogy of Fallot*— consists of the following (see Fig. 14-24A and B):

* Pulmonary stenosis (obstructed right ventricular outflow)
* Ventricular septal defect
* Dextroposition of the aorta (straddling or overriding both ventricles)
* Right ventricular hypertrophy

In these cardiac defects, the pulmonary trunk is usually small and there may be varying degrees of **pulmonary artery stenosis** as well.

AORTIC STENOSIS AND AORTIC ATRESIA

In **aortic valve stenosis,** the edges of the valve are usually fused to form a dome with a narrow opening. This defect may be present at birth or it may develop after birth (acquired). The valvular stenosis causes extra work for the heart and results in **hypertrophy (enlargement)** of the left ventricle and abnormal heart sounds **(heart murmurs).**

In *subaortic stenosis,* there is often a band of fibrous tissue just inferior to the aortic valve. The narrowing of the aorta results from persistence of tissue that normally degenerates as the valve forms. **Aortic atresia** is present when obstruction of the aorta or its valve is complete.

Figure 14–25 Pharyngeal arches and pharyngeal arch arteries. **A,** Left side of an embryo (approximately 26 days). **B,** Schematic drawing of this embryo showing the left pharyngeal arch arteries arising from the aortic sac, running through the pharyngeal arches, and terminating in the left dorsal aorta. **C,** An embryo (approximately 37 days) showing the single dorsal aorta and that most of the first two pairs of pharyngeal arch arteries have degenerated.

DERIVATIVES OF PHARYNGEAL ARCH ARTERIES

As the pharyngeal arches develop during the fourth week, they are supplied by **pharyngeal arch arteries** arising from the aortic sac (Fig. 14-25B). These arteries terminate in the dorsal aorta on the ipsilateral (same) side. Although six pairs of arch arteries usually develop, they are not present at the same time (see Fig. 14-25B and C).

13

14

Derivatives of First Pair of Pharyngeal Arch Arteries

The first pair of arteries largely disappears but remnants of them form part of the **maxillary arteries**, which supply the ears, teeth, and muscles of the eyes and face. They may also contribute to the formation of the external carotid arteries (see Fig. 14-25B).

Derivatives of Second Pair of Pharyngeal Arch Arteries

Dorsal parts of these arteries persist and form the stems of the small **stapedial arteries**; these small vessels run through the ring of the **stapes**, a small bone in the middle ear (see Chapter 17, Fig. 17-11C).

Derivatives of Third Pair of Pharyngeal Arch Arteries

Proximal parts of these arteries form the **common carotid arteries**, which supply structures in the head (Fig. 14-26D). Distal parts of these arteries join with the dorsal aortae to form the **internal carotid arteries**, which supply the middle ears, orbits, brain and its meninges, and pituitary gland.

Derivatives of Fourth Pair of Pharyngeal Arch Arteries

The *left fourth artery* forms part of the **arch of the aorta** (see Fig. 14-26C and D). The proximal part of the arch artery develops from the **aortic sac** and the distal part is derived from the **left dorsal aorta**. The *right fourth artery* becomes the proximal part of the **right subclavian artery**. The distal part of the right subclavian artery forms from the **right dorsal aorta** and **right seventh intersegmental artery**. The left subclavian artery is not derived from a pharyngeal arch artery; it forms from the **left seventh intersegmental artery** (see Fig. 14-26A). As development proceeds, differential growth shifts the origin of the left subclavian artery cranially. Consequently, it lies close to the origin of the *left common carotid artery* (see Fig. 14-26D).

Fate of Fifth Pair of Pharyngeal Arch Arteries

Approximately 50% of the time, the fifth pair of arch arteries consists of rudimentary vessels that soon degenerate, leaving no vascular derivatives. In other 50%, these arches do not develop.

Derivatives of Sixth Pair of Pharyngeal Arch Arteries

The **left sixth artery** develops as follows (see Fig. 14-26B and C):

- The proximal part of the artery persists as the proximal part of the left pulmonary artery.
- The distal part of the artery passes from the left pulmonary artery to the dorsal aorta and forms a prenatal shunt, the ductus arteriosus.

The **right sixth artery** develops as follows:

- The proximal part of the artery persists as the proximal part of the right pulmonary artery.
- The distal part of the artery degenerates.

The transformation of the sixth pair of arteries explains why the course of the **recurrent laryngeal nerves** differs on the two sides. These nerves supply the sixth pair of arches and hook around the sixth pair of arteries on their way to the developing larynx (Fig. 14-27A). *On the right*, because the distal part of the right sixth artery degenerates, the right recurrent laryngeal nerve moves superiorly and hooks around the proximal part of the right subclavian artery, the derivative of the fourth artery (see Fig. 14-27B). *On the left*, the left recurrent laryngeal nerve hooks around the **ductus arteriosus (DA)** formed by the distal part of the sixth artery. When this arterial shunt involutes after birth, the nerve remains around the **ligamentum arteriosum** (remnant of DA) and the arch of the aorta (see Fig. 14-27C).

COARCTATION OF AORTA

Aortic coarctation (constriction) occurs in approximately 10% of children with CHDs. Coarctation is characterized by an **aortic constriction** of varying length (Fig. 14-28). Most constrictions occur distal to the origin of the left subclavian artery, at the entrance of the DA (**juxtaductal coarctation**).

A classification system of preductal and postductal coarctations is commonly used; however, in 90% of cases, the coarctation is directly opposite the DA. **Coarctation** occurs two times as often in males as in females, and is associated with a **mitral (bicuspid) aortic valve** in 70% of cases (see Fig. 14-15B).

DOUBLE PHARYNGEAL ARCH ARTERY

This rare anomaly is characterized by a *vascular ring around the trachea and esophagus* (Fig. 14-29). The ring results from failure of the distal part of the right dorsal aorta to disappear (see Fig. 14-29A); as a result, right and left arches form. Usually, the right arch of the aorta is the larger one and it passes posterior to the trachea and esophagus (see Fig. 14-29B). If the compression is significant, it causes wheezing respirations that are aggravated by crying, feeding, and flexion of the neck.

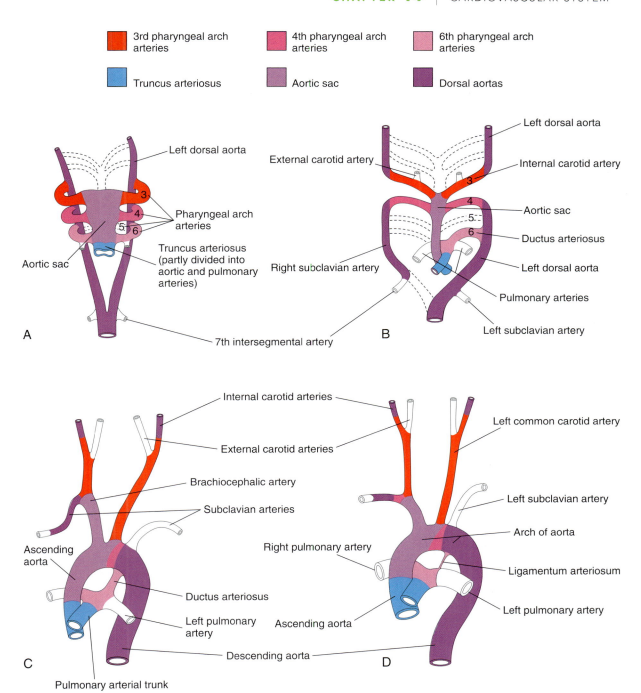

3rd pharyngeal arch arteries

4th pharyngeal arch arteries

6th pharyngeal arch arteries

Truncus arteriosus

Aortic sac

Dorsal aortas

A

Left dorsal aorta

Pharyngeal arch arteries

Aortic sac

Truncus arteriosus (partly divided into aortic and pulmonary arteries)

7th intersegmental artery

B

Left dorsal aorta

External carotid artery

Internal carotid artery

Aortic sac

Ductus arteriosus

Right subclavian artery

Left dorsal aorta

Pulmonary arteries

Left subclavian artery

C

Internal carotid arteries

External carotid arteries

Brachiocephalic artery

Subclavian arteries

Ascending aorta

Ductus arteriosus

Left pulmonary artery

Descending aorta

Pulmonary arterial trunk

D

Left common carotid artery

Left subclavian artery

Arch of aorta

Right pulmonary artery

Ligamentum arteriosum

Ascending aorta

Left pulmonary artery

Figure 14–26 Schematic drawings illustrating the arterial changes that result during transformation of the truncus arteriosus, aortic sac, pharyngeal arch arteries, and dorsal aortae into the adult arterial pattern. The vessels that are not colored are not derived from these structures. **A,** Pharyngeal arch arteries at 6 weeks; by this stage, the first two pairs of arteries have largely disappeared. **B,** Pharyngeal arch arteries at 7 weeks; the parts of the dorsal aortae and pharyngeal arch arteries that normally disappear are indicated with *broken lines*. **C,** Arterial arrangement at 8 weeks. **D,** Sketch of the arterial vessels of a 6-month-old neonate. Note that the ascending aorta and pulmonary arteries are considerably smaller in **C** than in **D.** This represents the relative flow through these vessels at the different stages of development. Observe the large size of the ductus arteriosus (DA) in **C** and that it is essentially a direct continuation of the pulmonary trunk. The DA normally becomes closed within the first few days after birth. Eventually the DA becomes the ligamentum arteriosum, as shown in **D.**

Figure 14–27   The relation of the recurrent laryngeal nerves to the pharyngeal arch arteries. **A,** At 6 weeks, showing that the recurrent laryngeal nerves are hooked around the sixth pair of pharyngeal arch arteries. **B,** At 8 weeks, showing that the right recurrent laryngeal nerve is hooked around the right subclavian artery, and the left recurrent laryngeal nerve is hooked around the ductus arteriosus and arch of the aorta. **C,** After birth, showing that the left recurrent laryngeal nerve is hooked around the ligamentum arteriosum and the arch of the aorta.

RIGHT ARCH OF AORTA

When the entire right dorsal aorta persists (Fig. 14-30A) and the distal part of the left dorsal aorta involutes, a right arch of the aorta results. There are two main types:

* *Right arch of the aorta without a retroesophageal component* (see Fig. 14-30B). The **ductus arteriosus** (ligamentum arteriosum) passes from the right pulmonary artery to the right arch of the aorta.
* *Right arch of the aorta with a retroesophageal component* (see Fig. 14-30C). Originally, a small left arch of the aorta probably involuted, leaving the right arch of the aorta posterior to the esophagus. The DA attaches to the distal part of the arch of the aorta and forms a ring that may constrict the esophagus and trachea.

ANOMALOUS RIGHT SUBCLAVIAN ARTERY

The right subclavian artery normally arises from the distal part of the arch of the aorta and passes posterior to the trachea and esophagus to supply the right upper limb (Fig. 14-31). A **retroesophageal right subclavian artery** occurs when the right fourth pharyngeal arch artery and the right dorsal aorta disappear cranial to the seventh intersegmental artery. As a result, the right subclavian artery forms from the right seventh intersegmental artery and the distal part of the right dorsal aorta. As development proceeds, differential growth shifts the origin of the right subclavian artery cranially, until it comes to lie close to the origin of the left subclavian artery.

Although an anomalous right subclavian artery is fairly common and always forms a vascular ring (see Fig. 14-31C), it is rarely clinically significant because the ring is usually not tight enough to constrict the esophagus and trachea very much.

PHARYNGEAL ARCH ARTERIAL BIRTH DEFECTS

Because of the many changes involved in the transformation of the embryonic pharyngeal arch system of arteries into the adult arterial pattern, it is understandable why defects may occur. Most defects result from the persistence of parts of the pharyngeal arch arteries that usually disappear or from the disappearance of parts that normally persist.

FETAL AND NEONATAL CIRCULATION

The fetal cardiovascular system is designed to serve prenatal needs (Fig. 14-32). Modifications at birth establish

13

14

Figure 14–28 **A,** Postductal coarctation of the aorta. **B,** Common routes of the collateral circulation that develop in association with postductal coarctation of the aorta. **C,** Preductal coarctation. *Arrows* indicate flow of blood. **D,** Preductal coarctation *(arrow)* in the aorta in an adult.

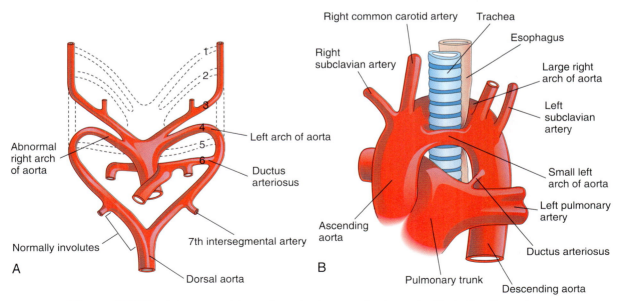

Figure 14–29 **A,** Drawing of the embryonic pharyngeal arch arteries illustrating the embryologic basis of the aorta (double arch of aorta). **B,** A large right arch of the aorta and a small left arch of the aorta arise from the ascending aorta and form a vascular ring around the trachea and esophagus. Observe that there is compression of the esophagus and trachea. The right common carotid and subclavian arteries arise separately from the large right arch of the aorta.

Figure 14–30 **A,** Sketch of the pharyngeal arch arteries showing normal involution of the distal portion of the left dorsal aorta. There is also persistence of the entire right dorsal aorta and the distal part of the right sixth pharyngeal arch artery. **B,** Right pharyngeal arch artery without a retroesophageal component. **C,** Right arch of the aorta with a retroesophageal component. The abnormal right arch of the aorta and ligamentum arteriosum (postnatal remnant of the ductus arteriosus) form a vascular ring that compresses the esophagus and trachea.

Figure 14–31 Sketches illustrating the possible embryologic basis for an abnormal origin of the right subclavian artery. **A,** The right fourth pharyngeal arch artery and the cranial part of the right dorsal aorta have involuted. As a result, the right subclavian artery forms from the right seventh intersegmental artery and the distal segment of the right dorsal aorta. **B,** As the arch of the aorta forms, the right subclavian artery is carried cranially *(arrows)* with the left subclavian artery. **C,** The abnormal right subclavian artery arises from the aorta and passes posterior to the trachea and esophagus.

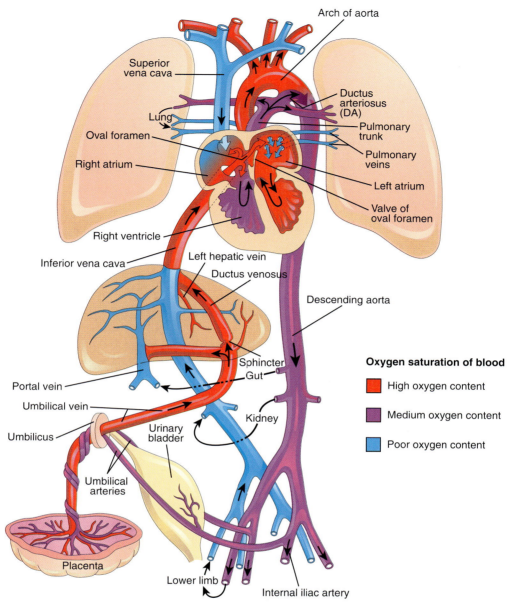

Figure 14–32 Fetal circulation. The colors indicate the oxygen saturation of the blood, and the *arrows* show the course of the blood from the placenta to the heart. The organs are not drawn to scale. A small amount of highly oxygenated blood from the inferior vena cava remains in the right atrium and mixes with poorly oxygenated blood from the superior vena cava. The medium-oxygenated blood then passes into the right ventricle. Observe that three shunts permit most of the blood to bypass the liver and lungs: (1) ductus venosus, (2) oval foramen, and (3) ductus arteriosus. The poorly oxygenated blood returns to the placenta for oxygen and nutrients through the umbilical arteries.

the neonatal pattern (Fig. 14-33). Good respiration in the neonatal period (1 to 28 days) is dependent on normal circulatory changes occurring at birth, which results in oxygenation of the blood occurring in the lungs when fetal blood flow through the placenta ceases. Before birth, the lungs do not provide gas exchange and the pulmonary vessels are vasoconstricted (narrow blood vessels). The three vascular structures most important in the transitional circulation are the ductus venosus, oval foramen, and DA (ductus arteriosus) (see Fig. 14-33).

Fetal Circulation

Highly oxygenated, nutrient-rich blood returns under high pressure from the placenta in the **umbilical vein** (see Fig. 14-32). On approaching the liver, approximately one half of the blood passes directly into the **ductus venosus**, a fetal vessel connecting the umbilical vein to the IVC; consequently this blood bypasses the liver. The other half of the blood in the umbilical vein flows into the sinusoids of the liver and enters the IVC through the **hepatic veins**. Blood flow through the ductus venosus is regulated by a

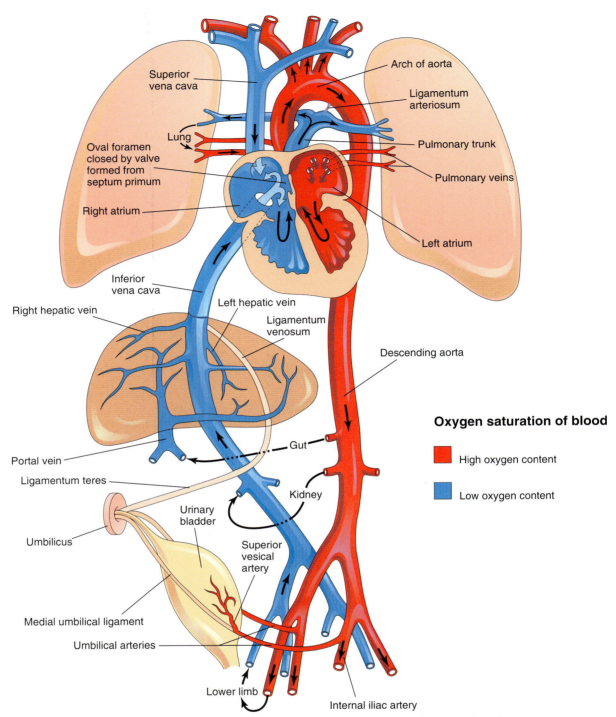

Figure 14–33 Neonatal circulation. The adult derivatives of the fetal vessels and structures that become nonfunctional at birth are shown. The *arrows* indicate the course of the blood in the infant. The organs are not drawn to scale. After birth, the three fetal shunts cease to function, and the pulmonary and systemic circulations become separated.

sphincter mechanism close to the umbilical vein. After a short course in the IVC, all of the blood enters the right atrium of the heart. Most blood from the IVC is directed by the **crista dividens**, through the **oval foramen** into the left atrium. There, it mixes with the relatively small amount of poorly oxygenated blood returning from the

lungs through the pulmonary veins. Fetal lungs use the oxygen from the blood instead of replenishing it. From the left atrium, the blood then passes to the left ventricle and leaves through the ascending aorta. The arteries to the heart, neck, head, and upper limbs receive well-oxygenated blood from the ascending aorta. *The liver also receives well-oxygenated blood from the umbilical vein.*

The small amount of well-oxygenated blood from the IVC in the right atrium mixes with poorly oxygenated blood from the SVC and coronary sinus and passes into the right ventricle. This blood, with medium oxygen content, leaves the heart through the pulmonary trunk. Because of the high pulmonary vascular resistance in fetal life, pulmonary blood flow is low. Approximately 10% of this blood flow goes to the lungs; most blood passes through the DA into the aorta to the fetal body. It then returns to the placenta through the umbilical arteries (see Fig. 14-32). Approximately 10% of blood from the ascending aorta enters the descending aorta to supply the viscera and the inferior part of the body. Most of the blood in the descending aorta passes into the umbilical arteries and is returned to the placenta for reoxygenation.

Transitional Neonatal Circulation

Important circulatory adjustments occur at birth, when the circulation of fetal blood through the placenta ceases and the infant's lungs expand and begin to function (see Fig. 14-33). *As soon as the fetus is born, the oval foramen, DA, ductus venosus, and umbilical vessels are no longer needed.* The sphincter in the ductus venosus constricts and all blood entering the liver passes through the hepatic sinusoids. This, combined with occlusion of the placental circulation, causes an immediate decrease in blood pressure in the IVC and right atrium.

Because of increased pulmonary blood flow, the pressure in the left atrium is higher than in the right atrium. The **increased left atrial pressure closes the oval foramen** by pressing the valve of the foramen against the septum secundum (see Fig. 14-33). The output from the right ventricle then flows entirely into the pulmonary circulation. Because pulmonary vascular resistance is lower than systemic vascular resistance, blood flow in the DA reverses, passing from the aorta to the pulmonary trunk.

The **DA begins to constrict at birth,** but for a few days there is often a small shunt of blood from the aorta to the pulmonary trunk in healthy, full-term neonates. In premature neonates and those with persistent hypoxia (decreased oxygen), the DA may remain open much longer. In full-term neonates, oxygen is the most important factor in controlling closure of the DA, and it appears to be mediated by *bradykinin (a substance released from the lungs)* and *prostaglandins that act on the smooth muscle in the wall of the DA.*

The **umbilical arteries constrict at birth,** preventing loss of the neonate's blood. The umbilical cord is not tied for a minute or so; consequently, blood flow through the umbilical vein continues, transferring fetal blood from the placenta to the neonate.

The change from the fetal to the adult pattern of blood circulation is not a sudden occurrence. Some changes occur with the first breath; others take place over hours and days. The closure of fetal vessels and the oval foramen is initially a functional change. Later, anatomical closure results from the proliferation of endothelial and fibrous tissues.

Derivatives of Fetal Vessels and Structures

Because of the changes in the cardiovascular system at birth, some vessels and structures are no longer required. Over a period of months, these fetal vessels form nonfunctional ligaments.

Umbilical Vein and Round Ligament of Liver

The intra-abdominal part of the *umbilical vein* eventually becomes the *round ligament of the liver (ligamentum teres)* (see Fig. 14-33). The umbilical vein remains patent for a considerable period and may be used for blood transfusions during the early neonatal period. These transfusions are often performed to prevent brain damage and death in neonates with anemia as a result of erythroblastosis fetalis.

Ductus Venosus and Ligamentum Venosum

The ductus venosus becomes the *ligamentum venosum*; however, its closure is more prolonged than that of the DA. The ligamentum venosum passes through the liver from the left branch of the portal vein to the IVC, to which it is attached (see Fig. 14-33).

Umbilical Arteries and Abdominal Ligaments

Most of the intra-abdominal parts of the umbilical arteries become the **medial umbilical ligaments** (see Fig. 14-33); the proximal parts of these vessels persist as the **superior vesical arteries,** which supply the urinary bladder.

Oval Foramen and Oval Fossa

The oval foramen normally closes functionally at birth (see Fig. 14-33). Anatomical closure occurs by the third month and results from tissue proliferation and adhesion of the septum primum to the left margin of the septum secundum. The septum primum forms the floor of the oval fossa. The inferior edge of the septum secundum forms a rounded fold, the border of the oval fossa, which marks the former boundary of the oval foramen (see Fig. 14-20).

Ductus Arteriosus and Ligamentum Arteriosum

Functional closure of the DA is usually completed 10 to 15 hours after birth. Anatomical closure of the DA and

PATENT DUCTUS ARTERIOSUS

Patent ductus arteriosus (PDA), a common birth defect, occurs two to three times more frequently in females than in males (Fig. 14-34B). Functional closure of the PDA usually occurs soon after birth; however, if it remains patent (open), aortic blood is shunted into the pulmonary artery. *PDA is the most common birth defect associated with maternal rubella infection during early pregnancy.* Preterm neonates and those born at high altitude may have PDA; this patency is the result of **hypoxia** (decrease of oxygen) and immaturity. The embryologic basis of PDA is failure of the DA to involute after birth and form the ligamentum arteriosum.

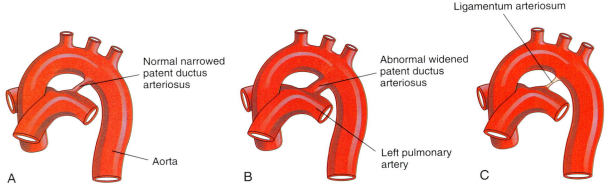

Figure 14–34 Closure of the ductus arteriosus (DA). **A,** The DA of a neonate. **B,** Abnormal patent DA in a 6-month-old infant. **C,** The ligamentum arteriosum in a 6-month-old infant.

formation of the ligamentum arteriosum usually occurs by the 12th postnatal week.

DEVELOPMENT OF THE LYMPHATIC SYSTEM

The lymphatic system begins to develop at the end of the sixth week. Studies have demonstrated that the precursor lymphatic endothelial cells are derived from the cardinal veins. Lymphatic vessels develop in a manner similar to that described for blood vessels, and they make connections with the venous system. The early lymphatic capillaries join each other to form a network of lymphatics. There are **six primary lymph sacs** present at the end of the embryonic period (Fig. 14-35A):

- Two *jugular lymph sacs* near the junction of the subclavian veins with the anterior cardinal veins (future internal jugular veins)
- Two *iliac lymph sacs* near the junction of the iliac veins with the posterior cardinal veins
- One *retroperitoneal lymph sac* in the root of the mesentery on the posterior abdominal wall
- One *cisterna chyli (chyle cistern)* located dorsal to the retroperitoneal lymph sac

Lymphatic vessels soon connect to the lymph sacs and pass along main veins: to the head, neck, and upper limbs from the **jugular lymph sacs**; to the lower trunk and lower limbs from the **iliac lymph sacs**; and to the primordial gut from the **retroperitoneal lymph sac** and the **cisterna chyli**. Two large channels (right and left thoracic ducts) connect the jugular lymph sacs with this cistern. Soon, a large anastomosis forms between these channels (see Fig. 14-35B).

The **thoracic duct** develops from:

- Caudal part of the right thoracic duct
- Anastomosis between the thoracic ducts and the cranial part of the left thoracic duct

The **right lymphatic duct** is derived from the cranial part of the right thoracic duct (see Fig. 14-35C). The thoracic duct and right lymphatic duct connect with the venous system at the **venous angle** between the internal jugular and subclavian veins (see Fig. 14-35B).

Development of Lymph Nodes

Except for the superior part of the **cisterna chyli,** the lymph sacs are transformed into groups of lymph nodes during the early fetal period. Mesenchymal cells invade each lymph sac and form a network of lymphatic channels, the primordia of the *lymph sinuses.* Other mesenchymal cells give rise to the capsules and connective tissue framework of the lymph nodes.

The **lymphocytes** are derived originally from **primordial stem cells** in the umbilical vesicle mesenchyme and later from the **liver and spleen.** The early lymphocytes eventually enter the **bone marrow,** where they divide to form *lymphoblasts.* The lymphocytes that appear in the lymph nodes before birth are derived from the thymus, a derivative of the third pair of pharyngeal pouches (see Chapter 10). Small lymphocytes leave the *thymus* and circulate to other lymphoid organs. Later, some mesenchymal cells in the lymph nodes also differentiate into lymphocytes.

BIRTH DEFECTS OF LYMPHATIC SYSTEM

Birth defects of the lymphatic system are uncommon. There may be diffuse swelling of a part of the body, termed **congenital lymphedema.** This condition may result from dilation of the primordial lymphatic channels, or from **congenital hypoplasia (underdevelopment)** of the lymphatic vessels. In **cystic hygroma,** large swellings usually appear in the inferolateral part of the neck, and consist of large, single or multilocular, fluid-filled cavities. **Hygromas** may be present at birth, but they often enlarge and become evident during later infancy. Hygromas are believed to arise from parts of a jugular lymph sac that are pinched off, or from lymphatic spaces that do not establish connections with the main lymphatic channels.

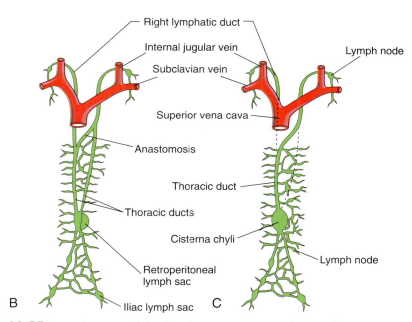

Figure 14–35 Development of the lymphatic system. **A,** Left side of a 7½ week embryo, showing the primary lymph sacs. **B,** Ventral view of the lymphatic system at 9 weeks, showing the paired thoracic ducts. **C,** Later in the fetal period, showing formation of the thoracic duct and right lymphatic duct.

Development of Spleen and Tonsils

The **spleen** develops from an aggregation of mesenchymal cells in the dorsal mesogastrium (see Chapter 12). The **palatine tonsils** develop from the endoderm of the second pair of pharyngeal pouches and nearby mesenchyme (see Chapter 10, Fig. 10-7). The **tubal tonsils** develop from aggregations of lymph nodules around the pharyngeal openings of the pharyngotympanic tubes. The **pharyngeal tonsils** (adenoids) develop from an aggregation of lymph nodules in the wall of the nasopharynx. The **lingual tonsil** develops from an aggregation of lymph nodules in the root of the tongue. Lymph nodules also develop in the mucosa of the respiratory and alimentary systems.

CLINICALLY ORIENTED QUESTIONS

1. A pediatrician diagnosed a heart murmur in a neonate. What does this mean? What causes this condition, and what does it indicate?

2. Are birth defects of the heart common? What is the most common congenital heart defect in neonates?

3. What are the causes of birth defects of the cardiovascular system? Can drugs taken by the mother during pregnancy cause cardiac defects? Could maternal alcohol abuse have caused the neonate's heart defect?

4. Can viral infections cause heart disease? If a mother had measles during pregnancy, could the neonate have a defect of the cardiovascular system? Can a pregnant woman be vaccinated to protect the unborn fetus against certain viruses?

5. In a neonate, the aorta arose from the right ventricle and the pulmonary artery arose from the left ventricle. The neonate died during the early neonatal period. What is this defect called and how common is this disorder? Can the condition be corrected surgically? If so, how is this done?

6. During a routine examination of 40-year-old identical twin sisters, it was found that one had a reversed heart. Is this a serious heart defect? How common is this among identical twins, and what causes this condition to develop?

The answers to these questions are at the back of this book.

Musculoskeletal System

SKELETAL SYSTEM

As the notochord and neural tube form in the third week, the *intraembryonic mesoderm* lateral to these structures thickens to form two longitudinal columns of **paraxial mesoderm** (Fig. 15-1*A* and *B*). Toward the end of the third week, these columns, located in the trunk (body), become segmented into blocks of mesoderm—**somites** (see Fig. 15-1*C*). Externally the somites appear as bead-like elevations along the dorsolateral surface of the embryo. Each somite differentiates into two parts (see Fig. 15-1*D* and *E*):

- The ventromedial part is the **sclerotome**; its cells form the vertebrae and ribs.
- The dorsolateral part is the **dermomyotome**; cells from its *myotome region* form **myoblasts** (primordial muscle cells), and those from its *dermatome* region form the **dermis** (fibroblasts).

The bones and connective tissue of the craniofacial structures are formed from mesenchyme in the head region that is derived from cranial **neural crest cells.**

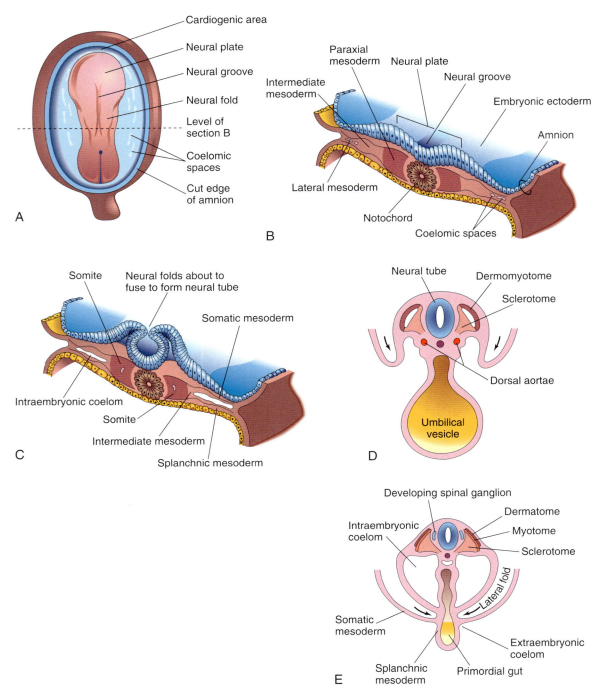

Figure 15–1 Illustrations of formation and early differentiation of somites. **A,** Dorsal view of an embryo of approximately 18 days. **B,** Transverse section of the embryo shown in **A,** illustrating the paraxial mesoderm from which the somites are derived. **C,** Transverse section of an embryo of approximately 22 days showing the appearance of the early somites. Note that the neural folds are about to fuse to form the neural tube. **D,** Transverse section of an embryo of approximately 24 days showing folding of the embryo in the horizontal plane *(arrows)*. The dermomyotome region of the somite gives rise to the dermatome and myotome. **E,** Transverse section of an embryo of approximately 26 days showing the dermatome, myotome, and sclerotome regions of the somite. The *arrows* in **D** and **E** indicate movement of the lateral body folds.

DEVELOPMENT OF CARTILAGE AND BONE

Histogenesis of Cartilage

Cartilage develops from mesenchyme during the fifth week. In areas where cartilage is to develop, the mesenchyme condenses to form **chondrification centers**. The mesenchymal cells differentiate into **chondroblasts**, which secrete collagenous fibrils and **extracellular matrix**. Subsequently, collagenous and or elastic fibers are deposited in the intercellular substance or **matrix**.

Three types of cartilage are distinguished according to the type of matrix that is formed:

- *Hyaline cartilage*, the most widely distributed type (e.g., in synovial joints)
- *Fibrocartilage* (e.g., in intervertebral discs)
- *Elastic cartilage* (e.g., in auricles of the external ears)

Histogenesis of Bone

Bone develops primarily in two types of connective tissue, mesenchyme and cartilage, but it can also develop in other connective tissues (e.g., the patella develops in a tendon). Most flat bones develop in mesenchyme within preexisting membranous sheaths; this type of osteogenesis is **intramembranous bone formation**. Mesenchymal models of most limb bones are transformed into cartilaginous bone models, which later become ossified by **endochondral bone formation**. Like cartilage, bone consists of cells and an organic intercellular substance—**bone matrix**, which comprises collagen fibrils embedded in an amorphous component.

Studies of cellular and molecular events that occur during embryonic bone formation suggest that osteogenesis and chondrogenesis are programmed early in development, and are independent processes under the influence of vascular events.

The Hox genes, bone morphogenetic proteins 5 and 7, and growth and differentiation factor 5—members of the transforming growth factor-β superfamily—as well as other signaling molecules, have been implicated as endogenous regulators of chondrogenesis and skeletal development.

Intramembranous Ossification

The mesenchyme condenses and becomes highly vascular; some cells differentiate into **osteoblasts** (bone-forming cells) and begin to deposit unmineralized matrix—**osteoid** (Fig. 15-2). *Wnt signaling is a key factor in osteoblast differentiation.* **Calcium phosphate** is then deposited in **osteoid tissue** as it is organized into bone. Osteoblasts are trapped in the matrix and become **osteocytes**. Spicules of bone soon become organized and coalesce into **lamellae** (layers).

Concentric lamellae develop around blood vessels, forming **osteons** (Haversian systems). Some osteoblasts remain at the periphery of the bone and continue to lay down lamellae, forming plates of compact bone on the surfaces. Between the **surface plates**, the intervening bone remains spiculated, or spongy. This spongy environment

Figure 15–2 Light micrograph of intramembranous ossification (×132). The trabeculae of the bone are being formed by osteoblasts lining their surface *(arrows)*. Observe that osteocytes are trapped in the lacunae *(arrowheads)* and that primordial osteons are beginning to form. The osteons (canals) contain blood capillaries. *(From Gartner LP, Hiatt JL: Color Textbook of Histology, 2nd ed. Philadelphia, Saunders, 2001.)*

is somewhat accentuated by the action of **osteoclasts** that reabsorb bone. In the interstices of the spongy bone, the mesenchyme differentiates into **bone marrow**. During fetal and postnatal life, continuous remodeling of bone occurs by the coordinated action of *osteoclasts* and *osteoblasts*.

Endochondral Ossification

Endochondral ossification (cartilaginous bone formation) is a type of bone formation that occurs in preexisting cartilaginous models (Fig. 15-3A to E). In a long bone, the **primary center of ossification** appears in the **diaphysis**, which forms the **shaft of a bone** (e.g., the humerus). Here the cartilage cells increase in size (hypertrophy), the matrix becomes calcified, and the cells die (see Fig. 15-3B). Concurrently, a thin layer of bone is deposited under the **perichondrium** surrounding the diaphysis; thus, the perichondrium becomes the **periosteum** (see Fig. 15-3A and B). Invasion of the vascular connective tissue by the blood vessels surrounding the periosteum breaks up the cartilage. Some invading progenitor cells differentiate into **hematopoietic cells** (blood cells of the bone marrow). This process continues toward the **epiphyses** (ends of the bones). The spicules (small needle-shaped body) of bone are remodeled by the action of osteoclasts and osteoblasts.

Lengthening of the long bones occurs at the diaphyseal-epiphyseal junction. The lengthening of bone depends on the **epiphyseal cartilage plates** (growth plates), whose chondrocytes proliferate and participate in endochondral

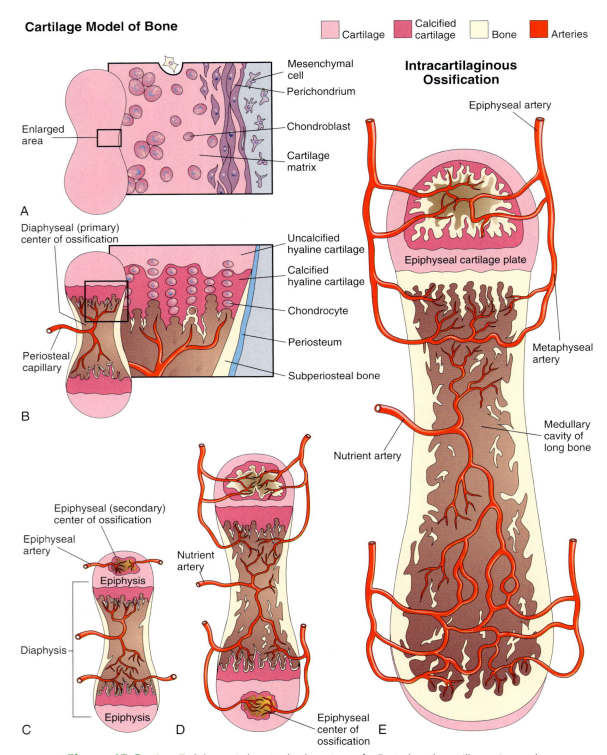

Figure 15–3   **A** to **E**, Schematic longitudinal sections of a 5-week embryo, illustrating endochondral ossification in a developing long bone.

bone formation (see Fig. 15-3*D* and *E*). Toward the **diaphysis**, the cartilage cells increase in size and the matrix becomes calcified. The spicules are isolated from each other by vascular invasion from the marrow or **medullary cavity of long bone** (see Fig. 15-3*E*). Bone is deposited on these spicules by osteoblasts; resorption of

this bone keeps the spongy bone masses relatively constant in length and enlarges the medullary cavity.

Ossification of limb bones begins at the end of the embryonic period (56 days after fertilization). Thereafter, it makes demands on the maternal supply of calcium and phosphorus beginning at approximately 8 weeks. At

RICKETS

Rickets is a disease in children attributable to **vitamin D deficiency**. This vitamin is required for calcium absorption by the intestine. The resulting calcium deficiency causes disturbances in ossification of the epiphyseal cartilage plates (i.e., they are not adequately mineralized) and there is disorientation of cells at the **metaphysis—the flared part of the diaphysis nearest the epiphysis** (see Fig. 15-3D). The limbs are shortened and deformed, with severe bowing of the limb bones. Rickets may also delay closure of the **fontanelles** (fibrous membranes) of the cranial bones in infants (see Fig. 15-8).

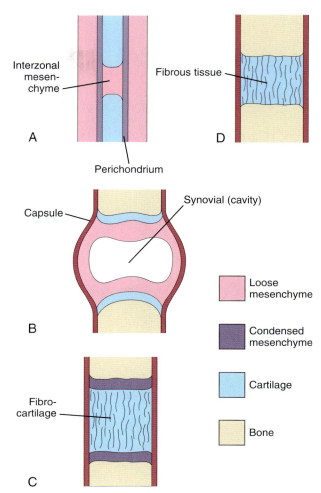

Figure 15–4 Development of joints during the sixth and seventh weeks. **A,** Condensed interzonal mesenchyme in the gap between the developing bones. This primordial joint may differentiate into a synovial joint (**B**), a cartilaginous joint (**C**), or a fibrous joint (**D**).

birth, the diaphyses are largely ossified, but most of the epiphyses are still cartilaginous. **Secondary ossification centers** appear in the epiphyses during the first few years after birth. The epiphyseal cartilage cells hypertrophy and there is invasion by vascular connective tissue. Ossification spreads radially and only the articular cartilage and **epiphyseal cartilage plate** remain cartilaginous (see Fig. 15-3E). Upon completion of growth, the cartilage plate is replaced by spongy bone; the epiphyses and diaphysis are united and no further elongation of the bone occurs.

In most bones, the epiphyses have fused with the diaphysis by the age of 20 years. Growth in the diameter of a bone results from deposition of bone at the **periosteum** (see Fig. 15-3B), and from resorption on the internal medullary surface. The rate of deposition and resorption is balanced to regulate the thickness of the compact bone and the size of the medullary cavity (Fig. 15-3E). The internal reorganization of bone continues throughout life.

DEVELOPMENT OF JOINTS

Joints begin to develop with the appearance of **condensed mesenchyme** during the sixth week (see Fig. 15-4A), and by the end of the eighth week, they resemble adult joints (see Fig. 15-4B).

Fibrous Joints

During the development of fibrous joints, the **interzonal mesenchyme** between the developing bones differentiates into dense fibrous tissue (see Fig. 15-4D). The sutures of the cranium are an example of fibrous joints (see Fig. 15-8).

Cartilaginous Joints

During the development of cartilaginous joints, the interzonal mesenchyme between the developing bones differentiates into **hyaline cartilage** (e.g., costochondral joints) or **fibrocartilage** (e.g., pubic symphysis) (see Fig. 15-4C).

Synovial Joints

During the development of synovial joints (e.g., knee joint), the interzonal mesenchyme between the developing bones differentiates as follows (see Fig. 15-4B):

- Peripherally, the interzonal mesenchyme forms the **joint capsular ligament** and other ligaments.
- Centrally, the mesenchyme disappears and the resulting space becomes the **joint cavity** or synovial cavity.
- Where the mesenchyme lines the joint capsule and articular surfaces, it forms the **synovial membrane**, which secretes synovial fluid.

DEVELOPMENT OF AXIAL SKELETON

The axial skeleton is composed of the cranium (skull), vertebral column, ribs, and sternum. During the fourth week, cells in the **sclerotomes** surround the neural tube (primordium of spinal cord) and notochord, the structure

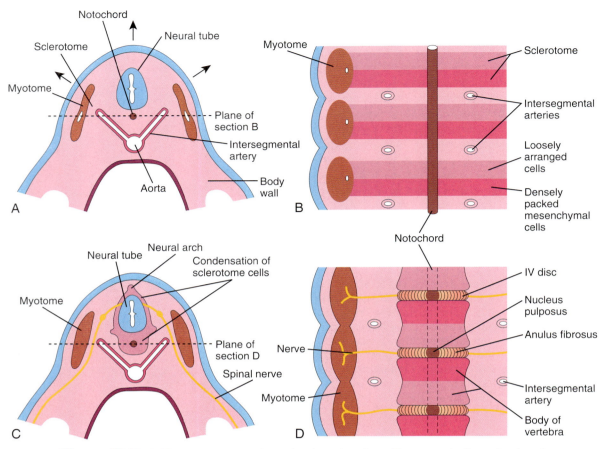

Figure 15–5   A, Transverse section through a 4-week embryo. The *arrows* indicate the dorsal growth of the neural tube and the simultaneous dorsolateral movement of the somite remnant, leaving behind a trail of sclerotomal cells. **B,** Diagrammatic frontal section of the same embryo showing that the condensation of sclerotomal cells around the notochord consists of a cranial area of loosely packed cells and a caudal area of densely packed cells. **C,** Transverse section through a 5-week embryo showing the condensation of sclerotomal cells around the notochord and neural tube, which forms a mesenchymal vertebra. **D,** Diagrammatic frontal section illustrating that the vertebral body forms from the cranial and caudal halves of two successive sclerotomal masses. The intersegmental arteries now cross the bodies of the vertebrae and the spinal nerves lie between the vertebrae. The notochord is degenerating, except in the region of the intervertebral disc, where it forms the nucleus pulposus.

around which the **primordia of the vertebrae** develop. This positional change of the sclerotomal cells is effected by differential growth of the surrounding structures and not by the migration of sclerotomal cells.

Development of Vertebral Column

During the precartilaginous or mesenchymal stage, mesenchymal cells from the **sclerotomes** are found in three main areas (Fig. 15-5A): around the notochord, surrounding the neural tube, and in the body wall. In a frontal section of a 4-week embryo, the **sclerotomes** appear as paired condensations of mesenchymal cells around the notochord (see Fig. 15-5B). Each sclerotome consists of loosely arranged cells cranially and densely packed cells caudally.

Some densely packed cells move cranially, opposite the center of the myotome, where they form the **intervertebral (IV) disc** (see Fig. 15-5C and D). *These cells express* PAX1, *a paired box gene.* The remaining densely packed cells fuse with the loosely arranged cells of the immediately caudal sclerotome to form the mesenchymal **centrum**, the primordium of a body of a vertebra. Thus, each centrum develops from two adjacent sclerotomes and becomes an intersegmental structure.

The spinal nerves now lie in close relationship to the IV discs, and the intersegmental arteries lie on each side of the vertebral bodies. In the thorax, the dorsal **intersegmental arteries** become the **intercostal arteries.** *Studies indicate that the regional development of the vertebral column is regulated along the anterior-posterior axis by homeobox* (HOX) *and paired box* (PAX) *genes.*

CHORDOMA

Remnants of the notochord may persist and form a **chordoma, a rare neoplasm (tumor)**. Approximately one third of these slowly growing, malignant tumors occur at the base of the cranium and extend to the nasopharynx (the part of the pharynx that lies above the soft palate).

Chordomas infiltrate bone and are difficult to remove. They also develop in the lumbosacral region. Surgical resection has provided long-term disease-free survival for many people.

Where it is surrounded by the developing vertebral bodies, the notochord degenerates and disappears. Between the vertebrae, the notochord expands to form the gelatinous center of the IV disc—the **nucleus pulposus** (see Fig. 15-5D). This nucleus is later surrounded by circularly arranged fibers that form the **anulus fibrosus**. The nucleus pulposus and anulus fibrosus together constitute the **IV disc**. The mesenchymal cells that surround the neural tube form the **neural arch**, the primordium of the **vertebral arch** (see Fig. 15-5C and Fig. 15-6D). The mesenchymal cells in the body wall form the **costal processes**, which form the ribs in the thoracic region.

Cartilaginous Stage of Vertebral Development

During the sixth week, **chondrification centers** appear in each mesenchymal vertebra (see Fig. 15-6A and B). At the end of the embryonic period, the two centers in each **centrum** fuse to form a cartilaginous centrum. Concomitantly, the centers in the neural arches fuse with each other and the centrum. The spinous and transverse processes develop from extensions of chondrification centers in the neural arch. Chondrification spreads until a cartilaginous vertebral column is formed.

Bony Stage of Vertebral Development

Ossification of typical vertebrae begins during the embryonic period and usually ends by the 25th year. There are two **primary ossification centers** in the centrum—ventral and dorsal (see Fig. 15-6C), which soon fuse to form one center. Three primary centers are present by the eighth week: one in the centrum and one in each half of the neural arch.

Ossification becomes evident in the **neural arches** during the eighth week. At birth, each vertebra consists of three bony parts connected by cartilage (see Fig. 15-6D). The bony halves of the **vertebral arch** usually fuse during the first 3 to 5 years. The arches first unite in

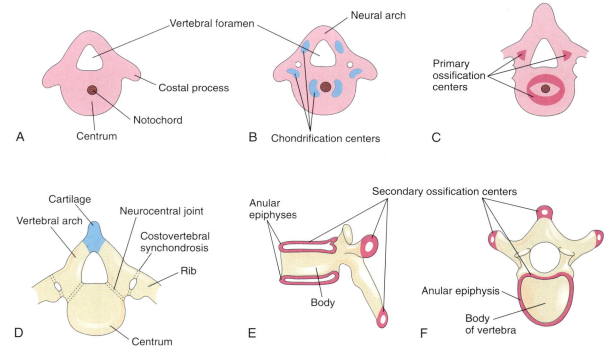

Figure 15–6 Stages of vertebral development. **A,** Mesenchymal vertebra at 5 weeks. **B,** Chondrification centers in a mesenchymal vertebra at 6 weeks. The neural arch is the primordium of the vertebral arch of the vertebra. **C,** Primary ossification centers in a cartilaginous vertebra at 7 weeks. **D,** Thoracic vertebra at birth consisting of three bony parts: vertebral arch, body of vertebra, and transverse processes. Note the cartilage between the halves of the vertebral arch and between the arch and the centrum (neurocentral joint). **E** and **F,** Two views of a typical thoracic vertebra at puberty showing the location of the secondary centers of ossification.

the lumbar region and union progresses cranially. The vertebral arch articulates with the **centrum** at cartilaginous **neurocentral joints,** which permit the vertebral arches to grow as the spinal cord enlarges. These joints disappear when the vertebral arch fuses with the centrum during the third to sixth years.

Five **secondary ossification centers** appear in the vertebrae after puberty (see Fig. 15-6E and F):

- One for the tip of the spinous process
- One for the tip of each transverse process
- Two *anular epiphyses,* one on the superior rim and one on the inferior rim of the vertebral body

The **vertebral body** is a composite of the anular epiphyses and the mass of bone between them. All secondary centers unite with the rest of the vertebrae at approximately 25 years of age. Variations in the ossification of vertebrae occur in C1 (atlas), C2 (axis), and C7 vertebrae, and in the lumbar vertebrae, sacrum, and coccyx.

Development of Ribs

The ribs develop from the mesenchymal **costal processes** of the thoracic vertebrae (see Fig. 15-6A). They become cartilaginous during the embryonic period and ossify during the fetal period. The original site of union of the costal processes with the vertebrae is replaced by **costovertebral synovial joints** (see Fig. 15-6D). Seven pairs of ribs (1–7)—**true ribs**—attach by their own cartilages to

---

VARIATIONS IN THE NUMBER OF VERTEBRAE

Most people have 7 cervical, 12 thoracic, 5 lumbar, and 5 sacral vertebrae. A few have one or two additional vertebrae or one less. An apparent extra (or absent) vertebra in one segment of the column may be compensated for by an absent (or extra) vertebra in an adjacent segment.

KLIPPEL-FEIL SYNDROME (BREVICOLLIS)

The main features of this syndrome are shortness of the neck, low hairline, restricted neck movements, fusion of cervical vertebral bodies, and abnormalities of the brainstem and cerebellum. In most cases, the number of cervical vertebral bodies is fewer than normal due to fusion of vertebrae before birth. In some cases, there is a lack of segmentation of several elements of the cervical region of the vertebral column. The number of cervical nerve roots may be normal but they are small, as are the intervertebral foramina. Persons with this syndrome may have other birth defects, including **scoliosis** (abnormal lateral and rotational curvature of the vertebral column) and urinary tract disorders.

---

the sternum. Five pairs of ribs (8–12)—**false ribs**—attach to the sternum through the cartilage of another rib or ribs. The last two pairs of ribs (11 and 12)—**floating ribs**—do not attach to the sternum.

Development of Sternum

A pair of vertical mesenchymal bands—**sternal bars**—develops ventrolaterally in the body wall. **Chondrification (conversion into cartilage)** occurs in these bars as they move medially. *They fuse craniocaudally in the median plane* to form cartilaginous models of the manubrium, sternebrae (segments of sternal body), and xiphoid process. Centers of ossification appear craniocaudally in the sternum before birth, except the ossification center for the xiphoid process, which appears during childhood. The xiphoid may never completely ossify.

Development of Cranium

The cranium (skull) develops from mesenchyme around the developing brain. The cranium consists of the:

- *Neurocranium,* the bones of the cranium enclosing the brain (brain box)
- *Viscerocranium,* the bones of the facial skeleton derived from the pharyngeal arches

Cartilaginous Neurocranium

Endochondral ossification of the neurocranium forms the bones of the base of the cranium. The ossification pattern of these bones has a definite sequence, beginning with the occipital bone, body of the sphenoid, and ethmoid bone. The **parachordal cartilage,** or basal plate, forms around the cranial end of the notochord (Fig. 15-7A), and fuses with the cartilages derived from the sclerotome regions of the occipital somites. This cartilaginous mass contributes to the **base of the occipital bone;** later, extensions grow around the cranial end of the spinal cord and form the boundaries of the **foramen magnum**—a large opening in the basal part of the occipital bone—(see Fig. 15-7C).

The **hypophyseal cartilage** forms around the developing pituitary gland and fuses to form the body of the sphenoid bone (see Fig. 15-7B). The *trabeculae cranii* fuse to form the body of the ethmoid bone, and the ala orbitalis forms the lesser wing of the sphenoid bone. Otic capsules develop around the otic vesicles, the primordia of the internal ears (see Chapter 17), and form the petrous and mastoid parts of the temporal bone. Nasal capsules develop around the nasal sacs (see Chapter 10) and contribute to the formation of the ethmoid bone.

Membranous Neurocranium

Membranous ossification occurs in the **head mesenchyme** at the sides and top of the brain, forming the **calvaria** (skullcap). During fetal life, the flat bones of the **calvaria** are separated by dense connective tissue membranes that form fibrous joints—the **sutures of the calvaria** (Fig. 15-8). Six large fibrous areas—**fontanelles**—are present where several sutures meet. The softness of the bones and their loose connections at the sutures enable the calvaria to undergo changes of shape during birth (**molding of**

Cartilaginous neurocranium	Membranous neurocranium	Cartilaginous viscerocranium	Membranous viscerocranium

Figure 15–7 Stages in the development of the cranium. The base of the developing cranium is viewed superiorly (**A** to **C**), and laterally (**D**). **A,** At 6 weeks showing the various cartilages that will fuse to form the chondrocranium. **B,** At 7 weeks after fusion of some of the paired cartilages. **C,** At 12 weeks showing the cartilaginous base of the cranium formed by the fusion of various cartilages. **D,** At 20 weeks indicating the derivation of the bones of the fetal cranium.

fetal cranium). The frontal bones become flat, the occipital bone is drawn out, and one parietal bone slightly overrides the other one. Within a few days after birth, the shape of the calvaria returns to normal.

Cartilaginous Viscerocranium

The cartilaginous viscerocranium is derived from the cartilaginous skeleton of the first two pairs of **pharyngeal arches** (see Chapter 10).

- The dorsal end of the first pharyngeal arch cartilage forms the malleus and incus of the middle ear.
- The dorsal end of the second pharyngeal arch cartilage forms a portion of the stapes of the middle ear and

styloid process of the temporal bone. Its ventral end ossifies to form the **lesser horn** of the hyoid bone.
- The third, fourth, and sixth pharyngeal arch cartilages form only in the ventral parts of the arches. The third arch cartilages form the greater horns of the hyoid bone.
- The fourth and sixth pharyngeal arch cartilages fuse to form the laryngeal cartilages, except for the epiglottis (see Chapter 10).

Membranous Viscerocranium

Membranous ossification occurs in the maxillary prominence of the first pharyngeal arch (see Chapter 10) and

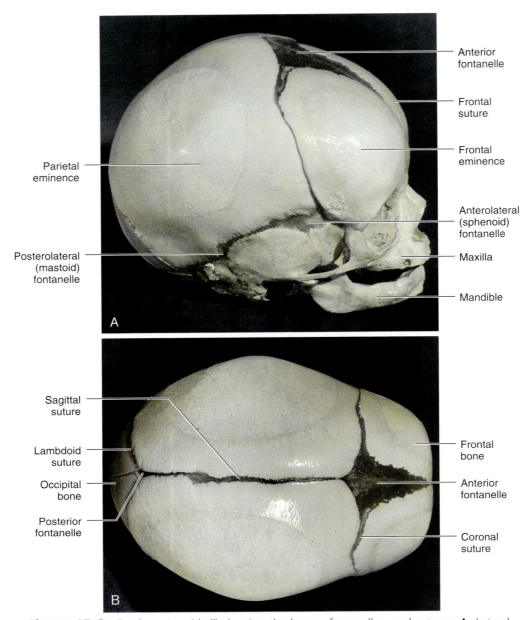

Figure 15–8   Fetal cranium (skull) showing the bones, fontanelles, and sutures. **A,** Lateral view. **B,** Superior view. The posterior and anterolateral fontanelles disappear within 2 or 3 months after birth because of the growth of the surrounding bones, but they remain as sutures for several years. The posterolateral fontanelles disappear in a similar manner by the end of the first year and the anterior fontanelle disappears by the end of the second year. The halves of the frontal bone normally begin to fuse during the second year, and the frontal suture is usually obliterated by the eighth year.

subsequently forms the squamous temporal, maxillary, and zygomatic bones. The **squamous temporal bones** become part of the neurocranium. The **mandibular prominence** forms the mandible. Some endochondral ossification occurs in the median plane of the chin and in the mandibular condyle.

Newborn Cranium

The cranium of a neonate is large in proportion to the rest of the skeleton, and the face is relatively small compared with the calvaria (roof of cranium). The small facial region of the cranium results from the small size of the jaws, the virtual absence of paranasal (air) sinuses, and underdevelopment of the facial bones.

Postnatal Growth of Cranium

After recovering from molding, the neonate's cranium is rather round and its bones are thin. The fibrous sutures permit the brain and calvaria to enlarge during infancy and childhood. The increase in size is greatest during the first 2 years, the period of most rapid postnatal growth of the brain. The calvaria continues to expand to conform to brain growth until approximately 16 years, after which its size usually increases slightly for 3 to 4 years because of thickening of its bones.

There is also rapid growth of the face and jaws, coinciding with eruption of the primary (deciduous) teeth. These facial changes are more marked after the secondary (permanent) teeth erupt (see Chapter 18). There is concurrent enlargement of the frontal and facial regions, associated with the increase in the size of the paranasal sinuses (e.g., the maxillary sinuses). Growth of these sinuses is important in adding resonance to the voice.

ACCESSORY RIBS

Accessory ribs, usually rudimentary, result from the development of costal processes from the cervical or lumbar vertebrae (see Fig. 15-6A). These processes usually form only in the thoracic region. The most common accessory rib is a **lumbar rib,** but it is usually clinically insignificant. A **cervical rib** occurs in 0.5% to 1% of people (Fig. 15-9A) and is often fused with the first rib; it is usually attached to the manubrium of the sternum or the seventh cervical vertebra. Accessory ribs may be unilateral or bilateral. *Pressure of a cervical rib on the brachial plexus of nerves, partly in the neck and axilla,* or on the subclavian artery often produces neurovascular symptoms (e.g., paralysis and anesthesia of the upper limb).

HEMIVERTEBRA

Usually developing vertebral bodies have two chondrification centers that soon unite. A hemivertebra results from failure of one of the chondrification centers to appear and subsequent failure of half of the vertebra to form. Hemivertebra is the most common cause of **congenital scoliosis** (lateral and rotational curvature) of the vertebral column (see Fig. 15-9B).

RACHISCHISIS

Rachischisis (cleft vertebral column) refers to vertebral abnormalities in a complex group of anomalies (**spinal dysraphism**) that primarily affect axial structures (Fig. 15-10). In affected neonates, the neural folds do not fuse, either because of faulty induction by the underlying notochord or because of a teratogenic agent.

ACRANIA

In acrania, the neurocranium is absent and there are major birth defects of the vertebral column that are incompatible with life (see Fig. 15-10). Acrania is associated with **meroencephaly** (partial absence of the brain), as well as **rachischisis** (extensive clefts in the vertebral arches of the vertebral column). Partial absence of the brain occurs in approximately 1 in 1000 births. Meroencephaly occurs when the cranial end of the neural tube does not close during the fourth week of development, resulting in subsequent failure of the calvaria to form.

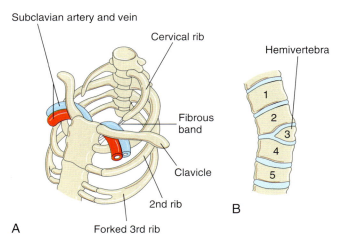

Figure 15–9 Vertebral and rib abnormalities. **A,** Cervical and forked ribs. Observe that the left cervical rib has a fibrous band that passes posterior to the subclavian vessels and attaches to the sternum. **B,** Anterior view of the vertebral column showing a hemivertebra. The right half of the third thoracic vertebra is absent. Note the associated lateral curvature (scoliosis) of the vertebral column.

Figure 15–10 Anterior **(A)** and posterior **(B)** views of a 20-week fetus with severe defects, including acrania (absence of calvaria), cervical rachischisis (extensive clefts in vertebral arches), cerebral regression (meroencephaly), and iniencephaly (defect in occiput—back of cranium).

Figure 15–11   Craniosynostosis. **A,** An infant with scapho-cephaly (long narrow head) resulting from premature closure of the sagittal suture. **B,** An infant with bilateral premature closure of the coronal suture—brachycephaly—resulting in a high, tower-like forehead. **C,** Cranium of a 9-month-old infant with scaphocephaly resulting from premature closure of the sagittal suture (sagittal synostosis; *double arrow*). Computed tomography reconstructed image.

CRANIOSYNOSTOSIS

Several birth defects result from prenatal fusion of the cranial sutures (Fig. 15-11). The cause of craniosynostosis is unclear but genetic factors appear to be important. *Homeobox gene (MSX2 and ALX4) mutations have been implicated in cases of craniosynostosis and other cranial defects.* These defects are much more common in males than in females, and they are often associated with other skeletal defects.

The type of cranial deformation produced depends on which sutures close prematurely. If the sagittal suture closes early, the cranium becomes elongated and wedge-shaped—**scaphocephaly** (see Fig. 15-11A and C). This type of cranial deformity constitutes approximately half of the cases of cra-niosynostosis. Another 30% of cases involve premature closure of the coronal suture, which results in a high, tower-like cranium—**brachycephaly** (see Fig. 15-11B). If the coronal suture closes prematurely on one side only, the cranium is twisted and asymmetrical, resulting in **plagio-cephaly.** Premature closure of the **frontal (metopic) suture** (see Fig. 15-8) results in a defect of the frontal bone and other defects—**trigonocephaly.**

DEVELOPMENT OF APPENDICULAR SKELETON

The appendicular skeleton consists of the pectoral and pelvic girdles and limb bones. During the sixth week, the **mesenchymal bone models in the limbs** undergo

BONE AGE

Bone age is a good index of general maturation. A radiolo-gist can determine bone age by assessing the ossification centers using two criteria:

* The time of appearance of calcified material in the diaphysis, epiphysis, or both is specific for each diaphysis and epiphysis and for each bone and sex.
* The disappearance of the dark line representing the epiphyseal cartilage plate indicates that the epiphysis has fused with the diaphysis.

Fusion of the diaphyseal-epiphyseal centers, which occurs at specific times for each epiphysis, happens 1 to 2 years earlier in females than in males. In the fetus, ultrasonography is used for the evaluation and measurement of bones.

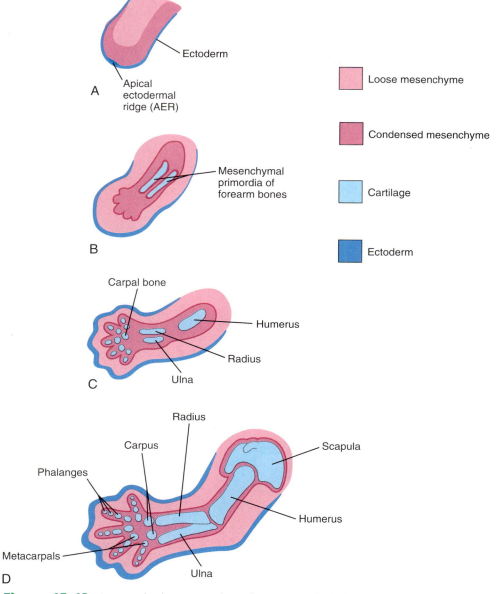

Figure 15–12   Longitudinal sections through an upper limb bud of a embryo showing development of the cartilaginous bones. **A,** At 28 days. **B,** At 44 days. **C,** At 48 days. **D,** At 56 days.

chondrification to form **hyaline cartilage bone models** (Fig. 15-12). The **clavicle** initially develops by intramembranous ossification and it later forms growth cartilages at both ends. The models of the pectoral girdle and upper limb bones appear slightly before those of the pelvic girdle and lower limb bones. The bone models appear in a proximodistal sequence. *The molecular mechanism of limb morphogenesis is regulated by specialized signaling centers along three axes of development (proximal/distal, ventral/dorsal, and anterior/posterior). Patterning in the developing limbs is controlled by Hox and other complex signaling pathways* (see Chapter 20).

Ossification begins in the long bones by the eighth week (see Fig. 15-3B and C). By 12 weeks, **primary ossification centers** have appeared in nearly all limb bones (Fig. 15-13). *The clavicles begin to ossify before any other bones in the body*, followed by the femurs. Virtually all primary centers of ossification (diaphyseal) are present at birth.

The centers for the distal end of the femur and the proximal end of the tibia usually appear during the last month of intrauterine life (34–38 weeks). The centers of the other bones appear after birth. The part of the bone ossified from the secondary center is the **epiphysis**. The bone formed from the primary center in the diaphysis does not fuse at the **epiphyseal cartilage plate** with that formed from the secondary centers in the epiphyses until the bone grows to its adult length (see Fig. 15-3E). This delay enables lengthening of the bone to continue until the final size is reached.

Parietal bone

Occipital bone

Cervical vertebrae

Scapula
Humerus

Thoracic vertebrae

Femur

Ilium

Frontal bone

Maxilla

Mandible

Metacarpals

Radius

Ulna
Ribs

Metatarsal bone

Tibia
Fibula

A

B

Figure 15–13 **A,** Alizarin-stained, 12-week fetus. **B,** Alizarin-stained, 20-week fetus. Observe the degree of progression of ossification from the primary centers of ossification, which are endochondral in the appendicular and axial parts of the skeleton, except for most of the cranial bones. Note that the carpus and tarsus are wholly cartilaginous at this stage, as are the epiphyses of all long bones.

GENERALIZED SKELETAL MALFORMATIONS

Achondroplasia is the most common cause of **dwarfism— short stature** (see Chapter 19, Fig. 19-9). It occurs in approximately 1 in 15,000 births. The limbs become bowed and short because of a disturbance of endochondral ossification at the epiphyseal cartilage plates, particularly of the long bones, during fetal life (Fig. 15-14). The trunk (of the body) is usually short, and the head is enlarged with a bulging forehead and a "scooped-out" nose (flat nasal bone).

Achondroplasia is an **autosomal dominant disorder,** and approximately 80% of cases arise from new mutations; the rate increases with paternal age. *The majority of cases are due to a point mutation (f.1,11,12) in the* FGFR3 *gene,* which results in magnification of the normal inhibiting effect of endochondral ossification, specifically in the zone of chondrocyte proliferation. This results in shortened bones, but does not affect growth of bone width (periosteal growth).

MUSCULAR SYSTEM

The muscular system develops from the **mesoderm,** except for the muscles of the iris, which develop from the **neuroectoderm.** Myoblasts—embryonic muscle cells—are derived from **mesenchyme.**

Figure 15–14 Radiograph of the skeletal system of a 2-year-old child with achondroplasia, showing proximal shortening of the femur with metaphyseal flaring.

HYPERPITUITARISM

Congenital infantile hyperpituitarism, which causes abnormally rapid growth in infancy, is rare. This condition may result in **gigantism** (excessive height and body proportions). In adults, hyperpituitarism results in **acromegaly** (enlargement of soft tissues, visceral organs, and bones of the face, hands, and feet). In acromegaly, the epiphyseal and diaphyseal centers of the long bones fuse, thereby preventing elongation of the bones. *Both gigantism and acromegaly result from an excessive secretion of growth hormone.*

Development of Skeletal Muscle

The myoblasts that form the skeletal muscles of the trunk are derived from the mesenchyme in the myotome regions of the somites. The limb muscles develop from **myogenic precursor cells** in the limb buds. Studies show that these cells originate from the ventral **dermomyotome of somites** in response to molecular signals from nearby tissues (Fig. 15-15). The myogenic precursor cells migrate into the limb buds, where they undergo epitheliomesenchymal transformation. The first indication of **myogenesis** (muscle formation) is the elongation of the nuclei and cell bodies of mesenchymal cells as they differentiate into myoblasts.

These **primordial muscle cells** soon fuse to form elongated, multinucleated, cylindrical structures—**myotubes**. *At the molecular level, these events are preceded by gene activation and expression of the MyoD family of muscle-specific basic helix-loop-helix transcription factors (MyoD, myogenin, Myf-5, and MRF4) in the precursor myogenic cells. It has been suggested that signaling molecules from the ventral neural tube (Shh), the notochord (Shh), the dorsal neural tube (Wnt, BMP-4), and the overlying ectoderm (Wnt, BMP-4) regulate the beginning of myogenesis and the induction of the myotome.*

Muscle growth results from the ongoing fusion of myoblasts and myotubes. **Myofilaments** develop in the cytoplasm of the myotubes during or after fusion of the myoblasts. Soon after that, **myofibrils** and other organelles characteristic of striated muscle cells develop. Because muscle cells are long and narrow, they are called **muscle fibers**. As the myotubes differentiate, they become invested with external laminae, which segregate them from the surrounding connective tissue. **Fibroblasts** produce the perimysium and epimysium layers of the fibrous sheath; the endomysium is formed by the external lamina, which is derived from the muscle fiber, and by reticular fibers.

Most skeletal muscle develops before birth, and almost all remaining muscles are formed by the end of the first year. The increase in the size of a muscle after the first year results from an increase in the diameter of the fibers

Figure 15–15 Progression of muscle progenitor cells toward formation of differentiated skeletal muscle. **A,** The progression of adult muscle satellite cells toward new muscle fiber formation. Myf5 is shown in red in the quiescent state to indicate that transcripts are present but not the protein. **B,** The progression of somitic cells toward myogenesis, showing how Pax3 activates target genes that regulate different stages of this process. Pax3 target genes are shown in red. *(From Buckingham M, Rigby PWJ: Gene regulatory networks and transcriptional mechanisms that control myogenesis. Dev Cell 28:225, 2014.)*

because of the formation of more myofilaments. Muscles increase in length and width to grow with the skeleton.

Myotomes

Each myotome part of a somite divides into a dorsal **epaxial division** and a ventral **hypaxial division** (Fig. 15-16). Each developing **spinal nerve** also divides and sends a branch to each division, with the **dorsal primary ramus** supplying the epaxial division and the **ventral primary ramus** supplying the hypaxial division. Some muscles, such as the intercostal muscles, remain segmentally arranged like the somites, but most myoblasts migrate away from the myotome and form nonsegmented muscles.

Derivatives of Epaxial Divisions of Myotomes

Myoblasts from the epaxial divisions of the myotomes form the segmental muscles of the main body axis, the

Figure 15–16 Transverse section of the embryo showing the epaxial and hypaxial derivatives of a myotome.

extensor muscles of the neck and vertebral column (Fig. 15-17). The embryonic extensor muscles that are derived from the sacral and coccygeal myotomes degenerate; their adult derivatives are the dorsal sacrococcygeal ligaments.

Derivatives of Hypaxial Divisions of Myotomes

Myoblasts from the hypaxial divisions of the cervical myotomes form the scalene, prevertebral, geniohyoid, and infrahyoid muscles (see Fig. 15-17A). Those from the thoracic myotomes form the lateral and ventral flexor muscles of the vertebral column, whereas the lumbar myotomes form the quadratus lumborum muscle. The muscles of the limbs, the intercostal muscles, and the abdominal muscles are also derived from the hypaxial division of the myotomes. The sacrococcygeal myotomes form the muscles of the pelvic diaphragm and probably the striated muscles of the anus and sex organs.

Pharyngeal Arch Muscles

Myoblasts from the pharyngeal arches form the muscles of mastication and facial expression as well as those of the pharynx and larynx (see Chapter 10). These muscles are innervated by the pharyngeal arch nerves.

Ocular Muscles

The mesoderm in the prechordal plate area is believed to give rise to three *preotic myotomes* from which myoblasts differentiate (see Fig. 15-17B). Groups of myoblasts, each supplied by its own cranial nerve (CN III, CN IV, or CN VI), form the extrinsic muscles of the eye.

Tongue Muscles

Myoblasts from the *occipital (postotic) myotomes* form the tongue muscles, which are innervated by the hypoglossal nerve (CN XII).

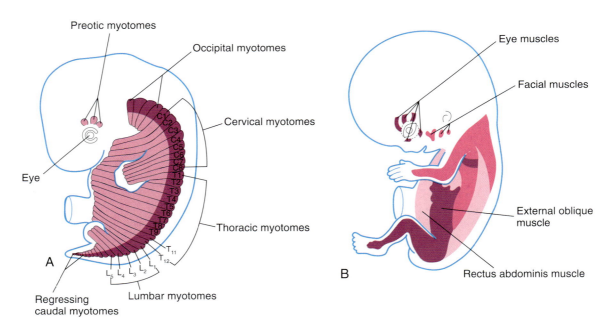

Figure 15–17 Illustrations of the developing muscular system. **A,** A 6-week embryo showing the myotome regions of the somites that give rise to most skeletal muscles. **B,** An 8-week embryo showing the developing trunk and limb musculature.

Limb Muscles

The musculature of the limbs develops from myoblasts surrounding the developing bones (see Fig. 15-16). The **precursor myogenic cells** in the limb buds originate from the somites. These cells are first located in the ventral part of the dermomyotome, and they are epithelial (see Fig. 15-1*D*). After **epitheliomesenchymal transformation**, the cells migrate into the primordium of the limb.

Development of Smooth Muscle

Some smooth muscle fibers differentiate from the **splanchnic mesenchyme** surrounding the endoderm of the primordial gut and its derivatives (see Fig. 15-1*E*). The smooth muscle in the walls of many blood and lymphatic vessels arises from the somatic mesoderm. The muscles of the iris (sphincter and dilator pupillae) and the **myoepithelial** cells in the mammary and sweat glands are believed to be derived from mesenchymal cells that originate from ectoderm.

The first sign of differentiation of smooth muscle is the development of elongated nuclei in spindle-shaped myoblasts. During early development, new myoblasts continue to differentiate from mesenchymal cells, but do not fuse; they remain mononucleated. During later development, the division of existing myoblasts gradually replaces the differentiation of new myoblasts in the production of new smooth muscle tissue. Filamentous, but nonsarcomeric, contractile elements develop in their cytoplasm, and the external surface of each differential cell acquires a surrounding external lamina. As smooth muscle fibers develop into sheets or bundles, they receive autonomic innervation; fibroblasts and muscle cells synthesize and lay down collagenous, elastic, and reticular fibers.

Development of Cardiac Muscle

The lateral splanchnic mesoderm gives rise to the mesenchyme surrounding the developing heart tube (see Chapter

Figure 15–18 Congenital muscular torticollis (wry neck) showing extensive involvement of the left sternocleidomastoid muscle in an infant at 2 months.

ACCESSORY MUSCLES

Accessory muscles occasionally develop. For example, an *accessory soleus muscle* is present in approximately 3% of the population. It has been suggested that the primordium of the soleus muscle may undergo early splitting to form an accessory soleus.

ANOMALIES OF MUSCLES

Any muscle in the body may occasionally be absent; common examples are the sternocostal head of the pectoralis major, the palmaris longus, the trapezius, the serratus anterior, and the quadratus femoris. Absence of the pectoralis major, often its sternal part, is usually associated with *syndactyly* (fusion of digits). This defect is part of the **Poland syndrome**, which also includes breast and nipple aplasia or hypoplasia, deficiencies of axillary hair and subcutaneous fat, and shortened arms and fingers.

The sternocleidomastoid muscle is sometimes injured at birth, resulting in **congenital torticollis**. There is fixed rotation and tilting of the head because of concomitant muscle fibrosis, as well as shortening of the sternocleidomastoid muscle on one side (Fig. 15-18). Although birth trauma is commonly considered a cause of congenital torticollis, this may also result from malpositioning in utero.

14). **Cardiac myoblasts** are derived from this mesenchyme by differentiation and growth of single cells, unlike striated skeletal muscle fibers, which develop by the fusion of cells. The myoblasts adhere to each other as in developing skeletal muscle, but the intervening cell membranes do not disintegrate; these areas of adhesion give rise to **intercalated discs**. Growth of cardiac muscle fibers results from the formation of new **myofilaments**. Late in the embryonic period, special bundles of muscle cells develop that have relatively few myofibrils and relatively larger diameters than typical cardiac muscle fibers. The cells develop from original trabeculated myocardium and have fast-conducting gap junctions and form the conducting system of the heart (Purkinje fibers) (see Chapter 14).

DEVELOPMENT OF LIMBS

Early Stages of Limb Development

The **limb buds** first appear toward the end of the fourth week as small elevations of the ventrolateral body wall

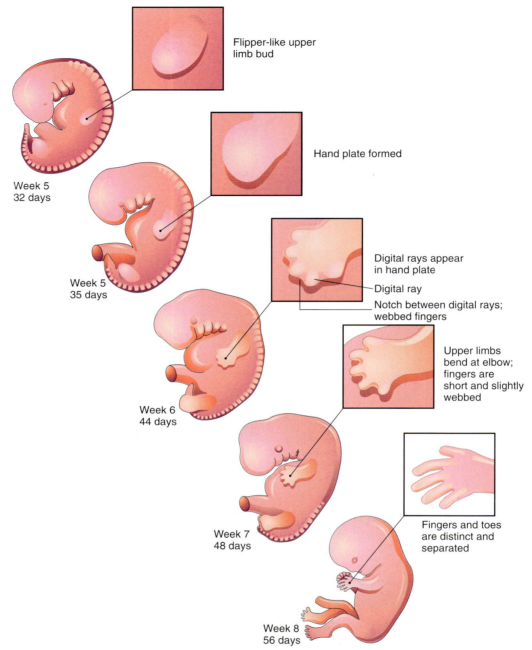

Flipper-like upper limb bud

Hand plate formed

Digital rays appear in hand plate

Digital ray

Notch between digital rays; webbed fingers

Upper limbs bend at elbow; fingers are short and slightly webbed

Fingers and toes are distinct and separated

Week 5
32 days

Week 5
35 days

Week 6
44 days

Week 7
48 days

Week 8
56 days

Figure 15–19 Development of the limbs of fetuses (32–56 days). Note that development of the upper limbs precedes that of the lower limbs.

(Fig. 15-19, week 5). Limb development begins with the activation of a group of mesenchymal cells in the lateral mesoderm. *The upper limb buds are visible by day 26 or 27*, whereas the lower limb buds appear 1 to 2 days later. Each limb bud consists of a mass of mesenchyme covered by ectoderm (see Fig. 15-12A and B). The mesenchyme is derived from the somatic layer of the lateral mesoderm.

The limb buds elongate by the proliferation of the mesenchyme. Although the early stages of limb development are alike for the upper and lower limbs (see Chapter 6, Fig. 6-11), there are distinct differences because of

their form and function. The **upper limb buds** develop opposite the caudal cervical segments, whereas the **lower limb buds** form opposite the lumbar and upper sacral segments.

At the apex of each limb bud, the ectoderm thickens to form an **apical ectodermal ridge** (AER) (see Fig. 15-12A). The AER, a specialized multilayered epithelial structure, interacts with the mesenchyme in the limb bud, promoting outgrowth of the bud *for which BMP is essential. Retinoic acid promotes the formation of the limb bud by inhibiting fibroblast growth factor (FGF8) signaling.* The AER exerts an inductive influence on the limb mesenchyme that initiates growth and development of the limbs in a proximodistal axis. Mesenchymal cells aggregate at the posterior margin of the limb bud to form a **zone of polarizing activity**. *Fibroblast growth factors from the AER activate the zone of polarizing activity, causing expression of sonic hedgehog (Shh), which controls the patterning of the limb along the anteroposterior axis.*

Expression of Wnt7 from the dorsal epidermis of the limb bud and engrailed-1 (En-1) from the ventral aspect is involved in specifying the dorsoventral axis. Curiously, the AER itself is maintained by inductive signals from Shh and Wnt7. The mesenchyme adjacent to the AER consists of undifferentiated, rapidly proliferating cells, whereas the mesenchymal cells proximal to it differentiate into blood vessels and cartilage bone models. *For cartilage formation, transforming growth factor-β (TGF-β) signaling plays a key role.* The distal ends of the limb buds eventually flatten into hand and foot plates (see Fig. 15-19).

By the end of the sixth week of development, mesenchymal tissue in the **hand plates** has condensed to form *finger buds*—**digital rays**—(see Fig. 15-19 and Fig. 15-20A to C), which outline the pattern of the digits. During the seventh week, similar condensations of mesenchyme in foot plates form *toe buds*—digital rays—(see Fig. 15-20G to I). At the tip of each digital ray, a part of the AER induces development of the mesenchyme into the mesenchymal primordia of the bones (phalanges) in the digits. The intervals between the digital rays are occupied by loose mesenchyme. Soon the intervening regions of mesenchyme undergo **apoptosis** *(programmed cell death)*, forming *notches between the digital rays* (see Fig. 15-19 and Fig. 15-20D and J). As this tissue breakdown progresses, separate digits are produced by the end of the eighth week of development (see Fig. 15-19). Molecular studies show that antagonism between retinoic acid and TGF-β control the interdigital cell apoptosis. Blocking of

cellular and molecular events during this process may account for webbing, or fusion, of the fingers or toes, a condition known as **syndactyly** (see Fig. 15-25C and D).

Final Stages of Limb Development

The mesenchyme in a limb bud gives rise to bones, ligaments, and blood vessels (see Fig. 15-12). As the limb buds elongate during the early part of the fifth week, mesenchymal models of the bones are formed by cellular aggregations (see Fig. 15-12A and B). **Chondrification centers** appear later in the fifth week. By the end of the sixth week, the entire limb skeleton is cartilaginous (see Fig. 15-12C and D).

Osteogenesis of the long bones begins in the seventh week from primary ossification centers in the diaphyses of the long bones. **Ossification centers** are present in all *long bones* by the 12th week. Primary ossification of the carpal (wrist) bones begins during the first year after birth.

From the **dermomyotome regions of the somites**, myogenic precursor cells also migrate into the limb bud and later differentiate into **myoblasts**, the precursors of muscle cells. As the long bones form, myoblasts aggregate and form a large muscle mass in each limb bud (see Fig. 15-16). In general, this muscle mass separates into dorsal (extensor) and ventral (flexor) components.

Early in the seventh week, the limbs extend ventrally and the preaxial and postaxial borders are cranial and caudal, respectively (see Fig. 15-22A and D). The *upper limbs rotate laterally* through 90 degrees on their longitudinal axes; thus, the future elbows point dorsally and the extensor muscles lie on the lateral and posterior aspects of the limb. The *lower limbs rotate medially* through almost 90 degrees; thus, the future knees face ventrally and the extensor muscles lie on the anterior aspect of the lower limb (Fig. 15-21A to D).

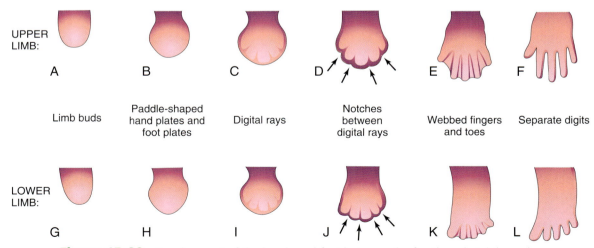

Figure 15–20 Development of the hands and feet between the fourth and eighth weeks. The early stages of limb development are similar, except that development of the hands precedes that of the feet by approximately 1 day. **A**, At 27 days. **B**, At 32 days. **C**, At 41 days. **D**, At 46 days. **E**, At 50 days. **F**, At 52 days. **G**, At 28 days. **H**, At 36 days. **I**, At 46 days. **J**, At 49 days. **K**, At 52 days. **L**, At 56 days. The *arrows* in **D** and **J** indicate the tissue breakdown processes that separate the fingers and toes.

Figure 15–21 Positional changes of the developing limbs of embryos. **A,** At approximately 48 days showing the limbs extending ventrally and the hand plates and foot plates facing each other. **B,** At approximately 51 days showing the upper limbs bent at the elbows and the hands curved over the thorax. **C,** At approximately 54 days showing the soles of the feet facing medially. **D,** At approximately 56 days. Note that the elbows now point caudally and the knees, cranially.

The radius and tibia are homologous bones, as are the ulna and fibula, just as the thumb and great toe are homologous digits. **Synovial joints** appear at the beginning of the fetal period, coinciding with functional differentiation of the limb muscles and their innervation.

Cutaneous Innervation of Limbs

Motor axons arising from the spinal cord enter the limb buds during the fifth week and grow into the dorsal and ventral muscle masses. **Sensory axons** enter the limb buds after the motor axons and use them for guidance. **Neural crest cells**, the precursors of Schwann cells, surround the motor and sensory nerve fibers in the limbs and *form the neurolemmal and myelin sheaths* (see Chapter 16).

A **dermatome** is the area of skin supplied by a single spinal nerve and its spinal ganglion. During the fifth week, the peripheral nerves grow from the developing **limb** (brachial and lumbosacral) **plexuses** into the mesenchyme of the limb buds (Fig. 15-22A and B). The spinal nerves are distributed in segmental bands, supplying both the dorsal and the ventral surfaces of the limb buds. As the limbs elongate, the cutaneous distribution of the spinal nerves migrates along the limbs and no longer reaches the surface in the distal part of the limbs. Although the original **dermatomal pattern** changes during growth of the limbs, an orderly sequence of distribution can still be recognized in the adult (see Fig. 15-22C and F). In the upper limb, the areas supplied by C5 and C6 adjoin the areas supplied by T2, T1, and C8, but the overlap between them is minimal at the ventral axial line.

Because there is overlapping of **dermatomes**, a particular area of skin is not exclusively innervated by a single segmental nerve. The limb dermatomes may be traced progressively down the lateral aspect of the upper limb and back up its medial aspect. A comparable distribution of dermatomes occurs in the lower limbs and may be traced down the ventral aspect and then up the dorsal aspect of the lower limb. When the limbs extend and

rotate, they carry their nerves with them; this explains the oblique course of the nerves arising from the brachial and lumbosacral plexuses.

Blood Supply of Limbs

The limb buds are supplied by branches of the **intersegmental arteries** (Fig. 15-23A), which arise from the dorsal aorta and form a fine capillary network throughout the mesenchyme. The primordial vascular pattern consists of a **primary axial artery** and its branches (see Fig. 15-23B and C), which drain into a peripheral marginal sinus. Blood in the sinus drains into a peripheral vein.

The vascular pattern changes as the limbs develop, chiefly as a result of vessels sprouting from existing vessels (**angiogenesis**). The new vessels coalesce with other sprouts to form new vessels. The primary axial artery becomes the **brachial artery** in the arm and the **ulnar and radial arteries** in the forearm, its terminal branches of the brachial artery (see Fig. 15-23B). As the digits form, the marginal sinus breaks up and the final venous pattern, represented by the basilic and cephalic veins and their tributaries, develops. In the thigh, the primary axial artery is represented by the **deep artery of the thigh** (profunda femoris artery). In the leg, the primary axial artery is represented by the anterior and posterior **tibial arteries** (see Fig. 15-23C).

CLEFT HAND AND CLEFT FOOT

In the rare *cleft hand or cleft foot* defects, one or more central digits are absent—ectrodactyly—resulting from failure of one or more digital rays to develop (Fig. 15-24A and B). The hand or foot is divided into two parts that oppose each other. The remaining digits are partially or completely fused (**syndactyly**).

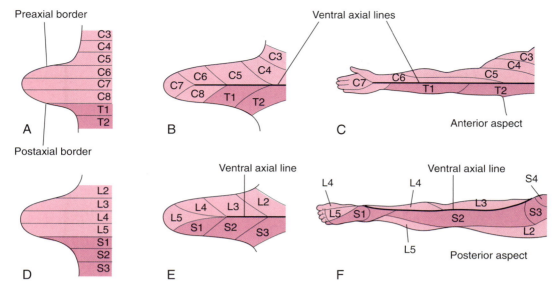

Figure 15-22 Development of the dermatomal patterns of the limbs. The axial lines indicate where there is no sensory overlap. **A** and **D,** Ventral aspect of the limb buds early in the fifth week. At this stage, the dermatomal patterns show the primordial segmental arrangement. **B** and **E,** Similar views later in the fifth week showing the modified arrangement of dermatomes. **C** and **F,** The dermatomal patterns in the adult upper and lower limbs. The primordial dermatomal pattern has disappeared, but an orderly sequence of dermatomes can still be recognized. In **F,** note that most of the original ventral surface of the lower limb lies on the back of the adult limb. This results from the medial rotation of the lower limb that occurs toward the end of the embryonic period. In the upper limb, the ventral axial line extends along the anterior surface of the arm and forearm. In the lower limb, the ventral axial line extends along the medial side of the thigh and knee, to the posteromedial aspect of the leg to the heel.

CONGENITAL ABSENCE OF RADIUS

In some people, the radius is partially or completely absent. The hand deviates laterally (radially), and the ulna bows with the concavity on the lateral side of the forearm. This defect results from failure of the mesenchymal primordium of the radius to form during the fifth week. Absence of the radius is usually caused by genetic factors.

POLYDACTYLY

Supernumerary digits are common (Fig. 15-25*A* and *B*). Often, the extra digit is incompletely formed and lacks proper muscular development, rendering it useless. If the hand is affected, the extra digit is most commonly medial or lateral rather than central. In the foot, the extra toe is usually on the lateral side. *Polydactyly is inherited as a dominant trait.*

SYNDACTYLY

This birth defect occurs approximately 1 in 2200 births. **Cutaneous syndactyly** (simple webbing of digits) is the most common limb defect (see Fig. 15-25*C*). It occurs more frequently in the foot than in the hand (see Fig. 15-25*C* and *D*). Syndactyly is most frequently observed between the third and fourth fingers, and between the second and third toes (see Fig. 15-25*D*). It is inherited as a simple dominant or simple recessive trait. Cutaneous syndactyly results from failure of the webs to degenerate between two or more digits. In some cases, there is **synostosis** (fusion of bones). **Osseous syndactyly** occurs when the notches between the digital rays do not develop during the seventh week; as a result, separation of the digits does not occur.

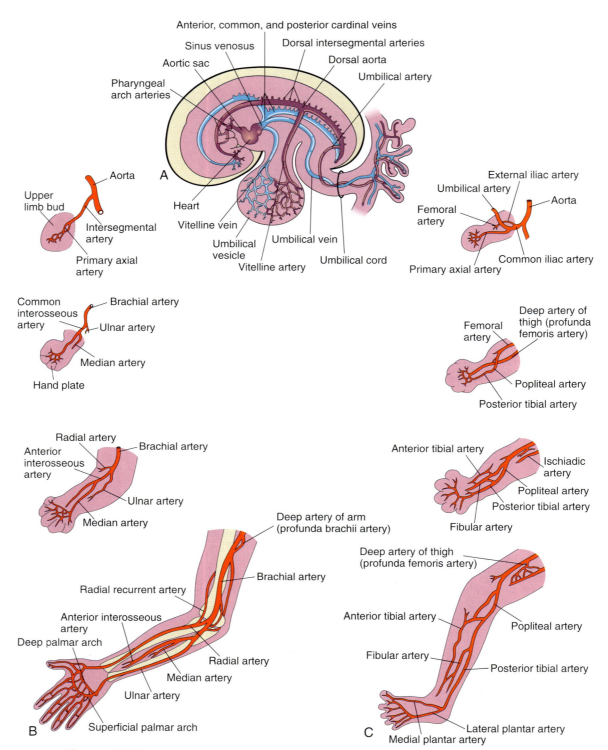

Figure 15–23 Development of the limb arteries. **A** and **B,** Development of the arteries in the upper limb. **C,** Development of the arteries in the lower limb.

Figure 15–24 Birth defects of the hands and feet. **A,** Ectrodactyly in a child. Note the absence of the central digits of the hands, resulting in split hands. **B,** A similar type of defect involving the feet. These limb defects can be inherited in an autosomal dominant pattern.

ARTHROGRYPOSIS

Arthrogryposis multiplex congenita refers to a heterogeneous group of musculoskeletal disorders characterized by multiple contractures, and immobility of two or more joints from birth. The incidence of this birth defect is 1 in 3000 live births; males are more affected in sex-linked cases. The causes may be both neurologic (central and peripheral nervous system defects), and non-neurologic (cartilaginous defects and restricted movement in utero).

CONGENITAL TALIPES

Talipes occurs at a rate of approximately 1 in 1000 births. **Talipes equinovarus,** the most common type, occurs approximately twice as frequently in males as in females. The sole of the foot is turned medially and the foot is inverted (Fig. 15-26). There is much uncertainty about the cause of talipes. Hereditary factors are involved in some cases, and it appears that environmental factors are involved in most cases. Talipes appears to follow a **multifactorial pattern of inheritance;** hence, any intrauterine position that results in abnormal positioning of the feet may cause talipes if the fetus is genetically predisposed to this deformity.

LIMB ANOMALIES

There are two main types of limb defects:
* **Amelia**—complete absence of a limb
* **Meromelia**—such as **hemimelia,** partial absence of a limb (e.g., absence of the fibula in the leg), and **phocomelia,** hands and feet are attached close to the body

Anomalies of the limbs originate at different stages of development. Suppression of limb bud development during the early part of the fourth week results in **amelia** (see Fig. 15-27A). Arrest or disturbance of the differentiation or growth of the limbs during the fifth week results in **meromelia** (see Fig. 15-27B and C). Some limb defects are caused by the following:
* **Genetic factors,** such as chromosomal abnormalities associated with trisomy 18 (see Chapter 19)

* **Mutant genes,** as in brachydactyly (shortness of digits) or osteogenesis imperfecta (connective tissue disorders). *Molecular studies have implicated gene mutation (HOX, BMP, SHH, WNT7, EN1, and others) in some cases of limb anomalies.*
* **Environmental factors,** such as teratogens (e.g., thalidomide)
* **Combination of genetic and environmental factors** *(multifactorial inheritance),* as in congenital dislocation of the hip
* **Vascular disruption and ischemia (diminished blood supply),** as in limb reduction defects

Figure 15–25 Types of digital birth defects. **A,** Polydactyly of the hands. **B,** Polydactyly of the foot. This condition results from the formation of one or more extra digital rays during the embryonic period. **C** and **D,** Various forms of syndactyly involving the fingers and toes. Cutaneous syndactyly **(C)** is probably caused by incomplete apoptosis (programmed cell death) in the tissues between the digital rays during embryonic life. **D,** Syndactyly of the second and third toes. In osseous syndactyly, the digital rays merge as a result of lack of apoptosis, causing fusion of the bones.

Figure 15–26 Neonate with bilateral talipes equinovarus deformities (club feet) illustrating the classic type of this birth defect, characterized by inversion and medial rotation of the soles of the feet.

Figure 15–27 Birth defects caused by maternal ingestion of thalidomide. **A,** Quadruple amelia (absence of the upper and lower limbs). **B,** Meromelia (partial absence) of the upper limbs; the limbs are represented by rudimentary stumps. **C,** Meromelia with rudimentary upper limbs attached directly to the trunk. *(From Lenz W, Knapp K: Foetal malformations due to thalidomide. Ger Med Mon 7:253, 1962.)*

CLINICALLY ORIENTED QUESTIONS

1. Occasionally, accessory ribs are associated with the seventh cervical vertebra and the first lumbar vertebra. Are these accessory ribs of clinical importance?

2. What vertebral defect can produce scoliosis? Define this condition. What is the embryologic basis of a vertebral defect?

3. What is meant by the term *craniosynostosis*? What results from this developmental abnormality? Give a common example and describe it.

4. A child presented with characteristics of Klippel-Feil syndrome. What are the main features of this condition? What vertebral defects are usually present?

5. A neonate was born with the prune-belly syndrome. What do you think would cause this birth defect? What urinary defect results from abnormal development of the anterior abdominal wall?

6. A boy presents with one nipple much lower than the other one. How would you explain the abnormally low position of the nipple to the parents?

7. An 8-year-old girl asked her doctor why the muscle on one side of her neck was so prominent. What would you tell her? What would happen if this is not treated?

8. After strenuous exercise, a young athlete complained of pain on the posteromedial aspect of his ankle. He was told that he had an accessory calf muscle. Is this possible? If so, what is the embryologic basis of this defect?

9. An infant had short limbs. His trunk was normally proportioned, but his head was slightly larger than normal. Both parents had normal limbs and these problems had never occurred in either of their families. Could the mother's ingestion of drugs during pregnancy have caused these abnormalities? If not, what would be the probable cause of these skeletal disorders? Could they occur again if the couple had more children?

10. A man has very short fingers (brachydactyly). He says that two of his relatives have short fingers, but none of his brothers or sisters have them. What are the chances that his children would have brachydactyly if his wife has normal digits?

11. A woman gave birth to a child with no right hand. She had taken a drug that contained doxylamine and dicyclomine to alleviate nausea during the 10th week of her pregnancy (8 weeks after fertilization). The woman is instituting legal proceedings against the company that makes the drug. Does this drug cause limb defects? If it does, could it have caused failure of the child's hand to develop?

12. An infant had syndactyly of the left hand and absence of the left sternal head of the pectoralis major muscle. The infant was otherwise normal, except that the nipple on the left side was approximately 2 inches lower than the other one. What is the cause of these defects? Can they be corrected?

13. What is the most common type of talipes? How common is it? What is the appearance of the feet of neonates born with this defect?

The answers to these questions are at the back of this book.

16

Nervous System

T he nervous system consists of three main regions:

- The **central nervous system** (CNS), which includes the brain and spinal cord and is protected by the cranium and vertebral column
- The **peripheral nervous system** (PNS), which includes the neurons outside the CNS; cranial nerves and ganglia and spinal nerves and ganglia, which connect the brain and spinal cord with peripheral structures
- The **autonomic nervous system** (ANS), which has parts in both the CNS and PNS and consists of the neurons that innervate smooth muscle, cardiac muscle, glandular epithelium, or combinations of these tissues

DEVELOPMENT OF NERVOUS SYSTEM

16   The first indications of the development of the nervous system appear during the third week as the **neural plate** and **neural groove** develop on the posterior aspect of the trilaminar embryo (Fig. 16-1*A*). The nervous system develops from the **neural plate**, a thickened area of embryonic ectoderm (see Fig. 16-1*A* and *B*). The notochord and paraxial mesoderm induce the overlying ectoderm to differentiate into the neural plate. Formation of the neural

251

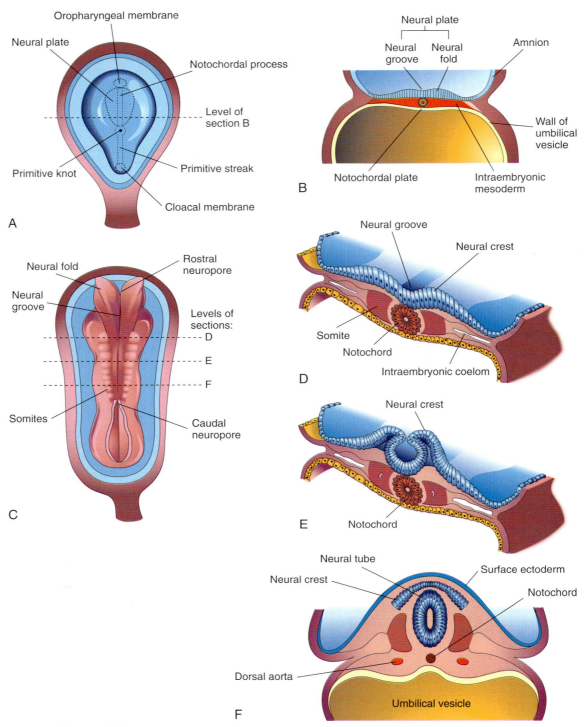

Figure 16–1 Illustrations of the neural plate and folding of it to form the neural tube. **A,** Dorsal view of an embryo of approximately 17 days, exposed by removing the amnion. **B,** Transverse section of the embryo showing the neural plate and early development of the neural groove and neural folds. **C,** Dorsal view of an embryo of approximately 22 days. The neural folds have fused opposite the fourth to sixth somites, but are open at both ends. **D** to **F,** Transverse sections of this embryo at the levels shown in **C** illustrating formation of the neural tube and its detachment from the surface ectoderm. Note that some neuroectodermal cells are not included in the neural tube, but remain between it and the surface ectoderm as the neural crest.

folds, neural crest, and neural tube is illustrated in Fig. 16-1*B* to *F*. The **neural tube** differentiates into the CNS, consisting of the brain and spinal cord. The **neural crest** gives rise to cells that form most of the PNS and ANS.

Neurulation—formation of the neural plate and neural tube—begins during the fourth week (22–23 days) in the region of the fourth to sixth pairs of somites (Fig. 16-1*C*). **Fusion of the neural folds** proceeds in cranial and caudal directions until only small areas of the neural tube remain open at both ends (Fig. 16-2*A* and *B*). At

these sites, the lumen of the neural tube—the **neural canal**—communicates freely with the amniotic cavity (see Fig. 16-2*C*). The cranial opening—the *rostral neuropore*—closes on approximately the 25th day and the *caudal neuropore* closes 2 days later (see Fig. 16-2*D*).

Closure of the neuropores coincides with the establishment of a vascular circulation for the neural tube. *Molecular studies show that syndecan4 and Vangl2 are involved in this process.* The neuroprogenitor cells of the walls of the neural tube proliferate to form the brain and spinal

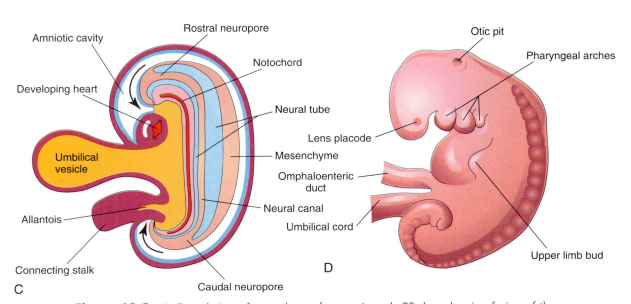

Figure 16–2   **A,** Dorsal view of an embryo of approximately 23 days showing fusion of the neural folds, which forms the neural tube. **B,** Lateral view of an embryo of approximately 24 days, showing the forebrain prominence and closing of the rostral neuropore. **C,** Diagrammatic sagittal section of the embryo showing the transitory communication of the neural canal with the amniotic cavity *(arrows)*. **D,** Lateral view of an embryo of approximately 27 days. Note that the neuropores shown in **B** are closed.

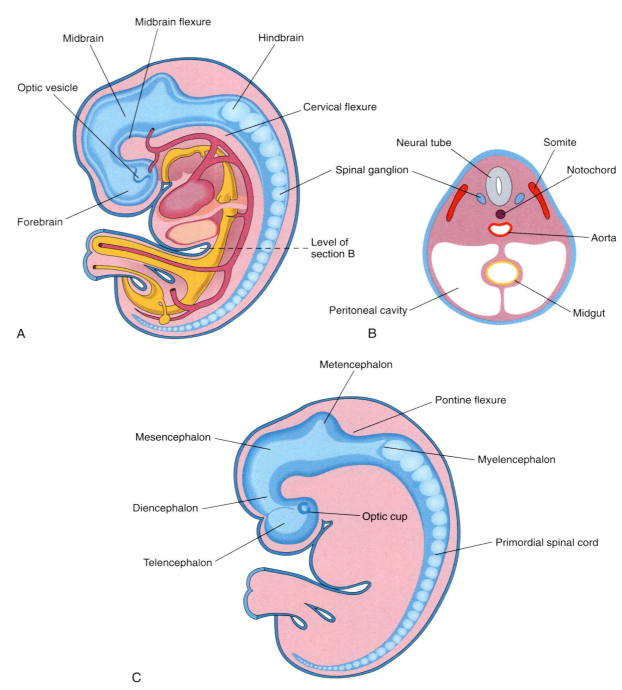

Figure 16–3   **A,** Schematic lateral view of an embryo of approximately 28 days showing the three primary brain vesicles: forebrain, midbrain, and hindbrain. Two flexures demarcate the primary divisions of the brain. **B,** Transverse section of the embryo, showing the neural tube that will develop into the spinal cord in this region. The spinal ganglia derived from the neural crest are also shown. **C,** Schematic lateral view of the central nervous system of a 6-week embryo showing the secondary brain vesicles and pontine flexure, which occurs as the brain grows rapidly.

cord (Fig. 16-3). The neural canal forms the ventricular system of the brain and central canal of the spinal cord. *The dorsoventral patterning of the neural tube appears to involve the sonic hedgehog (Shh) gene, Pax genes, bone morphogenetic proteins, and dorsalin, a transforming growth factor (TGF-β).*

DEVELOPMENT OF SPINAL CORD

The primordial spinal cord develops from the caudal part of the neural plate and caudal eminence. The neural tube caudal to the fourth pair of somites develops into the spinal cord (see Fig. 16-3). The lateral walls of the neural

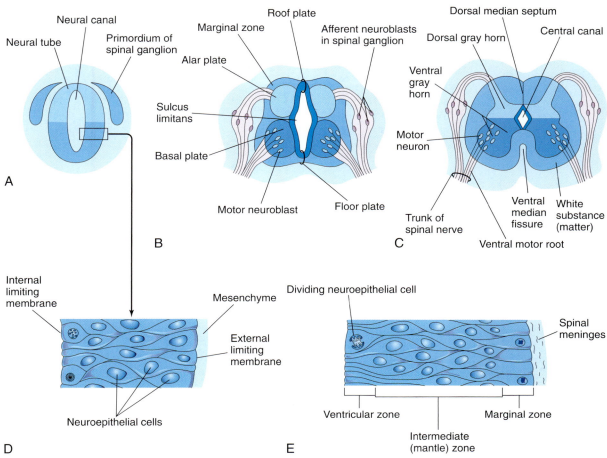

Figure 16–4 Illustrations of the development of the spinal cord. **A,** Transverse section of the neural tube of an embryo of approximately 23 days. **B** and **C,** Similar sections at 6 and 9 weeks, respectively. **D,** Section of the wall of the neural tube shown in **A. E,** Section of the wall of the developing spinal cord showing its three zones. In **A** to **C,** note that the neural canal of the neural tube is converted into the central canal of the spinal cord.

tube thicken and gradually reduce the size of the neural canal to a minute **central canal** (Fig. 16-4*A* to *C*). Initially, the wall of the neural tube is composed of a thick, pseudostratified, columnar **neuroepithelium** (see Fig. 16-4*D*).

These neuroepithelial cells constitute the **ventricular zone** (ependymal layer), which gives rise to all neurons and macroglial cells (macroglia) in the spinal cord (Fig. 16-5). Soon a **marginal zone** composed of the outer parts of the neuroepithelial cells is recognizable (see Fig. 16-4*E*). This zone gradually becomes the **white matter of the spinal cord** as axons grow into it from nerve cell bodies in the spinal cord, spinal ganglia, and brain.

Some dividing neuroepithelial cells in the ventricular zone differentiate into primordial neurons—**neuroblasts**. These embryonic cells form an **intermediate zone** (mantle layer) between the ventricular and marginal zones. *Neuroblasts become neurons* as they develop cytoplasmic processes (see Fig. 16-5).

The supporting cells of the CNS—the **glioblasts** (spongioblasts)—differentiate from the neuroepithelial cells, mainly after neuroblast formation has ceased. The glioblasts migrate from the ventricular zone into the intermediate and marginal zones. Some glioblasts become **astroblasts** and later **astrocytes**, whereas other glioblasts become oligodendroblasts and eventually **oligodendrocytes** (see Fig. 16-5). When neuroepithelial cells cease producing neuroblasts and glioblasts, they differentiate into ependymal cells, which form the **ependyma** (ependymal epithelium) lining the central canal of the spinal cord.

Microglia (microglial cells), which are scattered throughout the gray and white matter of the spinal cord, are small cells that are derived from **mesenchymal cells** (see Fig. 16-5). Microglial cells invade the CNS rather late in the fetal period, after it has been penetrated by blood vessels. Microglia originate in the bone marrow and are part of the mononuclear phagocytic cell population.

Proliferation and differentiation of neuroepithelial cells in the developing spinal cord produce thick walls and a thin roof plate and floor plate (see Fig. 16-4*B*). Differential thickening of the lateral walls of the spinal cord soon produces a shallow, longitudinal groove on each side, the **sulcus limitans** (see Fig. 16-4*B* and Fig. 16-6). This groove separates the dorsal part, the **alar plate,** from the ventral part, the **basal plate.** The alar and basal plates produce longitudinal bulges extending through most of the length of the developing spinal cord.

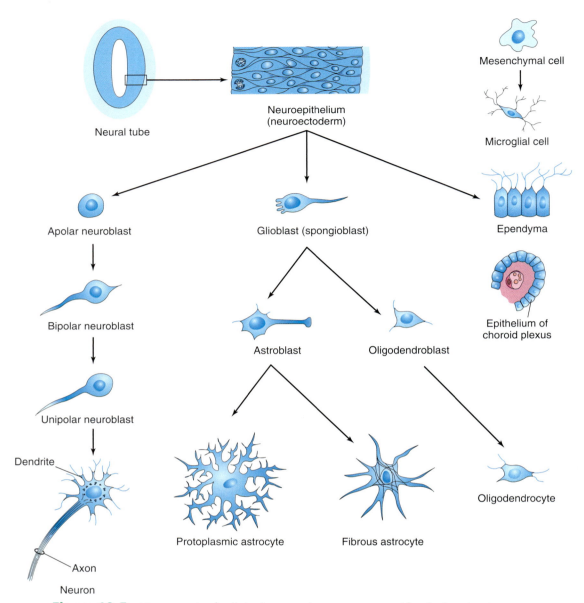

Figure 16–5 Histogenesis of cells in the central nervous system. After further development, the multipolar neuroblast *(lower left)* becomes a nerve cell or neuron. Neuroepithelial cells give rise to all neurons and macroglial cells. Microglial cells are derived from mesenchymal cells that invade the developing nervous system with blood vessels.

This regional separation is of fundamental importance because the alar and basal plates are later associated with afferent and efferent functions, respectively.

Cell bodies in the alar plates form the **dorsal gray columns** that extend the length of the spinal cord. In transverse sections, these columns are **dorsal gray horns** (Fig. 16-7). Neurons in these columns constitute afferent nuclei, which form the dorsal roots of the spinal nerves. As the alar plates enlarge, the **dorsal median septum** forms. Cell bodies in the basal plates form the ventral and lateral gray columns.

In transverse sections of the spinal cord, these columns are the **ventral gray horns** and **lateral gray horns**, respectively. Axons of the ventral horn cells grow out of the spinal cord and form the **ventral roots of the spinal nerves**

(see Fig. 16-7). As the basal plates enlarge, they bulge ventrally on each side of the median plane. As this occurs, the *ventral median septum* forms and a deep longitudinal groove—**the ventral median fissure**—develops on the ventral surface of the cord (see Fig. 16-4C).

Development of Spinal Ganglia

The unipolar neurons in the **spinal ganglia** (dorsal root ganglia) are derived from **neural crest cells** (see Fig. 16-7). The peripheral processes of the **spinal ganglion cells** pass in the spinal nerves to sensory endings in somatic or visceral structures (see Fig. 16-7). The central processes enter the spinal cord, constituting the **dorsal roots of the spinal nerves.**

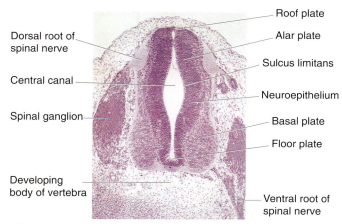

Roof plate

Dorsal root of spinal nerve

Alar plate

Sulcus limitans

Central canal

Neuroepithelium

Spinal ganglion

Basal plate

Floor plate

Developing body of vertebra

Ventral root of spinal nerve

Figure 16–6   Transverse section of an embryo (×100) at Carnegie stage 16 at approximately 40 days. The ventral root of the spinal nerve is composed of nerve fibers arising from neuroblasts in the basal plate (developing ventral horn of spinal cord), whereas the dorsal root is formed by nerve processes arising from neuroblasts in the spinal ganglion. *(From Moore KL, Persaud TVN, Shiota K: Color Atlas of Clinical Embryology, 2nd ed. Philadelphia, Saunders, 2000.)*

Development of Spinal Meninges

The meninges (membranous covering of the brain and spinal cord) develop from cells of the mesenchyme and neural crest cells during days 20 to 35. These cells migrate to surround the neural tube (primordium of brain and spinal cord) and form the primordial meninges (Fig. 16-8A and B). The external layer of these membranes thickens to form the **dura mater** (see Fig. 16-8A). The internal layer—the **pia mater** and **arachnoid mater (leptomeninges)**—is derived from neural crest cells. Fluid-filled spaces appear within the leptomeninges that soon coalesce to form the **subarachnoid space** (Fig. 16-9A). **Cerebrospinal fluid (CSF)** begins to form during the fifth week.

Positional Changes of Spinal Cord

The spinal cord in the embryo extends the entire length of the vertebral canal at 8 weeks (see Fig. 16-8A). The spinal nerves pass through the intervertebral foramina opposite their levels of origin. Because the vertebral column and dura mater grow more rapidly than the spinal cord, this positional relationship to the spinal nerves does not persist. The caudal end of the spinal cord in fetuses gradually comes to lie at relatively higher levels. In a 24-week-old, it lies at the level of the first sacral vertebra (see Fig. 16-8B).

The **spinal cord in the neonate** terminates at the level of the second or third lumbar vertebra (see Fig. 16-8C). In an adult, the **spinal cord** usually terminates at the inferior border of the first lumbar vertebra (see Fig. 16-8D). As a result, the spinal nerve roots, especially those of the lumbar and sacral segments, run obliquely from the spinal cord to the corresponding level of the vertebral column. The nerve roots inferior to the end of the cord—the **medullary cone** (*conus medullaris*)—form a sheaf of nerve roots—**cauda equina**—that arises from the lumbosacral enlargement (swelling) and medullary cone of the spinal cord (see Fig. 16-8C and D).

Although in adults the dura mater and arachnoid mater usually end at the S2 vertebra, the pia mater does not. Distal to the caudal end of the spinal cord, the pia mater forms a long, fibrous thread, the **filum terminale** (terminal filum), which indicates the original level of the caudal end of the embryonic spinal cord (see Fig. 16-8C and D). This filum extends from the medullary cone to the periosteum of the first coccygeal vertebra (see Fig. 16-8D).

Myelination of Nerve Fibers

Myelin sheaths surrounding the nerve fibers within the spinal cord begin to form during the late fetal period, and continue to form during the first postnatal year. In general, fiber tracts become myelinated at approximately the time they become functional. Motor roots are myelinated before sensory roots. The **myelin sheaths** are formed by **oligodendrocytes**. The myelin sheaths surrounding the axons of peripheral nerve fibers are formed by plasma membranes of the **neurolemma (sheath of Schwann cells)**. *Myelination of the nerve fibers is regulated by β_1 integrins and profilin 1 (Pfn1), a protein that plays an essential role in microfilament polymerization.* Neurolemma cells are derived from **neural crest cells** that migrate peripherally and wrap themselves around the axons of somatic motor neurons and preganglionic autonomic motor neurons as they pass out of the CNS (see Fig. 16-7). These cells also wrap themselves around the central and peripheral processes of the somatic and visceral sensory neurons, as well as around the axons of postsynaptic autonomic motor neurons.

BIRTH DEFECTS OF SPINAL CORD

Most defects result from failure of fusion of one or more neural arches of the developing vertebrae during the fourth week (see Fig. 16-9A). **Neural tube defects (NTDs)** affect the tissues overlying the spinal cord: meninges, neural arches, muscles, and skin (see Fig. 16-9B to D). Birth defects involving the **neural arches** are referred to as **spina bifida**. The term *spina bifida* denotes nonfusion of the halves of the embryotic neural arches.

SPINA BIFIDA OCCULTA

This NTD results from failure of the embryonic halves of the neural arch to grow normally and fuse in the median plane (see Fig. 16-9A). Spina bifida occulta occurs in vertebra L5 or S1 in approximately 10% of otherwise normal people. In its most minor form, the only evidence of its presence may be a small dimple with a tuft of hair arising from it (Fig. 16-10). Spina bifida occulta usually produces no clinical symptoms.

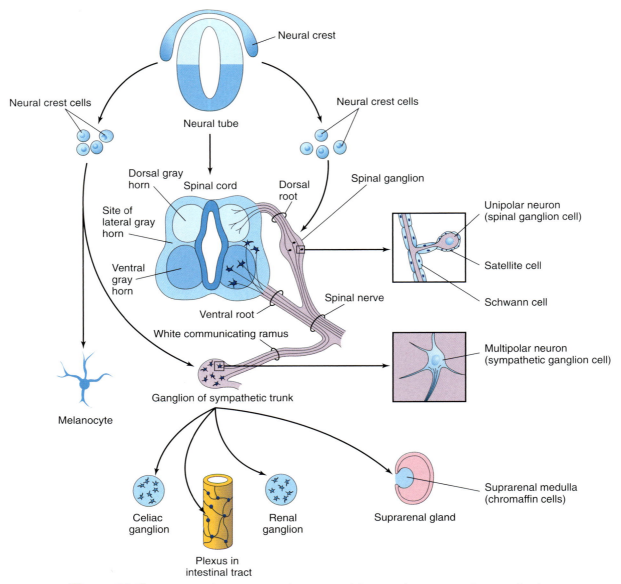

Figure 16–7 Diagrams showing some derivatives of the neural crest. Neural crest cells also differentiate into the cells in the afferent ganglia of cranial nerves and many other structures. The formation of a spinal nerve is also shown.

SPINA BIFIDA CYSTICA

Severe types of spina bifida involve protrusion of the spinal cord and/or meninges through defects resulting from failure of fusion of one or more neural arches of developing vertebrae during the fourth week (see Fig. 16-9A to D). These severe NTDs are referred to collectively as **spina bifida cystica** because of the cyst-like sac that is associated with these birth defects (see Figs. 16-9B to D and Fig. 16-11). Spina bifida cystica occurs in approximately 1 in 1000 births. When the sac contains meninges and CSF, the defect is called **spina bifida with meningocele** (see Fig. 16-9B). The spinal cord and spinal roots are in their normal position, but spinal cord defects may be present. If the spinal cord, nerve roots, or both are included in the sac, the defect is called **spina bifida with meningomyelocele** (Figs. 16-9C and 16-11). Spina bifida with meningomyelocele involving several vertebrae is often associated with partial absence of the brain—**meroencephaly** (Fig. 16-12).

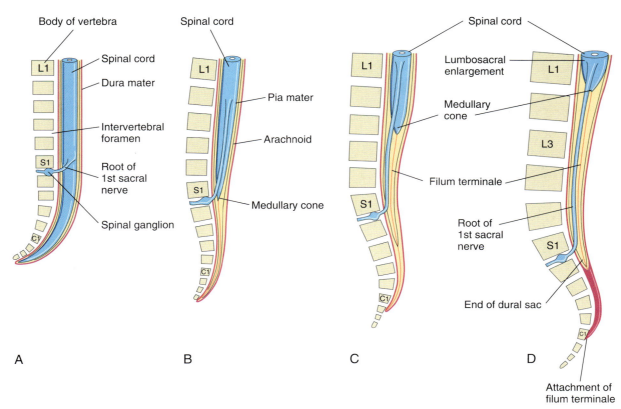

Body of vertebra

Spinal cord

Spinal cord

L1

Spinal cord
Dura mater
Intervertebral foramen
Root of 1st sacral nerve
Spinal ganglion

L1

Pia mater
Arachnoid
Medullary cone

Lumbosacral enlargement
Medullary cone
Filum terminale
Root of 1st sacral nerve
End of dural sac
Attachment of filum terminale

A　　　　**B**　　　　**C**　　　　**D**

Figure 16–8　Diagrams showing the position of the caudal end of the spinal cord in relation to the vertebral column and meninges at various stages of development. The increasing inclination of the root of the first sacral nerve is also shown. **A,** At 8 weeks. **B,** At 24 weeks. **C,** Neonate. **D,** Adult.

CAUSES OF NEURAL TUBE DEFECTS

Genetic, nutritional, and environmental factors play a role in the production of NTDs. Gene-gene and gene-environmental interactions are likely involved in most cases. Epidemiologic studies have shown that folic acid supplements (400 μg daily) taken at least 1 month before conception and continuing through the first trimester reduce the incidence of NTDs. Certain drugs increase the risk of NTD. For example, valproic acid, an anticonvulsant, causes NTDs in 1% to 2% of pregnant women if given during the fourth week of development, when the neural folds are fusing.

DEVELOPMENT OF BRAIN

The brain begins to develop in the third week when the neural plate and tube are developing from neuroectoderm (see Fig. 16-1). The **neural tube**, cranial to the fourth pair of somites, develops into the brain. Neural progenitor cells proliferate, migrate, and differentiate to form specific areas of the brain. Even before the neural folds are completely fused, three distinct primary brain vesicles are recognizable in the rostral end of the developing neural tube (Fig. 16-13). From rostral to caudal, these primary brain vesicles form the *forebrain* (prosencephalon), *midbrain* (mesencephalon), and *hindbrain* (rhombencephalon).

During the fifth week, the forebrain partly divides into two **secondary brain vesicles**—the *telencephalon* and *diencephalon*; the midbrain does not divide. The hindbrain partly divides into two vesicles, the *metencephalon* and *myelencephalon*. Consequently, there are five secondary brain vesicles.

Brain Flexures

The embryonic brain grows rapidly during the fourth week and bends ventrally with the head fold. The bending produces the **midbrain flexure** in the midbrain region and the **cervical flexure** at the junction of the hindbrain and spinal cord (Fig. 16-14A). Later, unequal growth of these flexures produces the **pontine flexure** in the opposite direction. This flexure results in thinning of the roof of the hindbrain (see Fig. 16-14C). The **sulcus limitans** extends cranially to the junction of the midbrain and forebrain, and the alar and basal plates are recognizable only in the midbrain and the hindbrain (see Figs. 16-14C).

Hindbrain

The *cervical flexure* demarcates the hindbrain from the spinal cord (see Fig. 16-14A). The *pontine flexure* divides

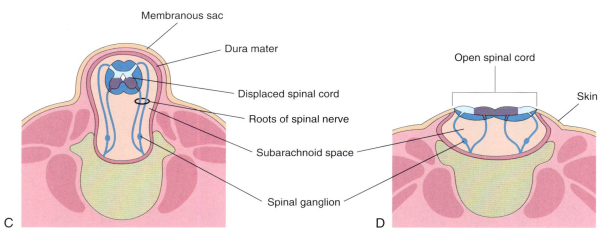

Figure 16–9 Diagrammatic sketches illustrating various types of spina bifida and the associated defects of the vertebral arches. **A,** Spina bifida occulta. Observe the unfused vertebral arch. **B,** Spina bifida with meningocele. **C,** Spina bifida with meningomyelocele. **D,** Spina bifida with myeloschisis. The types shown in **B** to **D** are referred to collectively as *spina bifida cystica* because of the cyst-like sac that is associated with them. *CSF,* Cerebrospinal fluid.

the hindbrain into caudal (myelencephalon) and rostral (metencephalon) parts. The *myelencephalon* becomes the **medulla oblongata**, whereas the *metencephalon* becomes the **pons** and **cerebellum**. The cavity of the hindbrain becomes the **fourth ventricle** and the **central canal** in the medulla (see Fig. 16-14*B* and *C*).

Myelencephalon

Neuroblasts from the alar plates in the myelencephalon migrate into the marginal zone and form isolated areas of gray matter: the **gracile nuclei** medially and the **cuneate nuclei** laterally (see Fig. 16-14*B*). These nuclei are associated with correspondingly named nerve tracts that enter the medulla from the spinal cord. The ventral area of the medulla contains a pair of fiber bundles—**pyramids**—that consist of corticospinal fibers descending from the developing cerebral cortex (see Fig. 16-14*B*).

The rostral part of the **myelencephalon** is wide and rather flat, especially opposite the pontine flexure (see Fig. 16-14*C* and *D*). As the pontine flexure forms, the walls of the medulla move laterally and the alar plates come to lie lateral to the basal plates (see Fig. 16-14*C*).

As the positions of the plates change, the motor nuclei generally develop medial to the sensory nuclei.

Neuroblasts in the basal plates of the medulla, like those in the spinal cord, develop into motor neurons. The neuroblasts form nuclei (groups of nerve cells) and organize into three cell columns on each side (see Fig. 16-14*D*). From medial to lateral, they are:

- The *general somatic efferent,* represented by neurons of the hypoglossal nerve
- The *special visceral efferent,* represented by neurons innervating muscles derived from the pharyngeal arches (see Chapter 10)
- The *general visceral efferent,* represented by some neurons of the vagus and the glossopharyngeal nerves

Neuroblasts in the alar plates of the medulla form neurons that are arranged in four columns on each side (see Fig. 16-14*D*). From medial to lateral, the columns are:

- The *general visceral afferent,* receiving impulses from the viscera
- The *special visceral afferent,* receiving taste fibers

- The *general somatic afferent*, receiving impulses from the surface of the head
- The *special somatic afferent*, receiving impulses from the ear

Some neuroblasts from the alar plates migrate ventrally and form the neurons in the **olivary nuclei** (see Fig. 16-14C and D).

Metencephalon

The walls of the metencephalon form the **pons** and **cerebellum**, and the cavity of the metencephalon forms the *superior part of the fourth ventricle* (Fig. 16-15A). As in the rostral part of the myelencephalon, the **pontine flexure**

Figure 16–10 A female child with a tuft of hair covering a small dimple (spinal defect) in the lumbosacral region, indicating the site of a spina bifida occulta.

Figure 16–11 The back of a neonate with a large lumbar meningomyelocele. The neural tube defect is covered with a thin membrane.

Figure 16–12 **A,** A fetus with meroencephaly. **B,** Magnetic resonance image of diamniotic-monochorionic twins, one with meroencephaly. Note the absent calvaria of the abnormal twin *(arrow)* and the amnion of the normal twin.

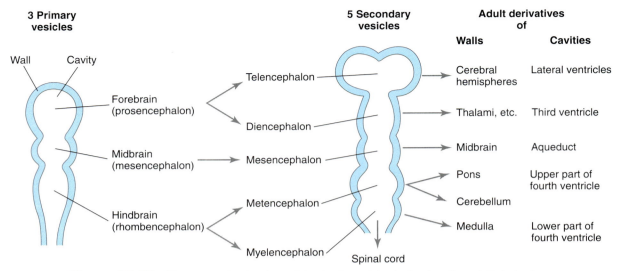

Figure 16–13 Diagrammatic sketches of the brain vesicles indicating the adult derivatives of their walls and cavities. The rostral part of the third ventricle forms from the cavity of the telencephalon; most of this ventricle is derived from the cavity of the diencephalon.

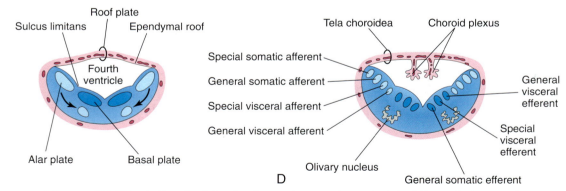

Figure 16–14 **A,** Sketch of the developing brain at the end of the fifth week showing the three primary divisions of the brain and the brain flexures. **B,** Transverse section of the caudal part of the myelencephalon (developing closed part of medulla). **C** and **D,** Similar sections of the rostral part of the myelencephalon (developing open part of medulla) showing the position and successive stages of differentiation of the alar and basal plates. The *arrows* in **C** show the pathway taken by the neuroblasts from the alar plates to form the olivary nuclei.

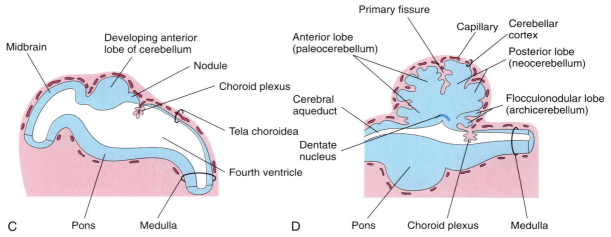

Figure 16–15 **A,** Sketch of the developing brain at the end of the fifth week. **B,** Transverse section of the metencephalon (developing pons and cerebellum) showing the derivatives of the alar and basal plates. **C** and **D,** Sagittal sections of the hindbrain at 6 and 17 weeks, respectively, showing successive stages in the development of the pons and cerebellum.

causes divergence of the lateral walls of the pons, which spreads the gray matter in the floor of the fourth ventricle (see Fig. 16-15B).

The **cerebellum** develops from the dorsal parts of the alar plates (see Fig. 16-15A and B). Initially, the **cerebellar swellings** project into the fourth ventricle (see Fig. 16-15B). As the swellings enlarge and fuse in the median plane, they overgrow the rostral half of the fourth ventricle and overlap the pons and medulla (see Fig. 16-15D). Some neuroblasts in the intermediate zone of the alar plates migrate to the marginal zone and differentiate into the neurons of the **cerebellar cortex**. Other neuroblasts from these plates give rise to the **central nuclei**, the largest of which is the **dentate nucleus** (see Fig. 16-15D). Cells from the alar plates also give rise to the **pontine nuclei**, the cochlear and vestibular nuclei, and the sensory nuclei of the trigeminal nerve.

Nerve fibers connecting the cerebral and cerebellar cortices with the spinal cord pass through the marginal layer of the ventral region of the metencephalon. This region of the brainstem is the pons (bridge) because of the robust band of nerve fibers that crosses the median plane (see Fig. 16-15C and D).

Choroid Plexuses and Cerebrospinal Fluid

The thin ependymal roof of the fourth ventricle is covered externally by *pia mater*. This vascular membrane, together with the ependymal roof, forms the **tela choroidea** of the fourth ventricle (see Fig. 16-15C and D). Because of the active proliferation of the pia mater, the tela choroidea invaginates the fourth ventricle, where it differentiates into the **choroid plexus**, infoldings of choroidal arteries of the pia mater (see Fig. 16-14C and Fig. 16-15C and D). Similar choroid plexuses develop in the roof of the third ventricle and in the medial walls of the lateral ventricles.

*The choroid plexuses secrete ventricular fluid, which becomes **cerebrospinal fluid**. Various signaling morphogens present in the CSF and choroid plexus are necessary for the development of the brain.* The thin roof of the fourth ventricle evaginates in three locations. These outpouchings rupture to form openings, the **median and lateral apertures**. These apertures permit CSF to enter the **subarachnoid space** from the fourth ventricle. Studies have shown that specific neurogenic molecules, such as retinoic acid, control the proliferation and differentiation of neuroprogenitor cells. Thus, the epithelium lining the choroid plexus is derived from neuroepithelium but the stroma develops from mesenchymal cells.

Midbrain

The midbrain (mesencephalon) undergoes less change than any other part of the developing brain. The neural canal narrows and becomes the **cerebral aqueduct** (see Fig. 16-15D), a canal that connects the third and fourth ventricles. **Neuroblasts** migrate from the alar plates of the midbrain into the **tectum** (roof), where they aggregate to form four large groups of neurons—the paired **superior and inferior colliculi** (Fig. 16-16B), which are concerned with visual and auditory reflexes, respectively. Neuroblasts from the basal plates appear to give rise to groups of neurons in the **tegmentum of the midbrain** (red nuclei, nuclei of the third and fourth cranial nerves, and reticular

nuclei). The **substantia nigra**, a broad layer of gray matter adjacent to the cerebral peduncle (see Fig. 16-16D and E), may also differentiate from the basal plate, but some authorities believe that it is derived from cells in the alar plate that migrate ventrally.

Fibers growing from the cerebrum (principal part of brain, including the diencephalon and cerebral hemispheres) form the **cerebral peduncles** anteriorly (see Fig. 16-16B). These peduncles become progressively more prominent as additional descending fiber groups (corticopontine, corticobulbar, and corticospinal) pass through the developing midbrain on their way to the brainstem and spinal cord.

Forebrain

As closure of the rostral neuropore occurs, two lateral outgrowths—**optic vesicles**—appear (see Fig. 16-3A), one on each side of the forebrain. The optic vesicles are the

Figure 16–16   **A,** Sketch of the developing brain at the end of the fifth week. **B,** Transverse section of the developing midbrain showing the early migration of cells from the basal and alar plates. **C,** Sketch of the developing brain at 11 weeks. **D** and **E,** Transverse sections of the developing midbrain at the level of the inferior and superior colliculi, respectively. *CN,* Cranial nerve.

Figure 16–17 **A,** External view of the brain at the end of the fifth week. **B,** Similar view at 7 weeks. **C,** Median section of this brain showing the medial surface of the forebrain and midbrain. **D,** Similar section at 8 weeks. **E,** Transverse section of the diencephalon showing the epithalamus dorsally, the thalamus laterally, and the hypothalamus ventrally.

primordia of the retinas and optic nerves (see Chapter 17). A second pair of diverticula soon arises more dorsally and rostrally, representing the **telencephalic vesicles** (see Fig. 16-16C). They are the primordia of the cerebral hemispheres, and their cavities become the **lateral ventricles** (Fig. 16-19B).

The rostral (anterior) part of the forebrain, including the primordia of the **cerebral hemispheres**, is the *telencephalon*; the caudal (posterior) part of the forebrain is

the **diencephalon**. The cavities of the telencephalon and diencephalon contribute to the formation of the **third ventricle** (Fig. 16-17D and E).

Diencephalon

Three swellings develop in the lateral walls of the third ventricle, which later become the *thalamus, hypothalamus, and epithalamus* (see Fig. 16-17C to E). The **thalamus** develops rapidly on each side and bulges into the

Figure 16–18   Diagrammatic sketches illustrating the development of the pituitary gland. **A,** Sagittal section of the cranial end of an embryo at approximately 36 days showing the hypophyseal diverticulum, an upgrowth from the stomodeum, and the neurohypophyseal diverticulum, a downgrowth from the forebrain. **B** to **D,** Successive stages of the developing pituitary gland. By 8 weeks, the diverticulum loses its connection with the oral cavity and is in close contact with the infundibulum and posterior lobe (neurohypophysis) of the pituitary gland. **E** and **F,** Later stages showing proliferation of the anterior wall of the hypophyseal diverticulum to form the anterior lobe (adenohypophysis) of the pituitary gland.

cavity of the third ventricle, eventually reducing it to a narrow cleft. The **hypothalamus** arises by the proliferation of neuroblasts in the intermediate zone of the diencephalic walls. A pair of nuclei, the **mammillary bodies,** form pea-sized swellings on the ventral surface of the hypothalamus (see Fig. 16-17C).

The **epithalamus** develops from the roof and dorsal part of the lateral wall of the diencephalon. Initially, the epithalamic swellings are large, but later they become relatively small (see Fig. 16-17C to E).

The **pineal gland** (pineal body) develops as a median diverticulum of the caudal part of the roof of the

diencephalon (see Fig. 16-17D). Proliferation of the cells in its walls soon converts it into a solid, cone-shaped gland.

The **pituitary gland** (*hypophysis*) is ectodermal in origin (Fig. 16-18 and Table 16-1). It develops from two sources:

- An upgrowth from the ectodermal roof of the stomodeum—the **hypophyseal diverticulum (Rathke pouch)**
- A downgrowth from the neuroectoderm of the diencephalon—the **neurohypophyseal diverticulum**

Table 16–1   Derivation and Terminology of Pituitary Gland

Oral Ectoderm

(Hypophyseal diverticulum from roof of stomodeum) ⟶ Adenohypophysis (glandular portion)

{ Pars anterior / Pars tuberalis / Pars intermedia }   Anterior lobe

Neuroectoderm

(Neurohypophyseal diverticulum from floor of diencephalon) ⟶ Neurohypophysis (nervous portion)

{ Pars nervosa / Infundibular stem / Median eminence }   Posterior lobe

This double embryonic origin of the pituitary gland explains why it is composed of two different types of tissue:

- The **adenohypophysis** (glandular part), or anterior lobe, arises from oral ectoderm.
- The **neurohypophysis** (nervous part), or posterior lobe, arises from neuroectoderm.

During the third week, a **hypophyseal diverticulum** projects from the roof of the stomodeum (primordial oral cavity) and lies adjacent to the floor (ventral wall) of the diencephalon (see Fig. 16-18A and B). By the fifth week, this diverticulum has elongated and constricted at its attachment to the oral epithelium, giving it a nipple-like appearance (see Fig. 16-18C). By this stage, it has come into contact with the **infundibulum** (derived from the neurohypophyseal diverticulum), a ventral downgrowth of the diencephalon (see Fig. 16-17C and D and Fig. 16-18). The stalk of the hypophyseal diverticulum gradually regresses (see Fig. 16-18C to E). The parts of the pituitary gland that develop from the ectoderm of the stomodeum—pars anterior, pars intermedia, and pars tuberalis—form the **adenohypophysis** (see Table 16-1).

Cells of the anterior wall of the hypophyseal diverticulum proliferate and give rise to the **pars anterior of the pituitary gland**. Later, an extension, the **pars tuberalis**, grows around the *infundibular stem* (see Fig. 16-18F). The extensive proliferation of the anterior wall of the hypophyseal diverticulum reduces its lumen to a narrow cleft (see Fig. 16-18E). Cells in the posterior wall of the hypophyseal diverticulum do not proliferate; they give rise to the thin, poorly defined **pars intermedia** (see Fig. 16-18F). The part of the pituitary gland that develops from the neuroectoderm of the brain (infundibulum) is the **neurohypophysis** (see Fig. 16-18B to F and Table 16-1). The infundibulum gives rise to the *median eminence, infundibular stem,* and *pars nervosa.*

Telencephalon
The telencephalon consists of a median part and two lateral diverticula, the **cerebral vesicles** (see Fig. 16-16C and Fig. 16-18A). These vesicles are the primordia of the **cerebral hemispheres**, which are identifiable at 7 weeks (Fig. 16-19A). The cavity of the median part of the telencephalon forms the extreme anterior part of the third ventricle. At first, the cerebral hemispheres are in wide communication with the cavity of the third ventricle

through the **interventricular foramina** (see Fig. 16-19B). As the cerebral hemispheres expand, they cover successively the diencephalon, midbrain, and hindbrain. The hemispheres eventually meet each other in the midline, flattening their medial surfaces.

The **corpus striatum** appears during the sixth week as a prominent swelling in the floor of each cerebral hemisphere (Fig. 16-20B). The floor of each hemisphere expands more slowly than its thin cortical walls because it contains the rather large corpus striatum; consequently, the cerebral hemispheres become C-shaped (Fig. 16-21).

The growth and curvature of the hemispheres also affect the shape of the lateral ventricles. They become roughly C-shaped cavities filled with CSF. The caudal end of each cerebral hemisphere turns ventrally and then rostrally, forming the **temporal lobe**; in so doing, it carries with it the ventricle (forming the **temporal horn**) and the choroid fissure (see Fig. 16-21). Here, the thin medial wall of the hemisphere is invaginated along the **choroid fissure** by the vascular pia mater to form the *choroid plexus of the temporal horn of the lateral ventricle* (see Fig. 16-20B and Fig. 16-21B).

As the cerebral cortex differentiates, fibers passing to and from it pass through the **corpus striatum** and divide it into the *caudate and lentiform nuclei.* This fiber pathway—the **internal capsule** (see Fig. 16-20C)—becomes C-shaped as the hemisphere assumes this form. The **caudate nucleus** becomes elongated and C-shaped, conforming to the outline of the lateral ventricle (see Fig. 16-21A to C). Its pear-shaped head and elongated body lie in the floor of the frontal horn and the body of the lateral ventricle; its tail makes a U-shaped turn to gain the roof of the temporal horn.

Cerebral Commissures
As the cerebral cortex develops, groups of nerve fibers—commissures—connect corresponding areas of the cerebral hemispheres with one another (see Fig. 16-20A). The most important of these commissures cross in the **lamina terminalis**, the rostral (anterior) end of the forebrain. This lamina extends from the roof plate of the diencephalon to the **optic chiasm (decussation or crossing of the fibers of the optic nerve)**.

The **anterior commissure** connects the olfactory bulb and related brain areas of one hemisphere with those of the opposite side. The **hippocampal commissure** connects the hippocampal formations. The **corpus callosum**, the largest cerebral commissure, connects the neocortical

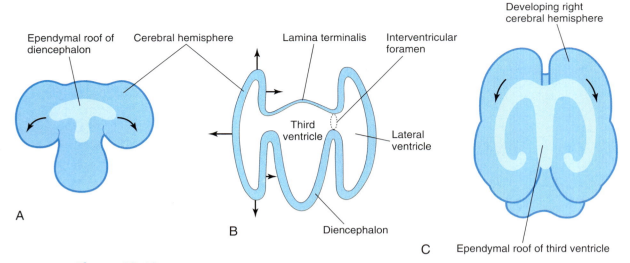

Figure 16–19 **A,** Sketch of the dorsal surface of the forebrain indicating how the ependymal roof of the diencephalon is carried out to the dorsomedial surface of the cerebral hemispheres. **B,** Diagrammatic section of the forebrain showing how the developing cerebral hemispheres grow from the lateral walls of the forebrain and expand in all directions until they cover the diencephalon. The rostral wall of the forebrain, the lamina terminalis, is very thin. **C,** Sketch of the forebrain showing how the ependymal roof is finally carried into the temporal lobes as a result of the C-shaped growth pattern of the cerebral hemispheres. The *arrows* indicate some of the directions in which the hemispheres expand.

areas (see Fig. 16-20*A*). The rest of the **lamina terminalis** becomes stretched to form the **septum pellucidum**, a thin plate of brain tissue.

At birth, the corpus callosum extends over the roof of the diencephalon. The **optic chiasm**, which develops in the ventral part of the lamina terminalis (see Fig. 16-20*A*), consists of fibers from the medial halves of the retinae, which cross to join the optic tract of the opposite side.

Initially, the surface of the hemispheres is smooth (Fig. 16-22); however, as growth proceeds, **sulci** (grooves between the gyri) and **gyri** (tortuous convolutions) develop (see Fig. 16-22). The sulci and gyri permit a considerable increase in the surface area of the cerebral cortex without requiring an extensive increase in cranial size. As each cerebral hemisphere grows, the cortex covering the external surface of the corpus striatum grows relatively slowly and is soon overgrown. This buried cortex, hidden from view in the depths of the **lateral sulcus** (fissure) of the cerebral hemisphere, is the **insula** (island).

CONGENITAL ANOMALIES OF BRAIN

Defects of the brain are common—approximately 3 per 1000 births. Most major birth defects, such as **meroencephaly** and **meningoencephalocele**, result from *defective closure of the rostral neuropore* **(neural tube defects [NTDs])** during the fourth week of development (Fig. 16-23*A*), and involve the overlying tissues (meninges and calvaria). Magnetic resonance imaging (MRI) is often used for evaluation of the fetal brain in pregnancies at risk for fetal defects (Fig. 16-24). The factors causing NTDs are genetic, nutritional, and/or environmental in nature.

PHARYNGEAL HYPOPHYSIS AND CRANIOPHARYNGIOMA

A remnant of the stalk of the hypophyseal diverticulum may persist and form a **pharyngeal hypophysis** in the roof of the oropharynx (see Fig. 16-18*E* and *F*). Occasionally, rare, benign tumors—**craniopharyngiomas**, formed from remnants of the stalk—develop in the pharynx or the basisphenoid (posterior part of sphenoid bone), but most often, they form in and/or superior to the sella turcica of the cranium (see Fig. 16-24).

CRANIUM BIFIDUM

Defects in the formation of the cranium (skull)—**cranium bifidum**—are often associated with birth defects of the brain, meninges, or both. Defects of the cranium usually involve the median plane of the calvaria. The defect is often in the squamous part of the occipital bone and may include the posterior part of the foramen magnum. When the defect is small, usually only the meninges herniate, and the defect is *cranial meningocele*. Cranium bifidum associated with herniation of the brain, meninges, or both occurs in approximately 1 in 2000 births. When the cranial defect is large, the meninges and part of the brain herniate, forming a *meningoencephalocele* (see Fig. 16-23*A* and *B*). If the protruding brain contains part of the ventricular system, the defect is a *meningohydroencephalocele* (see Fig. 16-23*C*).

Figure 16–20 **A,** Drawing of the medial surface of the forebrain of a 10-week embryo showing the diencephalic derivatives, the main commissures, and the expanding cerebral hemispheres. **B,** Transverse section of the forebrain at the level of the interventricular foramina showing the corpus striatum and choroid plexuses of the lateral ventricles. **C,** Similar section at approximately 11 weeks showing division of the corpus striatum into the caudate and lentiform nuclei by the internal capsule. The developing relationship of the cerebral hemispheres to the diencephalon is also illustrated.

MEROENCEPHALY

Meroencephaly (also called anencephaly, an inappropriate term) is a severe birth defect of the calvaria that results from failure of the rostral neuropore to close during the fourth week (see Fig. 16-12). As a result, the forebrain, midbrain, most of the hindbrain, and the calvaria are absent. **Meroencephaly** is a common lethal defect, occurring at least once in every 1000 births. It is two to four times more common in females than in males. Meroencephaly is usually associated with a multifactorial pattern of inheritance.

MICROCEPHALY

In microcephaly (a neurodevelopmental disorder), the calvaria and brain are small, but the face is of normal size. Affected infants are usually severely mentally challenged because the cranium and brain are underdeveloped. Microcephaly is the result of a reduction in brain growth. Some cases of **microcephaly** appear to be genetic (autosomal recessive); others are caused by environmental factors such as cytomegalovirus infection in utero (see Chapter 19). Exposure during the fetal period to large amounts of ionizing radiation, infectious agents, and certain drugs is a contributing factor in some cases.

A

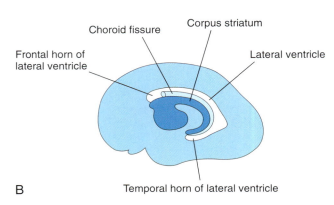

B

Figure 16–21 Schematic diagrams of the medial surface of the developing right cerebral hemisphere, showing the development of the lateral ventricle, choroid fissure, and corpus striatum. **A,** At 13 weeks. **B,** At 21 weeks. **C,** At 32 weeks.

C

16 weeks   22 weeks   27 weeks   40 weeks

Figure 16–22 Lateral and medial surfaces of human fetal brains at 16, 22, 27, and 40 weeks' gestation.

Defect in cranium at foramen magnum

Skin

Part of cerebellum

B

Defect at posterior fontanelle of skull

Ventricle

Dura mater

Part of occipital lobe

C

Skin

Figure 16–23 Cranium bifidum (bony defect of cranium) and herniation of the brain and meninges. **A,** Infant with a large meningoencephalocele in the occipital area. **B,** Meningoencephalocele, consisting of a protrusion of part of the cerebellum that is covered by meninges and skin. **C,** Meningohydroencephalocele, consisting of a protrusion of part of the occipital lobe that contains part of the posterior horn of a lateral ventricle.

Figure 16–24 Magnetic resonance image of a large craniopharyngioma (arrow).

HYDROCEPHALUS

An infant with hydrocephalus has a significant enlargement of the head, but the face is of normal size. Usually this defect is associated with mental deficiency. Hydrocephalus results from impaired circulation and absorption of CSF or, in unusual cases, from increased production of CSF. An excess of CSF is present in the ventricular system of the brain (Fig. 16-25). Impaired circulation of CSF often results from **congenital aqueductal stenosis** (narrow cerebral aqueduct). Blockage of CSF circulation results in dilation of the ventricles proximal to the obstruction and increased pressure on the cerebral hemispheres. This squeezes the brain between the ventricular fluid and calvaria. In infants, the internal pressure results in an accelerated rate of expansion of the brain and calvaria because the fibrous sutures of the calvaria are not fused.

Figure 16–25   **A,** An infant with hydrocephalus and a bilateral cleft palate. Hydrocephalus often produces thinning of the bones of the calvaria, prominence of the forehead, and atrophy of the cerebral cortex and white substance. **B,** Axial magnetic resonance image (transverse section through the brain) of a fetus with X-linked hydrocephalus at approximately 29 weeks' gestation, showing the massively enlarged ventricles (*) and thinned cortex (oval).

CHIARI MALFORMATION

Chiari malformation (CM) is a structural defect of the cerebellum. It is characterized by a tongue-like projection of the medulla and inferior displacement of the cerebellar tonsil through the foramen magnum into the vertebral canal. The posterior cranial fossa is usually abnormally small, thus causing pressure on the cerebellum and brainstem. This condition may lead to a type of noncommunicating hydrocephalus that obstructs the absorption and flow of CSF; as a result, the entire ventricular system is distended. CM can be diagnosed by MRI and, as a result, more cases are detected than in the past.

Several types of CM have been described. In *Type I*, the inferior part of the cerebellum herniates through the foramen magnum. This is the most commonly occurring form, usually asymptomatic, and detected often in adolescence. In *Type II*, also known as Arnold-Chiari malformation, there is herniation of cerebellar tissue and of the brainstem into the foramen magnum, often accompanied by occipital encephalocele and lumbar myelomeningocele (Fig. 16-26). In *Type III*, the most severe form, there is herniation of both the cerebellum and brainstem through the foramen magnum into the vertebral column with severe neurologic consequences. In *Type IV*, the cerebellum is either absent or underdeveloped—these infants do not survive.

DEVELOPMENT OF PERIPHERAL NERVOUS SYSTEM

The PNS consists of cranial, spinal, and visceral nerves and cranial, spinal, and autonomic ganglia. All sensory cells (somatic and visceral) of the PNS are derived from **neural crest cells**. The cell bodies of these sensory cells are located outside the CNS. The cell body of each afferent neuron is closely invested by a capsule of modified Schwann cells—*satellite cells* (see Fig. 16-7), which are derived from neural crest cells. This capsule is continuous with the **neurolemmal sheath of Schwann cells** that surround the axons of afferent neurons.

Neural crest cells in the developing brain migrate to form sensory ganglia only in relation to the trigeminal (CN V), facial (CN VII), vestibulocochlear (CN VIII), glossopharyngeal (CN IX), and vagus (CN X) nerves. Neural crest cells also differentiate into multipolar neurons of the *autonomic ganglia* (see Fig. 16-7), including ganglia of the sympathetic trunks that lie along the sides of the vertebral bodies; collateral, or prevertebral, ganglia in the plexuses of the thorax and abdomen (e.g., cardiac, celiac, and mesenteric plexuses); and parasympathetic, or terminal, ganglia in or near the viscera (e.g., submucosal, or Meissner, plexus).

Cells of the paraganglia—**chromaffin cells**—are also derived from the neural crest. The term *paraganglia* includes several widely scattered groups of cells that are similar in many ways to the medullary cells of the suprarenal glands. The cell groups largely lie retroperitoneally,

Figure 16–26 Arnold-Chiari type II malformation in a 23-week fetus. In situ exposure of the hindbrain shows cerebellar tissue well below the foramen magnum *(arrow).*

often in association with sympathetic ganglia. The carotid and aortic bodies also have small islands of chromaffin cells associated with them. These widely scattered groups of chromaffin cells constitute the **chromaffin system.**

Spinal Nerves

Motor nerve fibers arising from the spinal cord begin to appear at the end of the fourth week (see Fig. 16-4). The nerve fibers arise from cells in the *basal plates* of the developing spinal cord and emerge as a continuous series of rootlets along its ventrolateral surface. The fibers destined for a particular developing muscle group become arranged in a bundle, forming a **ventral nerve root** (see Fig. 16-6 and Fig. 16-7). The nerve fibers of the **dorsal nerve root** are derived from neural crest cells that migrate to the dorsolateral aspect of the spinal cord, where they differentiate into the cells of the **spinal ganglion** (see Fig. 16-7).

The central processes of the neurons in the spinal ganglion form a single bundle that grows into the spinal cord, opposite the apex of the dorsal horn of gray matter (see Fig. 16-4*B* and *C*). The distal processes of the spinal ganglion cells grow toward the ventral nerve root and eventually join it to form a **spinal nerve** (see Fig. 16-7).

As the limb buds develop, the nerves from the spinal cord segments opposite to them elongate and grow into the limbs. The nerve fibers are distributed to their muscles,

which differentiate from myogenic cells that originate from the somites (see Chapter 15). The skin of the developing limbs is also innervated in a segmental manner.

Cranial Nerves

Twelve pairs of cranial nerves form during the fifth and sixth weeks. They are classified into three groups according to their embryologic origins.

Somatic Efferent Cranial Nerves

The trochlear (CN IV), abducent (CN VI), hypoglossal (CN XII), and the greater part of the oculomotor (CN III) nerves are homologous with the ventral roots of the spinal nerves (Fig. 16-27*A*). The cells of origin of these nerves are located in the *somatic efferent column* (derived from the basal plates) of the brainstem. Their axons are distributed to the muscles derived from the head myotomes (preotic and occipital) (see Fig. 15-17*A*).

The **trochlear nerve** (CN IV) arises from nerve cells in the somatic efferent column in the posterior part of the midbrain. Although a motor nerve, it emerges from the brainstem dorsally and passes ventrally to supply the superior oblique muscle of the eye.

The **abducent nerve** (CN VI) arises from nerve cells in the basal plates of the metencephalon. It passes from its ventral surface to the posterior of the three preotic myotomes from which the lateral rectus muscle of the eye is thought to originate.

The **hypoglossal nerve** (CN XII) develops by fusion of the ventral root fibers of three or four occipital nerves (see Fig. 16-27*A*). Sensory roots, corresponding to the dorsal roots of the spinal nerves, are absent. The somatic motor fibers originate from the *hypoglossal nucleus.* These fibers leave the ventrolateral wall of the medulla in several groups—*hypoglossal nerve roots*—which converge to form the common trunk of CN XII (see Fig. 16-27*B*). They grow rostrally and eventually innervate the muscles of the tongue, which are derived from the occipital myotomes (see Fig. 15-17*A*).

The **oculomotor nerve** (CN III) supplies the superior, inferior, and medial recti and inferior oblique muscles of the eye.

Nerves of Pharyngeal Arches

Cranial nerves V, VII, IX, and X supply the embryonic pharyngeal arches; thus, the structures that develop from these arches are innervated by these cranial nerves (see Fig. 16-27*A* and Table 10-1).

The **trigeminal nerve** (CN V) is the nerve of the first pharyngeal arch, but it has an ophthalmic division that is not a pharyngeal arch component. *CN V is the principal sensory nerve for the head.* The cells of the large **trigeminal ganglion** are derived from the most anterior part of the neural crest. The central processes of the cells in this ganglion form the large sensory root of CN V, which enters the lateral part of the pons. The peripheral processes of cells in this ganglion separate into three large divisions (ophthalmic, maxillary, and mandibular nerves). Their sensory fibers supply the skin of the face as well as the lining of the mouth and nose. The *motor fibers of CN V arise from cells in the most anterior part of the special*

Figure 16–27 **A,** Schematic drawing of a 5-week embryo showing distribution of most of the cranial nerves, especially those supplying the pharyngeal arches. **B,** Schematic drawing of the head and neck of an adult showing the general distribution of most of the cranial nerves. *CN,* Cranial nerve.

visceral efferent column in the metencephalon. These fibers pass to the muscles of mastication and to other muscles that develop in the mandibular prominence of the first pharyngeal arch (see Table 10-1). The mesencephalic nucleus of CN V differentiates from cells in the midbrain.

The **facial nerve** (CN VII) is the nerve of the second pharyngeal arch. It consists mostly of motor fibers that arise principally from a nuclear group in the *special visceral efferent column* in the caudal part of the pons. These fibers are distributed to the *muscles of facial expression* and to other muscles that develop in the mesenchyme of the second pharyngeal arch (see Table 10-1). The small general visceral efferent component of CN VII terminates in the peripheral autonomic ganglia of the head. The sensory fibers of CN VII arise from the cells of the *geniculate ganglion*. The central processes of these cells enter the pons, and the peripheral processes pass to the greater superficial petrosal nerve and, via the chorda tympani nerve, to the taste buds in the anterior two thirds of the tongue.

The **glossopharyngeal nerve** (CN IX) is the nerve of the third pharyngeal arch. Its motor fibers arise from the special and, to a lesser extent, the general visceral efferent columns of the anterior part of the myelencephalon. CN IX forms from several rootlets that arise from the medulla just caudal to the developing internal ear. All the fibers from the special visceral efferent column are distributed to the stylopharyngeus muscle, which is derived from the mesenchyme in the third pharyngeal arch (see Table

10-1). The general efferent fibers are distributed to the otic ganglion from which postsynaptic fibers pass to the parotid and posterior lingual glands. The *sensory fibers of CN IX* are distributed as general sensory and special visceral afferent fibers (taste fibers) to the posterior part of the tongue.

The **vagus nerve** (CN X) is formed by fusion of the nerves of the fourth and sixth pharyngeal arches (see Table 10-1). The nerve of the fourth pharyngeal arch becomes the superior laryngeal nerve, which supplies the cricothyroid muscle and constrictor muscles of the pharynx. The nerve of the sixth pharyngeal arch becomes the recurrent laryngeal nerve, which supplies various laryngeal muscles.

The **spinal accessory nerve** (CN XI) arises from the cranial five or six cervical segments of the spinal cord (see Fig. 16-27A). The fibers of the traditional CN XI root are now considered to be part of CN X. These fibers supply the sternocleidomastoid and trapezius muscles.

Special Sensory Nerves

The **olfactory nerve** (CN I) arises from the olfactory organ. The olfactory cells are bipolar neurons that differentiate from cells in the epithelial lining of the primordial nasal sac. The axons of the olfactory cells are collected into 18 to 20 bundles around which the cribriform plate of the ethmoid bone develops. These unmyelinated nerve fibers end in the **olfactory bulb.**

The **optic nerve** (CN II) is formed by more than a million nerve fibers that grow into the brain from neuroblasts in the primordial retina. Because the optic nerve develops from the evaginated wall of the forebrain, it actually represents a fiber tract of the brain. Development of the optic nerve is described in Chapter 17.

The **vestibulocochlear nerve** (CN VIII) consists of two kinds of sensory fibers in two bundles; these fibers are known as *the vestibular and cochlear nerves*. The **vestibular nerve** originates in the semicircular ducts, and the **cochlear nerve** proceeds from the cochlear duct, in which the **spiral organ** (of Corti) develops (see Chapter 17). The bipolar neurons of the vestibular nerve have their cell bodies in the **vestibular ganglion**. The central processes of these cells terminate in the vestibular nuclei in the floor of the fourth ventricle. The bipolar neurons of the cochlear nerve have their cell bodies in the **spiral ganglion**. The central processes of these cells end in the ventral and dorsal *cochlear nuclei* in the medulla.

DEVELOPMENT OF AUTONOMIC NERVOUS SYSTEM

Functionally, the ANS can be divided into sympathetic (thoracolumbar) and parasympathetic (craniosacral) parts.

Sympathetic Nervous System

During the fifth week, neural crest cells in the thoracic region migrate along each side of the spinal cord, where they form paired cellular masses (ganglia) dorsolateral to the aorta (see Fig. 16-7). All these segmentally arranged **sympathetic ganglia** are connected in a bilateral chain by longitudinal nerve fibers. These ganglionated cords—**sympathetic trunks**—are located on each side of the vertebral bodies. Some neural crest cells migrate ventral to the aorta and form neurons in the **preaortic ganglia**, such as the celiac and mesenteric ganglia (see Fig. 16-7). Other neural crest cells migrate to the area of the heart, lungs, and gastrointestinal tract, where they form terminal ganglia in **sympathetic organ plexuses**, located near or within these organs.

After the sympathetic trunks have formed, axons of sympathetic neurons located in the **intermediolateral cell column** (lateral horn) of the thoracolumbar segments of the spinal cord pass through the ventral root of a spinal nerve and a **white ramus communicans** to a paravertebral ganglion (see Fig. 16-7). Here they may synapse with neurons or ascend or descend in the sympathetic trunk to synapse at other levels. Other presynaptic fibers pass through the **paravertebral ganglia** without synapsing, forming splanchnic nerves to the viscera. The postsynaptic fibers course through a **gray communicating branch (gray ramus communicans)**, passing from a sympathetic ganglion into a spinal nerve; hence, the sympathetic trunks are composed of ascending and descending fibers.

Parasympathetic Nervous System

The presynaptic parasympathetic fibers arise from neurons in the nuclei of the brainstem and in the sacral region of the spinal cord. The fibers from the brainstem leave through the oculomotor (CN III), facial (CN VII), glossopharyngeal (CN IX), and vagus (CN X) nerves. The **postsynaptic neurons** are located in the peripheral ganglia or in plexuses near or within the structure being innervated (e.g., pupil of eye and salivary glands).

 CLINICALLY ORIENTED QUESTIONS

1. Are neural tube birth defects hereditary? A woman had an infant with spina bifida cystica and her daughter had an infant with meroencephaly. Is the daughter likely to have another child with a neural tube defect? Can meroencephaly and spina bifida be detected early in fetal life?

2. Some say that pregnant women who are heavy drinkers may have infants who exhibit mental and growth deficiency. Is this true? There are reports of women who get drunk during pregnancy, yet have infants who seem to be normal. Is there a safe threshold for alcohol consumption during pregnancy?

3. A woman was told that cigarette smoking during pregnancy probably caused the slight mental deficiency of her infant. Was the woman correctly informed?

4. Do all types of spina bifida cause loss of motor function in the lower limbs? What treatments are there for infants with spina bifida cystica?

The answers to these questions are at the back of this book.

Development of Eyes and Ears

▶ DEVELOPMENT OF EYES AND RELATED STRUCTURES

17 The eyes are derived from four sources:

- Neuroectoderm of brain
- Surface ectoderm of head
- Mesoderm between the above layers
- Neural crest cells

Early eye development results from a series of inductive signals and is first evident at the beginning of the fourth week, when **optic grooves (sulci)** appear in the cranial neural folds (Fig. 17-1*A* and *B*). As the neural folds fuse, the optic grooves evaginate to form hollow diverticula—**optic vesicles**—that project from the wall of the forebrain into the adjacent mesenchyme (see Fig. 17-1*C*). Formation of the optic vesicles is induced by the mesenchyme adjacent to the developing brain. As the optic vesicles enlarge, their connections with the forebrain constrict to form hollow **optic stalks** (see Fig. 17-1*D*).

An inductive signal passes from the optic vesicles and stimulates the surface ectoderm to thicken and form **lens placodes**, the primordia of the lenses (see Fig. 17-1*C*). The placodes invaginate and sink deep to the surface ectoderm, forming **lens pits** (see Fig. 17-1*D* and Fig. 17-2). The edges of the pits approach and fuse to form spherical **lens vesicles** (see Fig. 17-1*F* and *H*), which soon lose their connection with the surface ectoderm.

As the lens vesicles develop, the **optic vesicles** invaginate to form double-walled **optic cups** (see Fig. 17-1*F* and Fig. 17-2), with the lens becoming infolded by the rim of the optic

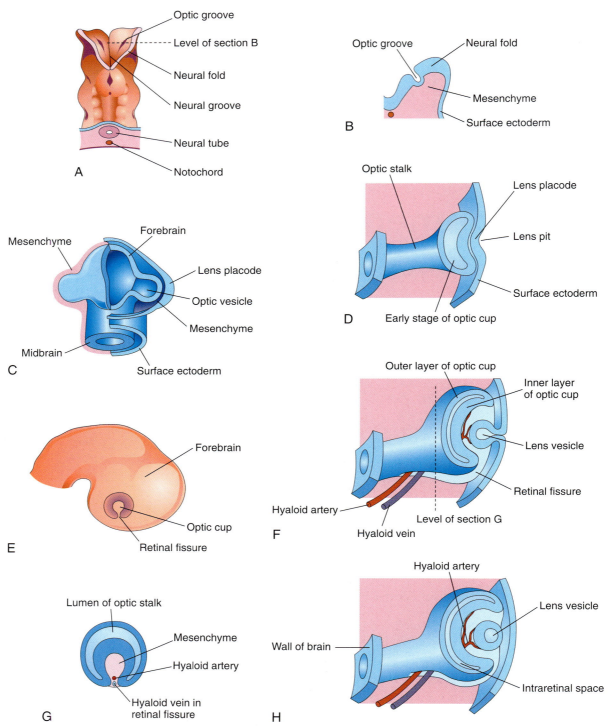

Figure 17–1   Illustrations of early stages of eye development. **A,** Dorsal view of the cranial end of an embryo at approximately 22 days, showing the optic grooves, the first indication of eye development. **B,** Transverse section of a neural fold showing the optic groove in it. **C,** Schematic drawing of the forebrain of an embryo at approximately 28 days, showing its covering layers of mesenchyme and surface ectoderm. **D, F,** and **H,** Schematic sections of the developing eye, illustrating successive stages in the development of the optic cup and lens vesicle. **E,** Lateral view of the brain of an embryo at approximately 32 days, showing the external appearance of the optic cup. **G,** Transverse section of the optic stalk, showing the retinal fissure and its contents. Note that the edges of the retinal fissure are growing together, thereby completing the optic cup and enclosing the central artery and vein of the retina in the optic stalk and cup.

Wall of optic stalk
(continuous with wall
of forebrain)

Cavity of optic
stalk (continuous with
cavity of forebrain)

Intraretinal space

Mesenchyme (primordium
of choroid and sclera)

Surface ectoderm

Lens pit

Inner layer of optic
cup (primordium of
neural retina)

Outer layer of optic
cup (primordium of
retinal pigment
epithelium)

Figure 17–2 Photomicrograph of a sagittal section of the eye of an embryo (×200) at approximately 32 days. Observe the primordium of the lens (invaginated lens placode), the walls of the optic cup (primordium of retina), and the optic stalk (primordium of the optic nerve). *(From Moore KL, Persaud TVN, Shiota K: Color Atlas of Clinical Embryology, 2nd ed. Philadelphia, Saunders, 2000.)*

cup (Fig. 17-3*A*). By this stage, the lens vesicles have entered the cavities of the optic cups (Fig. 17-4). Linear grooves—**retinal fissures (optic fissures)**—develop on the ventral surface of the optic cups and along the **optic stalks** (see Fig. 17-1*E* to *H* and Fig. 17-3*A* to *D*). The retinal fissures contain vascular mesenchyme from which the hyaloid blood vessels develop. The **hyaloid artery, a branch of the ophthalmic artery,** supplies the inner layer of the optic cup, the lens vesicle, and the mesenchyme in the optic cup (see Fig. 17-1*H* and Fig. 17-3). As the edges of the retinal fissure fuse, the hyaloid vessels are enclosed within the **primordial optic nerve** (see Fig. 17-3*C* to *F*). Distal parts of the hyaloid vessels eventually degenerate, but proximal parts persist as the **central artery** and **vein of the retina** (Fig. 17-5*D*). *Bone morphogenetic protein (BMP), sonic hedgehog (Shh), and fibroblast growth factor (FGF) are essential for signaling the optical vesicle and closure of the retinal fissure.*

Development of Retina

The retina develops from the walls of the **optic cup, an outgrowth of the forebrain** (see Fig. 17-1 and Fig. 17-2). The walls of the cup develop into two layers of the retina: the outer thin layer becomes the **pigment layer of the retina,** and the thick layer differentiates into the **neural retina.** The two retinal layers are separated by an **intraretinal space** (see Fig. 17-1*H* and Fig. 17-4), which is derived from the cavity of the optic cup. This space gradually disappears as the two layers of the retina fuse (see Fig. 17-5*D*). Because the optic cup is an outgrowth of the forebrain, the layers of the optic cup are continuous with the wall of the brain (see Fig. 17-1*H*).

DETACHMENT OF RETINA

This defect occurs when the inner and outer layers of the optic cup fail to fuse during the fetal period to form the retina and obliterate the intraretinal space (see Fig. 17-3 and Fig. 17-5). The separation of the neural and pigmented layers may be partial or complete. Retinal detachment may result from unequal rates of growth of the two retinal layers; as a result, the layers of the optic cup are not in perfect apposition. Although separated from the retinal pigment epithelium, the neural retina retains its blood supply (central artery of retina). Normally, the retinal pigment epithelium becomes firmly fixed to the choroid, but its attachment to the neural retina is not firm; hence, retinal detachment is not uncommon.

Under the influence of the developing lens, the inner layer of the optic cup proliferates to form a thick **neuroepithelium** (see Fig. 17-4). Subsequently, the cells of this layer differentiate into the **neural retina,** the light-sensitive region of the retina (see Fig. 17-7). This region contains **photoreceptors** (rods and cones) and the cell bodies of neurons (e.g., bipolar and ganglion cells). Because the optic vesicle invaginates as it forms the optic cup, the neural retina is "inverted"; that is, light-sensitive parts of the photoreceptor cells are adjacent to the retinal pigment epithelium. As a result, light must pass through the thickest part of the retina before reaching the photoreceptors; however, because, overall, the retina is thin and transparent, it does not form a barrier to light.

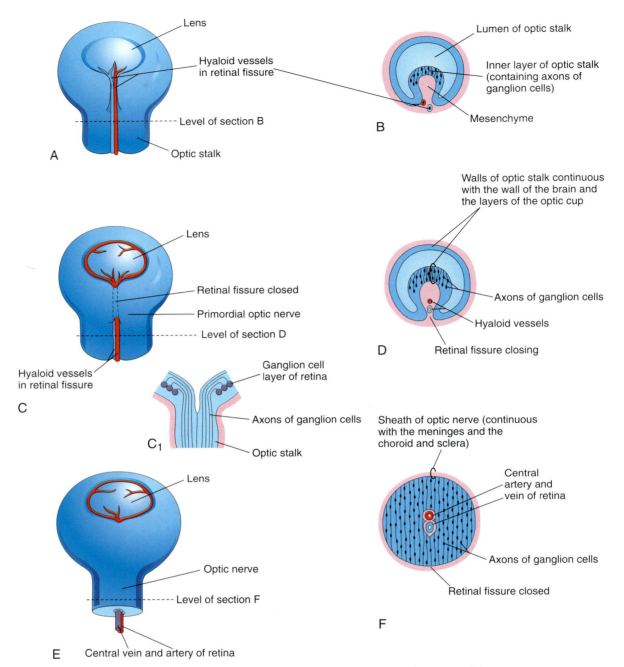

Figure 17–3 Illustrations of the closure of the retinal fissure and formation of the optic nerve. **A, C,** and **E,** Views of the inferior surface of the optic cup and optic stalk, showing progressive stages in the closure of the retinal fissure. **C₁,** Schematic sketch of a longitudinal section of a part of the optic cup and stalk, showing the optic disc and axons of the ganglion cells of the retina growing through the optic stalk to the brain. **B, D,** and **F,** Transverse sections of the optic stalk showing successive stages in the closure of the retinal fissure and formation of the optic nerve. Note that the lumen of the optic stalk is gradually obliterated as axons of ganglion cells accumulate in the inner layer of the optic stalk as the optic nerve forms.

Retinal pigment epithelium

Neuroepithelium

Optic nerve

Anterior lens epithelium

Branches of hyaloid artery

Lens fibers

Iris

Intraretinal space

Vitreous body

Surface ectoderm

Choroid

Sclera

Figure 17–4 Photomicrograph of a sagittal section of the eye of an embryo (×100) at approximately 44 days. Observe that it is the posterior wall of the lens vesicle that forms the lens fibers. The anterior wall does not change appreciably as it becomes the anterior lens epithelium. *(From Nishimura H [ed]: Atlas of Human Prenatal Histology. Tokyo, Igaku-Shoin, 1983.)*

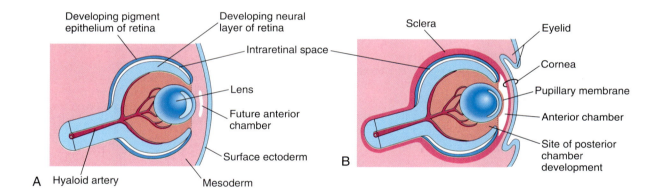

Developing pigment epithelium of retina

Developing neural layer of retina

Intraretinal space

Lens

Future anterior chamber

Surface ectoderm

A Hyaloid artery

Mesoderm

Sclera

Eyelid

Cornea

Pupillary membrane

Anterior chamber

B

Site of posterior chamber development

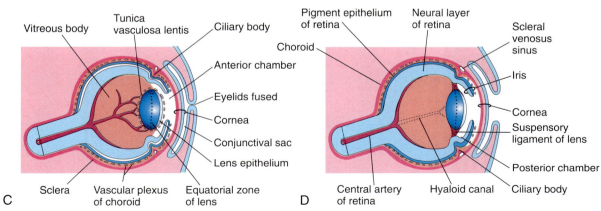

Vitreous body

Tunica vasculosa lentis

Ciliary body

Anterior chamber

Eyelids fused

Cornea

Conjunctival sac

Lens epithelium

C

Sclera

Vascular plexus of choroid

Equatorial zone of lens

Pigment epithelium of retina

Neural layer of retina

Choroid

Scleral venosus sinus

Iris

Cornea

Suspensory ligament of lens

Posterior chamber

D

Central artery of retina

Hyaloid canal

Ciliary body

Figure 17–5 Diagrammatic drawings of sagittal sections of the eye, showing successive developmental stages of the lens, retina, iris, and cornea. **A,** At 5 weeks. **B,** At 6 weeks. **C,** At 20 weeks. **D,** Neonate. Note that the retina and optic nerve are formed from the optic cup and optic stalk (see Fig. 17-1D).

The axons of the ganglion cells in the superficial layer of the neural retina grow proximally in the wall of the **optic stalk** to the brain (see Fig. 17-3A). The cavity of the stalk is gradually obliterated as the axons of the ganglion cells form the **optic nerve** (see Fig. 17-3F). *Myelination (formation of a myelin sheath) of the optic nerve fibers begins late in the fetal period and is completed by the 10th week after birth. Molecular studies have shown that the homeobox genes PAX6 and OTX2 regulate retinal differentiation and pigment formation, respectively.*

COLOBOMA OF RETINA

Retinal coloboma is a birth defect that is characterized by a localized gap in the retina, usually inferior to the optic disc. The defect is bilateral in most cases. A typical coloboma results from defective closure of the retinal fissure.

COLOBOMA OF IRIS

In infants, this birth defect in the inferior sector of the iris or pupillary margin gives the pupil a keyhole appearance (Fig. 17-6). The coloboma may be limited to the iris, or it may extend deeper and involve the ciliary body and retina. A typical coloboma *results from failure of closure of the retinal fissure* during the sixth week. The defect may be genetically determined, or it may be caused by environmental factors. A simple coloboma of the iris is frequently hereditary and is transmitted as an autosomal dominant characteristic.

Development of Choroid and Sclera

The mesenchyme surrounding the optic cup differentiates into an inner, vascular layer—the **choroid**—and an outer, fibrous layer—the **sclera** (see Fig. 17-5C and Fig. 17-7). At the rim of the optic cup, the choroid forms the cores of the **ciliary processes**, consisting chiefly of capillaries supported by delicate connective tissue.

Development of Ciliary Body

This body is a wedge-shaped extension of the **choroid** (see Fig. 17-5C and *D*). Its medial surface projects toward the

Figure 17–6   Coloboma of the left iris. Observe the defect in the inferior part of the iris (at the 6 o'clock position). The defect represents failure of fusion of the retinal fissure. *(From Guercio J, Martyn L: Congenital malformations of the eye and orbit. Otolaryngol Clin North Am 40(1):113, 2007. Copyright 2007, with permission from Elsevier.)*

Figure 17–7   Photomicrograph of a sagittal section of the eye of an embryo (×50) at approximately 56 days. Observe the developing neural retina and pigment layer of the retina. The large intraretinal space disappears when these two layers of the retina fuse. *(From Moore KL, Persaud TVN, Shiota K: Color Atlas of Clinical Embryology, 2nd ed. Philadelphia, Saunders, 2000.)*

lens, forming **ciliary processes**. The pigmented part of the ciliary epithelium is derived from the outer layer of the optic cup, which is continuous with the retinal pigment epithelium. The **nonvisual retina** is the nonpigmented ciliary epithelium, which represents the anterior prolongation of the neural retina, in which no neural elements develop. The smooth **ciliary muscle** is responsible for focusing the lens—and the connective tissue in the ciliary body. It develops from mesenchyme at the edge of the optic cup between the anterior scleral condensation and the ciliary pigment epithelium.

Development of Iris

The iris develops from the rim of the **optic cup**, which grows inward and partially covers the lens (see Fig. 17-5D). The epithelium of the iris represents both layers of the optic cup; it is continuous with the double-layered epithelium of the **ciliary body** and with the retinal pigment epithelium and neural retina. The connective tissue framework (stroma) of the iris is derived from neural crest cells that migrate into the iris. The **dilator pupillae** and **sphincter pupillae muscles** of the iris are derived from the *neuroectoderm of the optic cup*. These smooth muscles result from a transformation of epithelial cells into smooth muscle cells.

Development of Lens

The lens develops from the **lens vesicle**, a derivative of the surface ectoderm (see Fig. 17-1F and H). The anterior wall of the lens vesicle becomes the subcapsular **lens epithelium** (see Fig. 17-5C). The nuclei of the tall columnar cells that form the posterior wall of the lens vesicle undergo dissolution (dissolving). These cells lengthen considerably to form highly transparent epithelial cells, the **primary lens fibers**. As these fibers grow, they gradually obliterate the cavity of the lens vesicle (see Figs. 17-5A to C, Fig. 17-7, and Fig. 17-8). The rim of the lens—the **equatorial zone**—is located midway between the anterior and posterior poles of the lens. The cells in the equatorial zone are cuboidal; as they elongate, they lose their nuclei and become **secondary lens fibers** (see Fig. 17-8). These fibers are added to the external sides of the primary lens fibers. *Lens formation involves the expression of L-Maf (lens-specific Maf) and other transcription factors in the lens placode and vesicle. The transcription factors Pitx3 and GAT-3 are also essential for the formation of the lens.*

Although secondary lens fibers continue to form during adulthood and the lens increases in diameter as a result, the primary lens fibers must last a lifetime. The developing lens is supplied with blood by the distal part of the **hyaloid artery** (see Fig. 17-4 and Fig. 17-5); however, it becomes avascular in the fetal period when this part of the artery degenerates (see Fig. 17-5D). After this, the lens depends on diffusion from the **aqueous humor (watery fluid)** in the anterior chamber of the eye (see Fig. 17-5C), which bathes its anterior **surface**, and from the vitreous humor in other parts. The lens capsule is produced by the anterior lens epithelium. The **lens capsule** represents a greatly thickened basement membrane and has a lamellar structure. The former site of the **hyaloid artery** is indicated by the **hyaloid canal** in the vitreous body (see Fig. 17-5D); this canal is usually inconspicuous in the living eye.

The **vitreous body** forms within the cavity of the optic cup (see Fig. 17-4 and Fig. 17-5C). It is composed of **vitreous humor**, an avascular mass of transparent, gel-like, intercellular substance.

Development of Aqueous Chambers

The **anterior chamber of the eye** develops from a cleft-like space that forms in the mesenchyme located between the developing lens and cornea (see Fig. 17-5A to C and Fig. 17-8). The **posterior chamber of the eye** develops from a space that forms in the mesenchyme posterior to the developing iris and anterior to the developing lens (see Fig. 17-5D). After the lens is established, it induces the surface ectoderm to develop into the epithelium of the cornea and conjunctiva. When the **pupillary membrane** disappears (see Fig. 17-5B) and the pupil forms, the anterior and posterior chambers of the eye communicate with each other through the **scleral venous sinus** (see Fig. 17-5D). This vascular structure encircles the anterior chamber and allows aqueous humor to flow from the anterior chamber to the venous system.

PERSISTENCE OF HYALOID ARTERY

The distal part of the hyaloid artery normally degenerates as its proximal part becomes the central artery of the retina (see Fig. 17-5C and D). If part of the hyaloid artery persists distally, it may appear as a freely moving, nonfunctional vessel, or a worm-like structure projecting from the optic disc (see Fig. 17-3C), or as a fine strand traversing the vitreous body. In other cases, the hyaloid artery remnant may form a cyst.

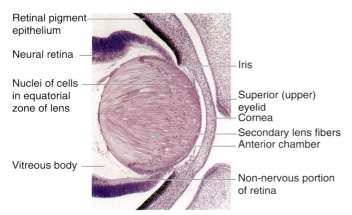

Retinal pigment epithelium

Neural retina

Nuclei of cells in equatorial zone of lens

Vitreous body

Iris

Superior (upper) eyelid
Cornea

Secondary lens fibers
Anterior chamber

Non-nervous portion of retina

Figure 17–8 Photomicrograph of a sagittal section of a portion of the developing eye of an embryo at approximately 56 days. Observe that the lens fibers have elongated and obliterated the cavity of the lens vesicle. *(From Moore KL, Persaud TVN, Shiota K: Color Atlas of Clinical Embryology, 2nd ed. Philadelphia, Saunders, 2000.)*

CONGENITAL GLAUCOMA

Intraocular tension in neonates (abnormal elevation of intraocular pressure) occurs because of an imbalance between the production of aqueous humor and its outflow. This imbalance may result from abnormal development of the **scleral venous sinus** (see Fig. 17-5*D*). Congenital glaucoma (present at birth) is usually genetically **heterogeneous**, but the condition may result from a rubella infection in the fetus during early pregnancy (see Chapter 19, Fig. 19-16*B*). It has been shown that the gene *CYP1B1* is responsible for the majority of cases of primary congenital glaucoma.

CONGENITAL CATARACTS

In this birth defect, the lens is opaque and frequently appears grayish white. Without treatment, blindness results. Many lens opacities are inherited, with dominant transmission being more common than recessive, or sex-linked, transmission. Some congenital cataracts are caused by teratogenic agents—particularly the **rubella virus** (see Chapter 19, Fig. 19-16*A*)—that affect the early development of the lenses. The lenses are vulnerable to the rubella virus between the fourth and seventh weeks, when primary lens fibers are forming. Physical agents, such as **radiation**, can also damage the lens and produce cataracts (see Chapter 19).

Development of Cornea

The cornea, induced by the lens vesicle, is formed from three sources, the:

- External corneal epithelium, derived from **surface ectoderm**
- **Mesenchyme**, derived from mesoderm, which is continuous with the developing sclera
- **Neural crest cells** that migrate from the lip of the optic cup (These cells also form the middle stroma layer of collagen-rich extracellular matrix.)

Development of Eyelids

The eyelids develop during the sixth week from mesenchyme derived from neural crest cells, and from two cutaneous folds of skin that grow over the cornea (see Fig. 17-5*B*). The eyelids adhere to one another during the 8th week and remain fused until the 26th to 28th weeks (see Fig. 17-5*C*). The **palpebral conjunctiva** lines the inner surface of the eyelids. The **eyelashes** and **glands** in the eyelids are derived from the surface ectoderm (see Chapter 18). The connective tissue and **tarsal plates (fibrous plates in the eyelids)** develop from mesenchyme in the developing eyelids. The *orbicularis oculi muscle* is derived from the mesenchyme in the second pharyngeal arch (see Chapter 10), and is supplied by its nerve (cranial nerve [CN] VII).

CONGENITAL PTOSIS OF EYELID

Drooping of the superior (upper) eyelids at birth is relatively common. **Ptosis (blepharoptosis)** may result from dystrophy of the **levator palpebrae superioris muscle**. Congenital ptosis occurs more rarely as a result of prenatal injury or **dystrophy** (defective nutrition) of the superior division of the **oculomotor nerve** (CN III), which supplies this muscle. Congenital ptosis may also be transmitted as an autosomal dominant trait. Severe ptosis can interfere with the development of normal sight and may need to be treated surgically.

COLOBOMA OF EYELID

This birth defect is characterized by a small notch in the superior eyelid; coloboma of the inferior (lower) eyelid is rare. **Palpebral colobomas** appear to result from local developmental disturbances in the formation and growth of the eyelids.

Development of Lacrimal Glands

The lacrimal glands are derived from a number of solid buds from the surface ectoderm. The buds branch and canalize to form **lacrimal excretory ducts** and alveoli of the glands. The **lacrimal glands** are small at birth and do not function fully until approximately 6 weeks; hence, neonates do not produce tears when they cry. Tears are often not produced when crying until 1 to 3 months.

DEVELOPMENT OF EARS

The ears are composed of external, middle, and internal anatomical parts. The external and middle parts regulate the transference of sound waves from the exterior to the internal ears, which convert the sound waves into nerve impulses. The internal ears are concerned with both hearing and balance.

Development of Internal Ears

The internal ears are the first of the three parts of the ears to develop. Early in the fourth week, a thickening of the surface ectoderm—the **otic placode**—appears on each side of the embryo at the level of the caudal part of the hindbrain (Fig. 17-9*A* and *B*). Inductive influences from the notochord and paraxial mesoderm stimulate the surface ectoderm to form the **otic placodes**. *Fibroblast growth factors (FGF-3 and FGF-10) may play a role in this process.* Each otic placode soon invaginates and sinks deep to the surface ectoderm into the underlying mesenchyme, forming an **otic pit** (see Fig. 17-9*C*). The edges of the pit come together and fuse to form an **otic vesicle** (see Fig. 17-9*D* and *E*). The vesicle soon loses its connection with the surface ectoderm, and a diverticulum grows

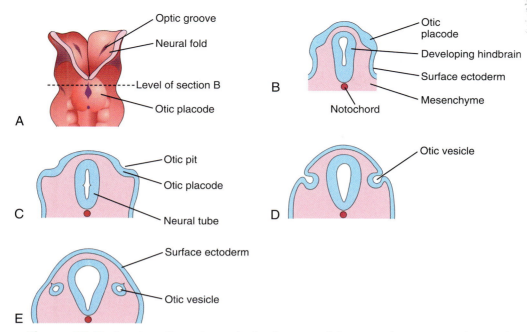

Figure 17–9 Drawings illustrating early development of the internal ear. **A,** Dorsal view of an embryo at approximately 22 days, showing the otic placodes. **B** to **E,** Schematic coronal sections illustrating successive stages in the development of otic vesicles.

from the vesicle and elongates to form the **endolymphatic duct** and **sac** (Fig. 17-10*A* to *E*). Two regions of the otic vesicles are visible:

- Dorsal utricular parts, from which the small endolymphatic ducts, utricles, and semicircular ducts arise
- Ventral saccular parts, which give rise to the saccules and cochlear ducts

Three disc-like diverticula grow out from the utricular parts of the **primordial membranous labyrinths.** Soon the central parts of these diverticula fuse and disappear (see Fig. 17-10*B* to *E*). The peripheral unfused parts of the diverticula become the **semicircular ducts,** which are attached to the utricle and are later enclosed in the **semicircular canals** of the **bony labyrinth.** Localized dilations, the **ampullae,** develop at one end of each semicircular duct (see Fig. 17-10*E*). Specialized receptor areas—**cristae ampullares**—differentiate in the ampullae and the utricle and saccule (maculae utricle and sacculi).

From the ventral saccular part of the otic vesicle, a tubular diverticulum—the **cochlear duct**—grows and coils to form the **membranous cochlea** (see Fig. 17-10*C* to *E*). A connection of the cochlea with the saccule, the **ductus reuniens,** soon forms. The **spiral organ** differentiates from cells in the wall of the cochlear duct (see Fig. 17-10*F* to *I*). Ganglion cells of the **vestibulocochlear nerve** (CN VIII) migrate along the coils of the membranous cochlea and form the **spiral ganglion.** Nerve processes extend from this ganglion to the spiral organ, where they terminate on the **hair cells.** The cells in the spiral ganglion retain their embryonic bipolar condition.

Inductive influences from the otic vesicle stimulate the mesenchyme around the otic vesicle to differentiate into a **cartilaginous otic capsule** (see Fig. 17-10*F*). The cartilaginous otic capsule later ossifies to form the **bony labyrinth** of the internal ear. *Retinoic acid and transforming growth factor β₁ may play a role in modulating epithelial-mesenchymal interaction in the internal ear and directing the formation of the otic capsule.*

As the membranous labyrinth enlarges, vacuoles appear in the cartilaginous otic capsule and soon coalesce to form the **perilymphatic space.** The membranous labyrinth is now suspended in **perilymph** (fluid in the perilymphatic space). The perilymphatic space, related to the cochlear duct, develops two divisions, the **scala tympani** and **scala vestibuli** (see Fig. 17-10*H* and *I*). The internal ear reaches its adult size and shape by the middle of the fetal period (20–22 weeks).

Development of Middle Ears

Development of the **tubotympanic recess** (Fig. 17-11*B*) from the first pharyngeal pouch is described in Chapter 10. The proximal part of the recess forms the **pharyngotympanic tube** (auditory tube). The distal part of the recess expands and becomes the **tympanic cavity** (see Fig. 17-11*C*), which gradually envelops the small bones of the middle ears—**auditory ossicles** (malleus, incus, and stapes), their tendons and ligaments, and the **chorda tympani nerve.**

These structures receive a virtually complete epithelial investment that is derived from neural crest cells and the endoderm. The neural crest cells undergo epithelial-mesenchymal transformation. An epithelial-type organizer, located at the tip of the tubotympanic recess, probably plays a role in the early development of the middle ear cavity by inducing programmed cell

Figure 17–10   Drawings of the otic vesicles showing the development of the membranous and bony labyrinths of the internal ear. **A** to **E,** Lateral views showing successive stages in the development of the otic vesicle into the membranous labyrinth from the fifth to eighth weeks. **A** to **D,** Diagrammatic sketches illustrating the development of a semicircular duct. **F** to **I,** Sections through the cochlear duct showing successive stages in the development of the spiral organ and the perilymphatic space from the 8th to 20th weeks.

death—**apoptosis.** The malleus and the incus develop from the cartilage of the first pharyngeal arch. The stapes has multiple origins. The head and crus are formed from neural crest cells. The outer boundary of the foot plate is mesenchymal in origin, while the inner ring is from neural crest cells. The **tensor tympani,** the muscle attached to the malleus, is derived from the mesenchyme in the first pharyngeal arch, and the **stapedius muscle** is derived from the second pharyngeal arch.

During the late fetal period, expansion of the **tympanic cavity** gives rise to the **mastoid antrum,** located in the temporal bone. The antrum is almost adult size at birth; however, *no mastoid cells are present in neonates.* By 2 years of age, the mastoid cells are well developed and produce conic projections of the temporal bones, the **mastoid processes.** The middle ear continues to grow through puberty.

Development of External Ears

The **external acoustic meatus,** the passage of the external ear leading to the tympanic membrane (eardrum), develops from the dorsal part of the first pharyngeal groove.

The ectodermal cells at the bottom of this tube proliferate to form a solid epithelial plate, the **meatal plug** (see Fig. 17-11C). Late in the fetal period, the central cells of this plug degenerate, forming a cavity that becomes the internal part of the external acoustic meatus (see Fig. 17-11D).

The primordium of the **tympanic membrane** is the first pharyngeal membrane, which separates the first pharyngeal groove from the first pharyngeal pouch (see Fig. 17-11A). The external covering of the tympanic membrane is derived from the surface ectoderm, whereas its internal lining is derived from the endoderm of the tubotympanic recess.

The **auricle (pinna), which projects from the side of the head,** develops from the mesenchymal proliferations in the first and second pharyngeal arches. Prominences—**auricular hillocks**—surround the first pharyngeal groove (Fig. 17-12A). As the auricle grows, the contribution of the first arch is reduced (see Fig. 17-12B to D). The **lobule** (earlobe) is the last part of the auricle to develop. The auricle is initially located at the base of the neck (see Fig. 17-12A and B). As the mandible develops, the auricles assume their normal position at the side of the head (see Fig. 17-12C and D).

Figure 17–11 Schematic drawings illustrating development of the external and middle parts of the ear. Observe the relationship of these parts of the ear to the otic vesicle, the primordium of the internal ear. **A,** At 4 weeks, illustrating the relation of the otic vesicle to the pharyngeal apparatus. **B,** At 5 weeks, showing the tubotympanic recess and pharyngeal arch cartilages. **C,** Later stage, showing the tubotympanic recess (future tympanic cavity and mastoid antrum) beginning to envelop the ossicles. **D,** Final stage of ear development showing the relationship of the middle ear to the perilymphatic space and external acoustic meatus. Note that the tympanic membrane develops from three germ layers: surface ectoderm, mesenchyme, and endoderm of the tubotympanic recess.

CONGENITAL DEAFNESS

Approximately 3 in every 1000 neonates have significant hearing loss. The deafness may be the result of maldevelopment of the sound-conducting apparatus of the middle and external ears, or of the neurosensory structures in the internal ear. *Enlargement of the vestibular aqueduct and endolymphatic duct is the most common congenital ear defect in children with hearing loss* (Fig. 17-13). This defect is typically bilateral and is an **autosomal recessive condition.**

Rubella infection during the critical period (fourth week) of development of the internal ear can cause maldevelopment of the spiral organ and deafness. **Congenital fixation of the stapes** results in conductive deafness in an otherwise normal ear. Failure of differentiation of the anular ligament, which attaches the base of the stapes to the oval window, results in fixation of the stapes to the bony labyrinth and loss of sound conduction.

AURICULAR ABNORMALITIES

Severe defects of the external ear are rare, but minor deformities are common and may serve as indicators of a specific pattern of congenital defects. For example, the auricles are often low-set and abnormal in shape in infants with **chromosomal syndromes,** such as trisomy 18 (see Chapter 19), and in infants affected by maternal ingestion of certain drugs (e.g., trimethadione).

AURICULAR APPENDAGES

These appendages (skin tags) are common and may result from the development of **accessory auricular hillocks** (Fig. 17-14). The appendages usually appear anterior to the auricle, more often unilaterally than bilaterally. The appendages, often with narrow pedicles, consist of skin but they may also contain some cartilage.

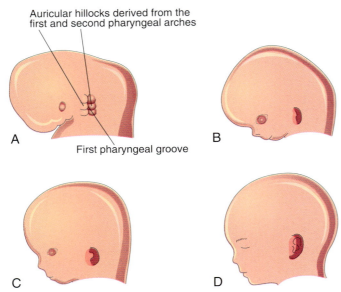

Figure 17–12   Illustration of the development of the auricle, the part of the external ear that is not within the head. **A,** At 6 weeks. Note that three auricular hillocks are located on the first pharyngeal arch and three are on the second arch. **B,** At 8 weeks. **C,** At 10 weeks. **D,** At 32 weeks.

Figure 17–13   Magnetic resonance image of a 5-year-old child demonstrating bilateral enlargement of the vestibular aqueduct and endolymphatic duct *(dashed arrow)*. Also note the cochlea *(solid arrow)*, the medulla *(M)*, and the cerebellum *(C)*.

MICROTIA

Microtia (a small or rudimentary auricle) results from suppressed mesenchymal proliferation (see Fig. 17-14). This defect often serves as an indicator of associated birth defects, such as an **atresia (absence of opening)** of the external acoustic meatus (80% of cases), and abnormalities of the middle ear. The cause can be both genetic and environmental.

PREAURICULAR SINUSES

Shallow, pit-like cutaneous sinuses are occasionally located anterior to the auricle (see Fig. 10-9D). These sinuses usually have pinpoint external openings. Some sinuses contain a vestigial cartilaginous mass. These defects are probably related to abnormal development of the auricular hillocks and defective closure of the dorsal part of the first pharyngeal groove. *Preauricular sinuses* are familial and are frequently bilateral. These sinuses may be associated with internal defects, such as deafness and kidney malformations.

Figure 17–14   A child with a rudimentary auricle **(microtia)** and a preauricular tag. She also has several other birth defects. The external acoustic meatus is also absent.

ATRESIA OF EXTERNAL ACOUSTIC MEATUS

Atresia (blockage) of the external acoustic meatus results from failure of the meatal plug to canalize—form a canal (see Fig. 17-11C). Usually the deep part of the canal is open but the superficial part is blocked by bone or fibrous tissue. Most cases are associated with the *first arch syndrome* (see Chapter 10). Often the auricle is also severely affected, and defects of the middle ear, internal ear, or both may be present. Atresia of the external acoustic meatus can occur bilaterally or unilaterally and usually results from autosomal dominant inheritance.

ABSENCE OF EXTERNAL ACOUSTIC MEATUS

Absence of the external acoustic meatus (canal) is rare (see Fig. 17-14). This defect results from failure of inward expansion of the first pharyngeal groove and failure of the meatal plug to disappear.

CLINICALLY ORIENTED QUESTIONS

1. If a woman has rubella during the first trimester of pregnancy, what are the chances that the eyes and ears of the fetus will be affected? What is the most common manifestation of late fetal rubella infection? If a pregnant woman is exposed to rubella, can it be determined if she is immune to the infection?

2. Is the purposeful exposure of young girls to rubella the best way for a woman to avoid rubella infection during pregnancy? If not, what can be done to provide immunization against rubella infection?

3. It has been reported that deafness and tooth defects occurring during childhood may result from fetal syphilis. Is this true? If so, how could this happen? Can these birth defects be prevented?

4. There are reports that blindness and deafness can result from herpesvirus infections. Is this true? If so, which herpesvirus is involved? What are the affected infant's chances of normal development?

5. It has been reported that methyl mercury exposure in utero can cause mental deficiency, deafness, and blindness. The article cited the eating of contaminated fish as the cause of the abnormalities. How might these birth defects be caused by methyl mercury?

The answers to these questions are at the back of this book.

Integumentary System

T he integumentary system consists of the skin and its appendages: sweat glands, nails, hairs, sebaceous glands, and arrector muscles of hairs. The system also includes the mammary glands and teeth.

DEVELOPMENT OF SKIN AND APPENDAGES

The skin, the outer protective covering of the body, is a complex organ system and is the body's largest organ. The skin consists of two layers (epidermis and dermis) that are derived from two different germ layers (Fig. 18-1): the ectoderm and mesoderm.

- The **epidermis** is a superficial epithelial tissue that is derived from **surface embryonic ectoderm.**
- The **dermis,** underling the epidermis, is a deep layer composed of dense, irregularly arranged connective tissue that is derived from **mesenchyme.**

Ectodermal (epidermal) and mesenchymal (dermal) interactions involve mutual inductive mechanisms. The embryonic skin at 4 to 5 weeks consists of a single layer of surface ectoderm overlying the mesoderm (see Fig. 18-1A).

Epidermis

The **primordium of the epidermis** is the surface ectoderm (see Fig. 18-1A). The cells in this layer proliferate and form a layer of squamous epithelium, the **periderm,** and a **basal layer** (see Fig. 18-1B). The cells of the periderm continually undergo **keratinization** (formation of a horny layer) and **desquamation** (shedding of the cuticle in scales) and are replaced by cells arising from the basal layer. The exfoliated peridermal cells form part of a white, greasy

291

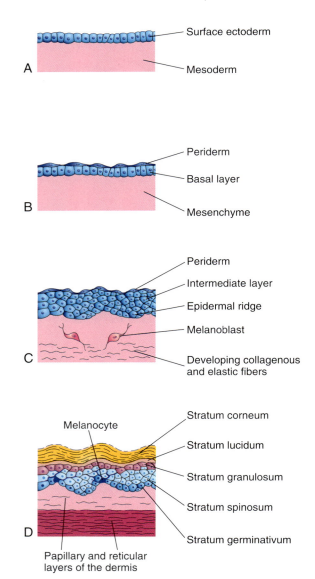

Figure 18–1   Illustrations of the successive stages of skin development. **A,** At 4 weeks. **B,** At 7 weeks. **C,** At 11 weeks. The cells of the periderm continually undergo keratinization and desquamation. Exfoliated peridermal cells form part of the vernix caseosa. **D,** Neonate. Note the melanocytes in the basal layer of the epidermis and the way their processes extend between the epidermal cells to supply them with melanin.

substance—**vernix caseosa**—that covers the fetal skin (Fig. 18-2). The vernix protects the developing skin from constant exposure to amniotic fluid containing urine, bile salts, and sloughed cells.

The **basal layer of the epidermis** becomes the **stratum germinativum** (see Fig. 18-1D), which produces new cells that are displaced into the more superficial layers. By 11 weeks, cells from the stratum germinativum have formed an **intermediate layer** (see Fig. 18-1C). Replacement of the peridermal cells continues until approximately the 21st week; thereafter, the **periderm disappears** and the **stratum corneum** forms from the **stratum lucidum** (see Fig. 18-1D).

DISORDERS OF KERATINIZATION

Ichthyosis is a general term for a group of skin disorders resulting from **excessive keratinization** (keratin formation). The skin is characterized by dryness and scaling, which may involve the entire body surface (Fig. 18-3). **Harlequin ichthyosis** results from a rare keratinizing disorder that is inherited as an autosomal recessive trait and caused by a mutation in the *ABCA12* gene. The skin is markedly thickened, ridged, and cracked. Most of the affected neonates require intensive care, and even so, 70% die early. A **collodion neonate** is covered by a thick, taut membrane that resembles collodion or parchment. This membrane cracks with the first respiratory efforts and begins to fall off in large sheets. Complete shedding of membranes may take several weeks, occasionally leaving normal-appearing skin.

Proliferation of cells in the **stratum germinativum** also produces **epidermal ridges**, which extend into the developing dermis (see Fig. 18-1C). These ridges begin to appear in embryos at 10 weeks and are permanently established by the 17th week. The pattern of epidermal ridges that develops on the surface of the palms of the hands and the soles of the feet is determined genetically, and constitutes the basis for examining fingerprints (**dermatoglyphics**) in criminal investigations and medical genetics. Abnormal chromosome complements affect the development of ridge patterns; for example, approximately 50% of neonates with Down syndrome have distinctive ridge patterns on their hands and feet that are of diagnostic value.

Late in the embryonic period, **neural crest cells** migrate into the mesenchyme in the developing dermis and differentiate into **melanoblasts** (see Fig. 18-1B and C). Later, these cells migrate to the **dermoepidermal junction** and differentiate into melanocytes (see Fig. 18-1D). The **melanocytes** begin producing **melanin** before birth and distribute it to the epidermal cells. After birth, increased amounts of melanin are produced in response to ultraviolet light. The relative content of melanin in the melanocytes accounts for the different colors of skin. *Molecular studies indicate that melanocyte-stimulating hormone cell surface receptor and melanosomal P-protein determine the degree of pigmentation by regulating tyrosinase levels and activity.*

Dermis

The dermis develops from mesenchyme underlying the surface ectoderm (see Fig. 18-1A and B). Most of the mesenchyme that differentiates into the connective tissue of the dermis originates from the somatic layer of the lateral mesoderm. By 11 weeks, the mesenchymal cells have begun to produce collagenous and elastic connective tissue fibers (see Fig. 18-1C). As the **epidermal ridges** form, the dermis projects into the epidermis, forming **dermal papillae**. Capillary loops develop in some of the

| Week 4 | Week 5 | Week 12 | Week 14 | Week 16 | Week 20 | Weeks 23–28 |

Layers of epidermis
- Stratum corneum
- Stratum lucidum
- Stratum granulosum
- Stratum spinosum
- Stratum germinativum
- Melanocyte
- Dermis
- Sweat duct
- Secreting cell of sweat gland

Hair bud
Hair bulb
Migrating melanocytes
Bud of sweat gland
Sebaceous gland
Mesenchymal cells
Collagen
Primordium of sebaceous gland
Developing sweat gland
Hair shaft
Epidermal root sheath
Arrector muscle of hair
Blood vessels
Hair papilla
Dermal root sheath
Bulb of hair follicle
Elastin fibers
Fat cells

Figure 18–2 Drawing of the successive stages in the development of hairs, sebaceous glands, and arrector muscles of hair. Note that the sebaceous gland develops as an outgrowth from the side of the hair follicle.

ANGIOMAS OF SKIN

These vascular anomalies are defects in which transitory and/or surplus blood or lymphatic vessels persist. Those composed of blood vessels may be mainly arterial, venous, or **cavernous** angiomas. Similar lesions that are composed of lymphatics are called **cystic lymphangiomas**, or **cystic hygromas**. True angiomas are benign tumors of endothelial cells, usually composed of solid or hollow cords; the hollow cords contain blood.

Nevus flammeus denotes a flat, pink or red, flame-like blotch that often appears on the posterior surface of the neck. A **port-wine stain hemangioma** is a larger, darker angioma than a nevus flammeus and is nearly always anterior or lateral on the face, neck, or both.

The blood vessels in the dermis differentiate from mesenchyme (vasculogenesis). As the skin grows, new capillaries grow out from the primordial vessels (**angiogenesis**). Some capillaries acquire muscular coats through the differentiation of myoblasts developing in the surrounding mesenchyme, and they become arterioles, arteries, venules, and veins. By the end of the **first trimester**, the blood supply of the fetal dermis is well established.

Development of Glands

The glands of skin include eccrine and apocrine sweat glands, sebaceous glands, and mammary glands. They are derived from the epidermis and grow into the dermis (see Fig. 18-2).

Sebaceous Glands

Most sebaceous glands develop as buds from the sides of the developing **epidermal root sheaths** of the hair follicles (see Fig. 18-2). The buds grow into the surrounding connective tissue and branch to form the primordia of the **alveoli** (hollow sacs) and their associated ducts. The central cells of the alveoli break down, forming an oily secretion—**sebum;** this substance is released into the hair

dermal ridges and provide nourishment for the epidermis. Sensory nerve endings form in other ridges. The developing **afferent nerve fibers** apparently play an important role in the spatial and temporal sequence of dermal ridge formation.

Figure 18–3 A child with severe keratinization of the skin (ichthyosis) from the time of birth. This particular defect has an autosomal dominant inheritance pattern.

ALBINISM

In *generalized albinism*, an autosomal recessive trait, the skin, hairs, and retina lack pigment; however, the iris usually shows some pigmentation. **Albinism** occurs when the melanocytes do not produce melanin because of a lack of the enzyme tyrosinase. In *localized albinism*—piebaldism—an autosomal dominant trait, there is a lack of melanin in patches of skin, hair, or both.

DEVELOPMENT OF HAIRS

Hairs begin to develop during the 9th to 12th weeks, but they do not become easily recognizable until approximately the 20th week (see Fig. 18-2). Hairs are first recognizable on the eyebrows, upper lip, and chin. A hair follicle begins as a proliferation of the stratum germinativum of the epidermis and extends into the underlying dermis. The **hair bud** soon becomes a club-shaped hair bulb. The epithelial cells of the hair bulb constitute the **germinal matrix**, which later produces the hair. The **hair bulb** is soon invaginated by a small mesenchymal **hair papilla** (see Fig. 18-2). The peripheral cells of the developing hair follicle form the **epidermal root sheath,** and the surrounding mesenchymal cells differentiate into the **dermal root sheath**. As cells in the germinal matrix proliferate, they are pushed toward the surface, where they **keratinize** to form **hair shafts**. The hair grows through the epidermis on the eyebrows and the upper lip by the end of the 12th week.

The first hairs—**lanugo**—are fine, soft, and lightly pigmented. Lanugo begins to appear toward the end of the 12th week and is plentiful by 17 to 20 weeks. These hairs help to hold the vernix on the skin. Lanugo is replaced during the perinatal period by coarser hairs that persist over most of the body. In the axillary and pubic regions, the lanugo is replaced at puberty by even coarser **terminal hairs**. In males, similar coarse hairs also appear on the face and often on the chest.

Melanoblasts migrate into the hair bulbs and differentiate into **melanocytes**. The melanin produced by these cells is transferred to the hair-forming cells in the germinal matrix several weeks before birth. The relative content of melanin accounts for different hair colors. **Arrector muscles of hairs,** small bundles of smooth muscle fibers, differentiate from the mesenchyme surrounding the hair follicle and attach to the dermal root sheath and the papillary layer of the dermis (see Fig. 18-2). The arrector muscles are poorly developed in the hairs of the axilla and in certain parts of the face. The hairs forming the eyebrows and eyelashes (cilia) have no arrector muscles.

follicle and passes to the surface of the skin. It mixes with desquamated peridermal cells to form **vernix caseosa**. Sebaceous glands, independent of the hair follicles (e.g., in the glans penis and labia minora), develop in a similar manner as buds from the epidermis that invade the dermis.

Sweat Glands

Eccrine sweat glands develop as epidermal downgrowths—**cellular buds**—into the underlying mesenchyme (see Fig. 18-2). As a bud elongates, its end coils to form the primordium of the secretory part of the gland. The epithelial attachment of the developing gland to the epidermis forms the **primordium of the sweat duct**. The central cells of the primordial ducts degenerate, forming a lumen. The peripheral cells of the secretory part of the gland differentiate into *myoepithelial* and *secretory cells* (see Fig. 18-2). The myoepithelial cells are believed to be specialized smooth muscle cells that assist in expelling sweat from the glands. Eccrine sweat glands begin to function shortly after birth.

Apocrine sweat glands develop from downgrowths of the stratum germinativum of the epidermis that give rise to the hair follicles (see Fig. 18-2). As a result, the ducts of these glands open into the upper part of the hair follicles, superficial to the openings of the sebaceous glands. These glands are mostly confined to the axillary, pubic, and perineal regions and the areolae surrounding the nipples. Secretion from the glands does not begin until puberty.

DEVELOPMENT OF NAILS

Toenails and fingernails begin to develop at the tips of the digits (fingers and toes) at approximately 10 weeks

Figure 18–4 Successive stages in the development of a fingernail. **A,** The first indication of a nail is a thickening of the epidermis, the nail field, at the tip of the finger. **B,** As the nail plate develops, it slowly grows toward the tip of the finger. **C,** The fingernail normally reaches the end of the digit by 32 weeks.

(Fig. 18-4). Development of the **fingernails** precedes that of the **toenails** by approximately 4 weeks. The primordia of the nails appear as thickened areas, or fields, of the epidermis at the tip of each digit. Later, these **nail fields** migrate onto the dorsal surface (see Fig. 18-4*A*), carrying their innervation from the ventral surface. The nail fields are surrounded laterally and proximally by folds of epidermis—**nail folds.**

Cells from the proximal nail fold grow over the nail field and keratinize to form the **nail plate** (see Fig. 18-4*B*). At first, the developing nail is covered by superficial layers of epidermis, the **eponychium** (see Fig. 18-4*C*). These layers degenerate, exposing the nail, except at its base, where it persists as the **cuticle.** The skin under the free margin of the nail is the **hyponychium** (see Fig. 18-4*C*). The fingernails reach the fingertips at approximately 32 weeks; the toenails reach the toe tips at approximately 36 weeks.

DEVELOPMENT OF MAMMARY GLANDS

Mammary glands are modified and highly specialized types of sweat glands. **Mammary buds** begin to develop during the sixth week as solid downgrowths of the epidermis into the underlying mesenchyme (Fig. 18-5*C*). These changes occur in response to an inductive influence from the mesenchyme. The mammary buds develop from **mammary crests,** which are thickened strips of ectoderm extending from the axillary to the inguinal regions (see Fig. 18-5*A*). The **mammary crests** appear during the fourth week but normally persist only in the pectoral area where the breasts develop (see Fig. 18-5*B*). Each primary mammary bud soon gives rise to several secondary mammary buds that develop into the **lactiferous ducts** and their branches (see Fig. 18-5*D* and *E*). Canalization of these buds is induced by maternal sex hormones entering the fetal circulation. This process continues until late gestation and, by term, 15 to 20 lactiferous ducts have formed. The fibrous connective tissue and fat of the mammary gland develop from the surrounding mesenchyme.

During the late fetal period, the epidermis at the site of origin of the **primordial mammary gland** becomes depressed, forming a shallow **mammary pit**

GYNECOMASTIA

The rudimentary mammary glands in males normally undergo no postnatal development. **Gynecomastia** refers to excessive development of male mammary tissue. It occurs in most male neonates because of stimulation of the mammary glands by maternal sex hormones. This effect disappears in a few weeks. During mid-puberty, approximately two thirds of males have varying degrees of **hyperplasia** (enlargement) of the breasts. Approximately 80% of males with *Klinefelter syndrome* have gynecomastia (see Chapter 19, Fig. 19-7).

SUPERNUMERARY BREASTS AND NIPPLES

An extra breast (**polymastia**) or nipple (**polythelia**) is an inheritable condition, which occurs in approximately 0.2% to 5.6% of the female population. **Supernumerary nipples** are also relatively common in males; they are often mistaken for moles. Polythelia is often found in association with other congenital defects, including renal and urinary tract anomalies. Less commonly, **supernumerary breasts** or nipples appear in the axillary or abdominal regions of females. In these positions, the nipples or breasts arise from extra mammary buds that develop along the mammary crests (see Fig. 18-5*A* and *B*).

(see Fig. 18-5*C* and *E*). The nipples are poorly formed and depressed in neonates. Soon after birth, the nipples usually rise from the mammary pits because of proliferation of the surrounding connective tissue of the **areola** (see Fig. 18-5*F*). The mammary glands develop similarly and are of the same structure in both sexes. In females, the glands enlarge rapidly during puberty, mainly because of fat and other connective tissue development in the breasts under the influence of estrodiol. Growth of the duct and lobe systems also occurs because of the increased levels of circulating **estrogen** and progesterone.

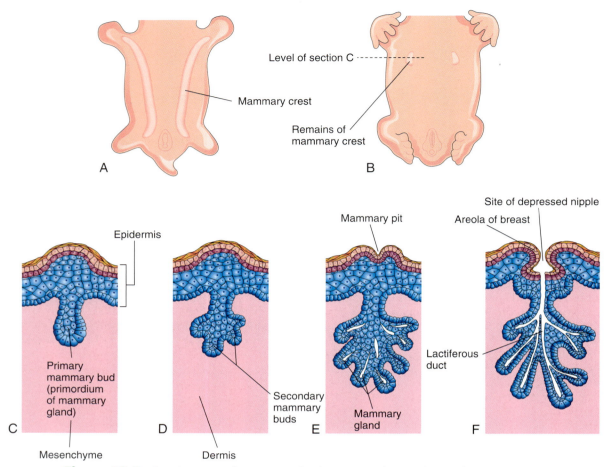

Figure 18–5 Development of mammary glands. **A,** Ventral view of an embryo at approximately 28 days showing the mammary crests. **B,** Similar view at 6 weeks showing the remains of these crests. **C,** Transverse section of a mammary crest at the site of a developing mammary gland. **D to F,** Similar sections showing successive stages of breast development between the 12th week and birth.

DEVELOPMENT OF TEETH

Two sets of teeth normally develop: the primary dentition, or **deciduous teeth**, and the secondary dentition, or **permanent teeth**. Teeth develop from the oral ectoderm, mesenchyme, and neural crest cells. The **enamel** is derived from ectoderm of the oral cavity; all other tissues differentiate from the surrounding mesenchyme and neural crest cells. *Expression of homeobox MSX and Dlx genes as well as BMP, Tnf, Wnt, Shh, and Fgf in the migrating neural crest cells, as well as in the ectoderm and mesenchyme, is essential for the initiation of tooth development. Wnt/β-catenin signaling also regulates many stages of tooth development.*

Odontogenesis (tooth development) is initiated by the inductive influence of the **neural crest–induced mesenchyme** on the overlying ectoderm. The first tooth buds appear in the anterior mandibular region; later tooth development occurs in the anterior maxillary region and progresses posteriorly in both jaws. Tooth development continues for years after birth (Table 18-1). The first indication of tooth development is a thickening of the oral epithelium, a derivative of the surface ectoderm seen during the sixth week. These U-shaped bands—**dental laminae**—follow the curves of the primordial jaws (Fig. 18-6*A* and Fig. 18-7*A*).

Bud Stage of Tooth Development

Each dental lamina (see Fig. 18-6*A*) develops 10 centers of proliferation from which **tooth buds** grow into the underlying mesenchyme (see Fig. 18-6*B* and Fig. 18-7*B*). These buds develop into the **deciduous teeth**, which are shed during childhood (see Table 18-1). There are 10 tooth buds in each jaw, one for each deciduous tooth. The tooth buds for the **permanent teeth** begin to appear at approximately 10 weeks from deep continuations of the dental laminae (see Fig. 18-7*D*). The permanent molars have no deciduous predecessors; they develop as buds from posterior extensions of the **dental laminae**. The tooth buds for the permanent teeth appear at different times, mostly during the fetal period. The buds for the second and third permanent molars develop after birth.

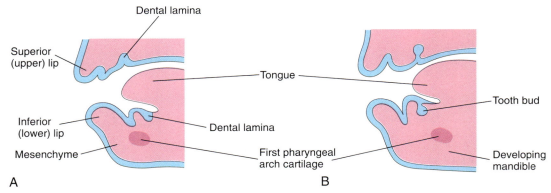

Figure 18–6 Sketches of sagittal sections through the developing jaws, illustrating early development of the teeth. **A,** Early in the sixth week, showing the dental laminae. **B,** Later in the sixth week, showing tooth buds arising from the laminae.

TOOTH	USUAL ERUPTION TIME	SHEDDING TIME
Table 18–1 The Order and Usual Time of Eruption of Teeth and the Time of Shedding of Deciduous Teeth		
Deciduous		
Medial incisor	6–8 mo	6–7 yr
Lateral incisor	8–10 mo	7–8 yr
Canine	16–20 mo	10–12 yr
First molar	12–16 mo	9–11 yr
Second molar	20–24 mo	10–12 yr
Permanent		
Medial incisor	7–8 yr	
Lateral incisor	8–9 yr	
Canine	10–12 yr	
First premolar	10–11 yr	
Second premolar	11–12 yr	
First molar	6–7 yr	
Second molar	12 yr	
Third molar	13–25 yr	

Data from Moore KL, Dalley AF, Agur AMR: Clinically Oriented Anatomy, 6th ed. Baltimore, Williams & Wilkins, 2010.

Cap Stage of Tooth Development

As each tooth bud is invaginated by mesenchyme—the **primordium of the dental papilla and dental follicle**—the bud becomes cap-shaped (see Fig. 18-7C). The ectodermal part of the developing tooth, the **enamel organ**, eventually produces **enamel**. The internal part of each cap-shaped tooth, the **dental papilla**, is the primordium of the dental pulp. Together, the dental papilla and enamel organ form the **tooth germ** (primordial tooth). The outer cell layer of the enamel organ is the **outer enamel epithelium**, whereas the inner cell layer lining the "cap" is the **inner enamel epithelium** (see Fig. 18-7D).

The central core of loosely arranged cells between the layers of enamel epithelium is the **enamel reticulum (stellate reticulum)** (see Fig. 18-7E). As the enamel organ and dental papilla develop, the mesenchyme surrounding the

developing tooth condenses to form the **dental sac**, a vascularized capsular structure (see Fig. 18-7E). The dental sac is the primordium of the **cement** and **periodontal ligament**. The cement is the bone-like, rigid connective tissue covering the root of the tooth. The periodontal ligament is derived from neural crest cells. It is a specialized vascular connective tissue that surrounds the root of the tooth, separating it from and attaching it to the **alveolar bone** (see Fig. 18-7G).

Bell Stage of Tooth Development

As the enamel organ differentiates, the developing tooth becomes bell-shaped (see Fig. 18-7D and Fig. 18-8). The mesenchymal cells in the dental papilla adjacent to the inner enamel epithelium differentiate into **odontoblasts**, which produce **predentin** and deposit it adjacent to the epithelium. Later, the predentin calcifies and becomes **dentin**. As the dentin thickens, the odontoblasts regress toward the center of the dental papilla; however, their cytoplasmic processes—**odontoblastic processes**—remain embedded in the dentin (see Fig. 18-7F and I). Enamel is the hardest tissue in the body. It overlies the yellowish dentin, the second hardest tissue in the body, and protects it from being fractured.

Cells of the *inner enamel epithelium* differentiate into **ameloblasts**, which produce enamel in the form of prisms (rods) over the dentin. As the enamel increases, the ameloblasts regress toward the *outer enamel epithelium*. The **root of the tooth** begins to develop after dentin and enamel formation is well advanced. The inner and outer enamel epithelia come together at the neck of the tooth, where they form a fold, the **epithelial root sheath** (see Fig. 18-7F). This sheath grows into the mesenchyme and initiates root formation. The odontoblasts adjacent to the epithelial root sheath form dentin that is continuous with that of the crown. As the dentin increases, it reduces the pulp cavity to a narrow **root canal** through which the vessels and nerves pass. The inner cells of the dental sac differentiate into **cementoblasts**, which produce cement that is restricted to the root. Cement is deposited over the dentin of the root and meets the enamel at the neck of the tooth.

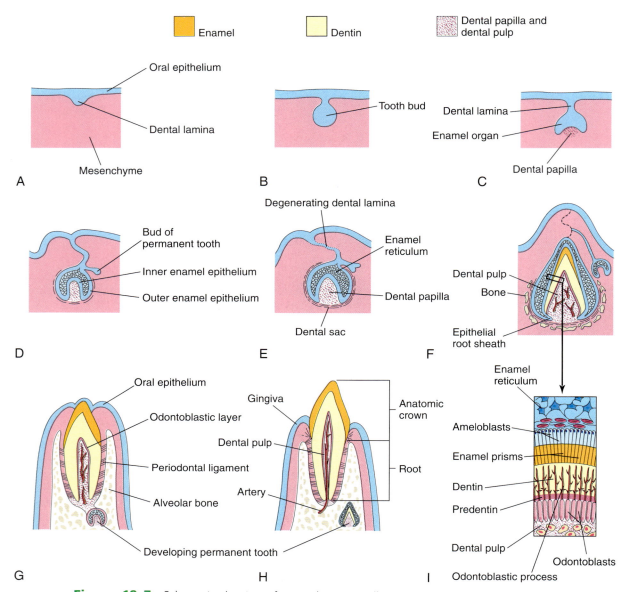

Figure 18–7 Schematic drawing of sagittal sections illustrating successive stages in the development and eruption of an incisor tooth. **A,** At 6 weeks, showing the dental lamina. **B,** At 7 weeks, showing the tooth bud developing from the dental lamina. **C,** At 8 weeks, showing the cap stage of tooth development. **D,** At 10 weeks, showing the early bell stage of a deciduous tooth and the bud stage of a permanent tooth. **E,** At 14 weeks, showing the advanced bell stage of tooth development. Note that the connection (dental lamina) of the tooth to the oral epithelium is degenerating. **F,** At 28 weeks, showing the enamel and dentin layers. **G,** At 6 months postnatally, showing early tooth eruption. **H,** At 18 months postnatally, showing a fully erupted deciduous incisor tooth. The incisor tooth now has a well-developed crown. **I,** Section through a developing tooth, showing ameloblasts (enamel producers) and odontoblasts (dentin producers).

As the teeth develop and the jaws ossify, the outer cells of the dental sac also become active in bone formation. Each tooth soon becomes surrounded by bone, except over its crown. The tooth is held in its **alveolus** (bony socket) by the strong **periodontal ligament**, a derivative of the dental sac (see Fig. 18-7G and H). Some fibers of this ligament are embedded in the cement of the root; other fibers are embedded in the bony wall of the alveolus. The periodontal ligament is located between the cement of the root and the bony alveolus.

Tooth Eruption

As the **deciduous teeth** develop, they begin a continuous slow movement toward the oral cavity (see Fig. 18-7F and G). The **mandibular teeth** usually erupt before the maxillary teeth, and female's teeth usually erupt sooner. A child's dentition contains **20 deciduous teeth**. As the root of the tooth grows, its crown gradually erupts through the oral epithelium. The part of the oral mucosa around the erupted crown becomes the **gingiva** (gum). Usually, eruption of the deciduous teeth occurs between 6 and 24 months after birth (see Table 18-1). The mandibular medial incisors—or **central incisors**—usually erupt 6 to 8 months after birth, but this process may not begin until 12 or 13 months in some children. Despite this, all 20 deciduous teeth are usually present by the end of the second year in healthy children.

The **permanent teeth** develop in a manner similar to that described for deciduous teeth. As a permanent tooth grows, the root of the corresponding deciduous tooth is gradually resorbed by **osteoclasts**. Consequently, when the deciduous tooth is shed, it consists only of the crown and the cervical, or uppermost, part of the root. The permanent teeth usually begin to erupt during the sixth year and continue to appear until early adulthood (Fig. 18-9; see also Table 18-1).

ENAMEL HYPOPLASIA

Defective enamel formation causes pits, fissures, or both in the enamel of teeth (Fig. 18-10). These defects result from temporary disturbances of enamel formation. Various factors may injure ameloblasts (source of enamel), such as nutritional deficiency, tetracycline therapy, and infectious diseases. **Rickets** arising during the critical period of permanent tooth development (6–12 weeks) is the most common cause of enamel hypoplasia. Rickets, a disease in children who are deficient in vitamin D, is characterized by disturbance of ossification of the epiphyseal cartilages and disorientation of cells at the metaphysis—section of bone between the epiphysis and diaphysis (see Chapter 15, Fig. 15-3).

VARIATIONS OF TOOTH SHAPE

Abnormally shaped teeth are relatively common. Occasionally there are spherical masses of enamel—**enamel pearls**—attached to the tooth (see Fig. 18-10E). They are formed by **aberrant groups of ameloblasts**. In other cases, the maxillary lateral incisor teeth may have a slender, tapered shape (peg-shaped incisors). **Congenital syphilis** affects the differentiation of the permanent teeth, resulting in incisors with central notches.

Figure 18–8 Photomicrograph of a section of the crown and neck of a tooth (×17). Observe the enamel (*E*), dentin (*D*), dental pulp (*P*), and odontoblasts (*O*). (*From Gartner LP, Hiatt JL: Color Textbook of Histology, 2nd ed. Philadelphia, Saunders, 2001.*)

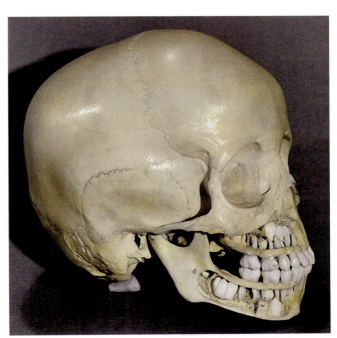

Figure 18–9 Cranium of a 4-year-old child. Bone has been removed from the jaws to show the relation of the developing permanent teeth to the erupted deciduous teeth.

Figure 18–10 Common tooth anomalies. **A,** Amelogenesis imperfecta. **B,** Dentinogenesis imperfecta. **C,** Tetracycline-stained teeth. **D,** Midline supernumerary tooth (*M, mesiodens*), located near the root apex of the central incisor. **E,** Molar tooth with an enamel pearl *(arrow).*

NUMERIC ABNORMALITIES OF TEETH

One or more **supernumerary teeth** may develop, or the normal number of teeth may not form (see Fig. 18-10*D*). Supernumerary teeth usually develop in the area of the maxillary incisors and may disrupt the position and eruption of normal teeth. The extra teeth commonly erupt posterior to the normal teeth. In **partial anodontia**, one or more teeth are absent. Congenital absence of one or more teeth is often a familial trait. In **total anodontia**, no teeth develop; this very rare condition is usually associated with **congenital ectodermal dysplasia** (disorders involving tissues that are ectodermal in origin).

MACRODONTIA

Macrodontia (a single large tooth) is a condition caused by the union of two adjacent tooth germs. The crowns of the two teeth can be partially or completely fused. The same applies to roots. Occasionally, a tooth bud divides or two buds partially fuse to form fused teeth. This condition is commonly observed in the mandibular incisors of the primary dentition, but it can also occur in the permanent dentition.

AMELOGENESIS IMPERFECTA

In amelogenesis imperfecta, the tooth enamel is soft and friable because of **hypocalcification** (deficient calcification), and the teeth are yellow to brown in color (see Fig. 18-10*A*). Mutational defects of the gene that encodes for enamel, dentin, and mineralization are likely involved. The teeth are covered with only a thin layer of abnormally formed enamel through which the color of the underlying dentin is visible, giving the teeth a darkened appearance. This rare autosomal dominant condition affects approximately 1 in 700 to 1 in 8000 children.

DENTINOGENESIS IMPERFECTA

Dentinogenesis imperfecta is relatively common in Caucasian children (see Fig. 18-10*B*). In affected children, the teeth are brown to gray-blue, with an opalescent sheen. This is caused by failure of the odontoblasts to differentiate normally, producing poorly calcified dentin. Both deciduous and permanent teeth are usually involved. The enamel tends to wear down rapidly, exposing the dentin. This defect is inherited as an autosomal dominant trait.

DISCOLORED TEETH

Foreign substances discolor the teeth if they are incorporated into the developing enamel and dentin. The **hemolysis** associated with **hemolytic disease** of the neonate (see Chapter 8) may produce blue to black discoloration of the teeth. *All tetracyclines are extensively incorporated into the teeth*. The critical period of risk is from approximately 14 weeks of fetal life to the 10th postnatal month for deciduous teeth, and from approximately 14 weeks of fetal life to the 16th postnatal year for permanent teeth. **Tetracyclines** produce brownish-yellow discoloration (mottling) and enamel hypoplasia because they interfere with the metabolic processes of the ameloblasts (see Fig. 18–10C). The enamel is completely formed on all but the third molars by approximately 8 years of age. For this reason, *tetracyclines should not be administered to pregnant women or to children younger than 8 years.*

CLINICALLY ORIENTED QUESTIONS

1. A neonate was reportedly born without skin. Is this possible? If so, could such an infant survive?

2. A dark-skinned person presented with patches of white skin on the face, chest, and limbs. He even had a white forelock. What is this condition called, and what is its developmental basis? Is there any treatment for these skin defects?

3. Some males have enlarged breasts at birth. Is this an indication of abnormal sex development?

4. A girl developed a breast in the axilla during puberty. She also had an extra nipple on her chest. What is the embryologic basis for these birth defects?

5. A neonate was born with two teeth. Would they be normal teeth? Is this a common occurrence? Are they usually extracted?

The answers to these questions are at the back of this book.

Human Birth Defects

B *irth defects (anomalies)* are developmental disorders present at birth. As a global problem, it has been estimated that almost 8 million children worldwide are born with a serious birth defect. Birth defects are the leading cause of infant mortality (fetal outcome) and may be structural, functional, metabolic, behavioral, or hereditary. A **birth defect** is a structural abnormality of any type; however, *not all variations are anomalies.* There are four clinically significant types of birth defects: malformation, disruption, deformation, and dysplasia.

- **Malformation:** A morphologic defect of an organ, part of an organ, or larger region of the body resulting from an intrinsically abnormal developmental process.
- **Disruption:** A morphologic defect of an organ, part of an organ, or larger region of the body resulting from the extrinsic breakdown of, or an interference with, an originally normal developmental process.
- **Deformation:** An abnormal form, shape, or position of a part of the body caused by mechanical force.
- **Dysplasia:** An abnormal organization of cells into tissue(s) and its morphologic result(s)— a process and consequence of dyshistogenesis.

TERATOLOGY: STUDY OF ABNORMAL DEVELOPMENT

Teratology is the branch of science that studies the causes, mechanisms, and patterns of abnormal development. A fundamental concept in teratology is that certain stages of embryonic development are more vulnerable to disruption than others (see Fig. 19-11).

303

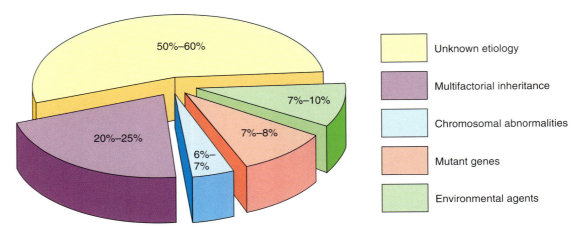

Figure 19–1 Graphic illustration of the causes of human birth defects. Note that the causes of most defects are unknown and that 20% to 25% of them are caused by a combination of genetic and environmental factors (multifactorial inheritance).

More than 20% of infant deaths in North America are attributable to birth defects. Major structural anomalies are observed in approximately 3% of neonates. Additional defects may only be detected after birth. The incidence of birth defects approaches 6% in 2-year-old infants and 8% in 5-year-old children.

The causes of birth defects may be **genetic factors**, such as chromosomal abnormalities, as well as **environmental factors**, such as drugs. However, many common defects are the result of **multifactorial inheritance**; that is, they are caused by genetic and environmental factors acting together. Moreover, epigenetic mechanisms may also be involved. For 50% to 60% of birth defects, the etiology (causes of disease) is unknown (Fig. 19-1). Birth defects may be single or multiple and of major or minor clinical significance.

Single minor defects are present in approximately 14% of neonates. Defects of the external ears, for example, are of no serious medical significance, but they indicate the possible presence of associated major defects. For example, the presence of a single umbilical artery alerts a clinician to the possible presence of cardiovascular and renal anomalies.

Major defects are much more common in early embryos (10%–15%), but most of them abort spontaneously during the first 6 weeks. **Chromosomal abnormalities** are present in more than 50% to 60% of spontaneously aborted embryos.

BIRTH DEFECTS CAUSED BY GENETIC FACTORS*

Numerically, *genetic factors are the most important cause of birth defects.* It has been estimated that they cause

*The authors are grateful to Dr. A. E. Chudley, MD, FRCPC, FCCMG, Medical Director, Program in Genetics and Metabolism; Professor of Pediatrics and Child Health; and Professor, Department of Biochemistry and Medical Genetics, University of Manitoba, Winnipeg, Manitoba, Canada, for his assistance with the preparation of this section on genetic disorders.

approximately one third of all defects (see Fig. 19-1). Any mechanism as complex as mitosis or meiosis may occasionally malfunction; thus, *chromosomal aberrations are common and are present in 6% to 7% of zygotes.* Many early embryos never undergo normal cleavage to become blastocysts. The changes may affect the sex chromosomes, the autosomes, or both. Persons with chromosomal abnormalities usually have characteristic phenotypes, such as the physical characteristics of infants with Down syndrome (see Fig. 19-4).

Numerical Chromosomal Abnormalities

Numerical aberrations of chromosomes usually result from **nondisjunction**, an error in cell division in which a chromosome pair or two chromatids of a chromosome do not disjoin during mitosis or meiosis. As a result, the chromosome pair or chromatids pass to one daughter cell, while the other cell receives neither (Fig. 19-2). Nondisjunction may occur during maternal or paternal gametogenesis (see Chapter 2). The chromosomes in somatic

INACTIVATION OF GENES

During embryogenesis, one of the two X chromosomes in female somatic cells is randomly inactivated and appears as a mass of **sex chromatin**. Inactivation of the genes on one X chromosome in the somatic cells of female embryos occurs during implantation.

X-inactivation is important clinically because it means that each cell from a carrier of an X-linked disease has the mutant gene causing the disease, either on the active X chromosome or on the inactivated X chromosome that is represented by sex chromatin. Uneven X-inactivation in monozygotic twins is one reason given for discordance in a variety of birth defects. The genetic basis for discordance is that one twin preferentially expresses the paternal X and the other, the maternal X.

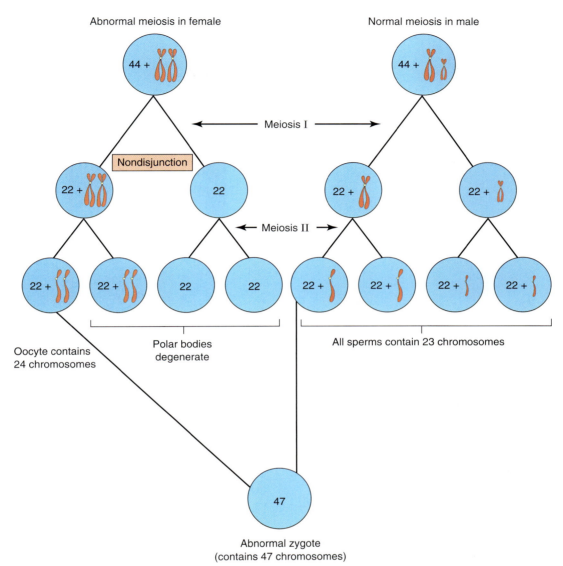

Abnormal meiosis in female   Normal meiosis in male

Meiosis I

Nondisjunction

Meiosis II

Oocyte contains
24 chromosomes

Polar bodies
degenerate

All sperms contain 23 chromosomes

Abnormal zygote
(contains 47 chromosomes)

Figure 19–2 Diagram showing nondisjunction of sex chromosomes during the first meiotic division of a primary oocyte, resulting in an abnormal oocyte with 24 chromosomes. Subsequent fertilization by a normal sperm produces a zygote with 47 chromosomes—aneuploidy—a deviation from the human diploid number of 46.

TURNER SYNDROME

Approximately 1% of female embryos with monosomy X (45,X) survive (chromosome count 45 and only one X chromosome). The incidence of 45,X—or **Turner syndrome**—in neonate females is approximately 1 in 8000 live births. Half of the affected individuals have 45,X; the other half have a variety of abnormalities affecting a sex chromosome. *The phenotype of Turner syndrome is female* (Fig. 19-3). **Phenotype** refers to the morphologic characteristics of an individual, as determined by the genotype and environment in which it is expressed. Secondary sexual characteristics do not develop in 90% of girls with Turner syndrome, necessitating hormone replacement therapy.

The monosomy X chromosomal abnormality is the most common cytogenetic abnormality observed in live-born neonates and fetuses that abort spontaneously; it accounts for approximately 18% of all spontaneous abortions caused by chromosomal abnormalities. In approximately 75% of cases, it is the paternal X chromosome that is missing.

Figure 19–3   Turner syndrome in a 14-year-old girl. Note the classic features of the syndrome: short stature; webbed neck; absence of sexual maturation; broad chest with widely spaced nipples; and lymphedema swelling of the hands and feet.

(body) cells are normally paired. The *homologous chromosomes* making up a pair are homologs. Normal females have 22 pairs of autosomes plus two X chromosomes, whereas normal males have 22 pairs of autosomes plus one X and one Y chromosome.

Trisomy

If three chromosomes of one type are present instead of the usual pair, the abnormality is called *trisomy*. Trisomies are the most common abnormalities of chromosome number. The usual cause of this numerical error is **meiotic nondisjunction of chromosomes** (see Fig. 19-2), resulting in a gamete with 24 instead of 23 chromosomes and, subsequently, a zygote with 47 chromosomes.

Trisomy of autosomes is associated mainly with three syndromes (Table 19-1):

Figure 19–4   A child with Down syndrome (trisomy 21). Note the round face, up-slanted palpebral fissures, and short digits with incurving of the fifth digit (clinodactyly).

ANEUPLOIDY AND POLYPLOIDY

Changes in chromosome number result in either aneuploidy or polyploidy. **Aneuploidy** is any deviation from the diploid number of 46 chromosomes. An *aneuploid* is an individual or a cell that has a chromosome number that is not an exact multiple of the haploid number of 23 (e.g., 45 or 47). *The principal cause of aneuploidy is nondisjunction during cell division* (see Fig. 19-2), resulting in an unequal distribution of one pair of homologous chromosomes to the daughter cells. One cell has two chromosomes and the other has neither chromosome of the pair. As a result, the embryo's cells may be *hypodiploid* (e.g. 45,X, or *Turner syndrome*) (see Fig. 19-3) or *hyperdiploid*, usually 47, as in trisomy 21 or *Down syndrome* (Fig. 19-4). Embryos with **monosomy**—missing a chromosome—usually die. Monosomy of an autosome is extremely uncommon, and approximately 99% of embryos lacking a sex chromosome (45,X) abort spontaneously.

- Trisomy 21, or Down syndrome (see Fig. 19-4)
- Trisomy 18, or Edwards syndrome (Fig. 19-5)
- Trisomy 13, or Patau syndrome (Fig. 19-6)

Infants with trisomy 13 and trisomy 18 are severely malformed and mentally challenged. They usually die early in infancy. More than 50% of **trisomic embryos**

Table 19-1   Trisomy of Autosomes

CHROMOSOMAL ABERRATION/SYNDROME	INCIDENCE	USUAL MORPHOLOGIC CHARACTERISTICS	FIGURE
Trisomy 21 (Down syndrome)*	1:800	Mental deficiency; brachycephaly; flat nasal bridge; upward slant to palpebral fissures; protruding tongue; simian crease; clinodactyly of fifth digit; congenital heart defects	19-4
Trisomy 18 (Edwards syndrome)[†]	1:8000	Mental deficiency; growth retardation; prominent occiput; short sternum; ventricular septal defect; micrognathia; low-set, malformed ears; flexed digits; hypoplastic nails; rocker-bottom feet	19-5
Trisomy 13 (Patau syndrome)[†]	1:25,000	Mental deficiency; severe central nervous system malformations; sloping forehead; malformed ears; scalp defects; microphthalmia; bilateral cleft lip or palate; polydactyly; posterior prominence of heels	19-6

*The importance of this disorder in the overall problem of mental deficiency is indicated by the fact that persons with Down syndrome represent 10% to 15% of institutionalized, mentally defective individuals. The incidence of trisomy 21 at fertilization is greater than that at birth; however, 75% of affected embryos are spontaneously aborted and at least 20% are stillborn.
[†]Infants with this syndrome rarely survive beyond 6 months of age.

Figure 19–5 Female neonate with trisomy 18. Note the growth retardation, clenched fists with characteristic positioning of the fingers (second and fifth digits overlapping the third and fourth), short sternum, and narrow pelvis.

Figure 19–6 Female neonate with trisomy 13. Note the bilateral cleft lip; low-set, malformed ears; and polydactyly (extra digits). A small omphalocele (herniation of viscera into the umbilical cord) is also present.

spontaneously abort early. *Trisomy of the autosomes occurs with increasing frequency as maternal age increases* (Table 19-2).

Trisomy of the sex chromosomes is a common condition (Table 19-3); however, because no characteristic physical findings are seen in infants or children, this defect is not usually detected before puberty (Fig. 19-7). The diagnosis is best established by chromosomal and molecular analysis.

MOSAICISM

A person who has at least two cell lines with *two or more different genotypes* (genetic constitutions) is a **mosaic**. Either the autosomes or sex chromosomes may be involved. Usually, the birth defects are less serious than in persons with monosomy or trisomy (e.g., features of the Turner syndrome are not as evident in 45,X/46,XX mosaic females as in the usual 45,X females). **Mosaicism** usually results from nondisjunction during early cleavage of the zygote (see Chapter 3). Mosaicism resulting from loss of a chromosome by *anaphase lagging* also occurs; the chromosomes separate normally, but one of them is delayed in its migration and is eventually lost.

TRIPLOIDY

The most common type of polyploidy is **triploidy** (69 chromosomes). **Triploid fetuses have severe intrauterine growth restriction** (IUGR), with a disproportionately small trunk as well as other defects. Triploidy can result if the second polar body does not separate from the oocyte during the second meiotic division (see Chapter 2); more likely, however, triploidy results when an oocyte is fertilized by two sperms (**dispermy**) almost simultaneously. Triploidy occurs in approximately 2% of embryos but most of them abort spontaneously. Triploid fetuses account for approximately 20% of chromosomally abnormal miscarriages.

TETRAPLOIDY

Doubling of the diploid chromosome number to 92 (tetraploidy) probably occurs during the first cleavage division. Division of this abnormal zygote would subsequently result in an embryo with cells containing 92 chromosomes. **Tetraploid embryos** abort very early; often, all that is recovered is an empty chorionic sac.

Table 19–2	Incidence of Down Syndrome in Neonates
MATERNAL AGE (YEARS)	**INCIDENCE**
20–24	1:1400
25–29	1:1100
30–34	1:700
35	1:350
37	1:225
39	1:140
41	1:85
43	1:50
45+	1:25

Structural Chromosomal Abnormalities

Most abnormalities of chromosome structure result from **chromosome breakage**, followed by reconstitution in an abnormal combination (Fig. 19-8). Chromosome breakage may be induced by various environmental factors, such as irradiation, drugs, chemicals, and viruses. The resulting abnormality in chromosome structure depends on what happens to the broken pieces. The only two aberrations of chromosome structure that are likely to be transmitted from parent to child are *structural rearrangements*, such as inversion and translocation.

Figure 19–7 A teenage boy with Klinefelter syndrome (XXY trisomy). Note the presence of developed breasts; approximately 40% of males with this syndrome have gynecomastia (excessive development of the male mammary glands) and small testes.

Table 19–3	Trisomy of Sex Chromosomes			
CHROMOSOME COMPLEMENT*	**SEX**	**INCIDENCE†**	**USUAL CHARACTERISTICS**	
47,XXX	Female	1:1000	Normal appearance; usually fertile; 15%–25% have mild mental deficiency	
47,XXY	Male	1:1000	Klinefelter syndrome; small testes; hyalinization of seminiferous tubules; aspermatogenesis; often tall, with disproportionately long lower limbs; intelligence is less than in normal siblings; gynecomastia in approximately 40%	
47,XYY	Male	1:1000	Normal appearance; usually tall	

*The numbers designate the total number of chromosomes, including the sex chromosomes (shown after the comma).
†Data from Nussbaum RL, McInnes RR, Willard HF: Thompson & Thompson Genetics in Medicine, 7th ed. Philadelphia, Saunders, 2007.

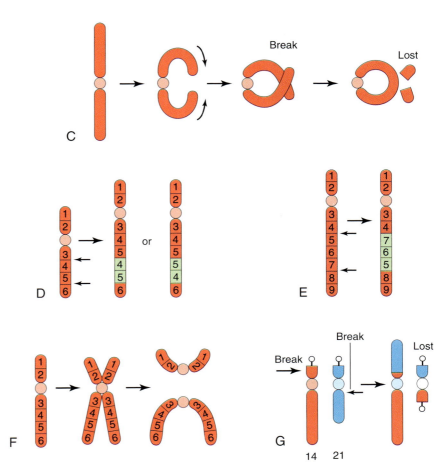

Figure 19–8 Diagrams illustrating various structural abnormalities of chromosomes. **A,** Reciprocal translocation. **B,** Terminal deletion. **C,** Ring chromosome. **D,** Duplication. **E,** Paracentric inversion. **F,** Isochromosome. **G,** Robertsonian translocation. *Arrows* indicate how the structural abnormalities are produced. *(Modified from Nussbaum RL, McInnes RR, Willard HE: Thomson & Thompson Genetics in Medicine, 6th ed. Philadelphia, Saunders, 2004.)*

Translocation

Translocation is the transfer of a piece of one chromosome to a nonhomologous chromosome. If two nonhomologous chromosomes exchange pieces, it is called a *reciprocal translocation* (see Fig. 19-8A). Translocation does not necessarily cause abnormal development. Persons with a translocation between chromosome 21 and chromosome 14, for example (see Fig. 19-8G), are phenotypically normal. Such persons are called *balanced translocation carriers*. They have a tendency, independent of age, to produce germ cells with an abnormal translocation chromosome. Between 3% and 4% of persons with Down syndrome have **translocation trisomies**; that is, the extra chromosome 21 is attached to another chromosome.

Deletion

When a chromosome breaks, a portion of it may be lost (see Fig. 19-8B). A partial terminal deletion from the short arm of chromosome 5 causes **cri du chat syndrome**. Affected neonates have a weak, cat-like cry at birth; growth delay with microcephaly (abnormally small head); hypertelorism (wide-set eyes); low-set ears; and micrognathia (a small jaw). They are severely mentally challenged (retardation) and have congenital heart disease.

A **ring chromosome** is a type of deletion chromosome from which both ends have been lost and the broken ends have rejoined to form a ring-shaped chromosome (see Fig. 19-8C). **Ring chromosomes** are very rare, but they have been found for all chromosomes. These abnormal

DUPLICATIONS

Duplications may be manifested as a duplicated part of a chromosome located within a chromosome (see Fig. 19-8*D*), as a duplicated part attached to a chromosome, or as a separate fragment. *Duplications are more common than deletions, and they are less harmful because no loss of genetic material occurs.* Duplication may involve part of a gene, a whole gene, or a series of genes.

INVERSION

Inversion is a chromosomal aberration in which a segment of a chromosome is reversed. *Paracentric inversion* is confined to a single arm of the chromosome (see Fig. 19-8*E*), whereas *pericentric inversion* involves both arms and includes the centromere. Carriers of **pericentric inversions** are at risk for having offspring with birth defects because of unequal crossing over and malsegregation at meiosis.

ISOCHROMOSOMES

The abnormality resulting in **isochromosomes** occurs when the centromere divides transversely instead of longitudinally (see Fig. 19-8*F*). An *isochromosome* is a chromosome in which one arm is missing and the other is duplicated. It appears to be the *most common structural abnormality of the X chromosome.* Persons with this chromosomal abnormality are often short in stature and have other stigmata of the Turner syndrome. These characteristics are related to the loss of an arm of an X chromosome.

chromosomes have been described in persons with Turner syndrome, trisomy 18, and other abnormalities.

Birth Defects Caused by Mutant Genes

Between 7% and 8% of birth defects are caused by **gene defects** (see Fig. 19-1). A **mutation** usually involves a loss or a change in the function of a gene, and is any permanent, heritable change in the sequence of genomic DNA. Because a random change is unlikely to lead to an improvement in development, *most mutations are deleterious and some are lethal.* The *mutation rate* can be increased by a number of environmental agents, such as large doses of radiation. Birth defects resulting from gene mutations are inherited according to **mendelian laws** (the laws of inheritance of single-gene traits that form the basis of the science of genetics); consequently, predictions can be made about the probability of their occurrence in the affected person's children and other relatives.

An example of a *dominantly inherited birth defect* is **achondroplasia**—abnormality in conversion of cartilage to bone—(Fig. 19-9), which results from a *mutation of*

Figure 19–9 A young boy with achondroplasia. Note the short stature, short limbs and fingers, normal length of the trunk, relatively large head, prominent forehead, and depressed nasal bridge.

the complementary DNA in the fibroblast growth factor receptor 3 gene on chromosome 4p. Other birth defects are attributable to *autosomal recessive inheritance.* Autosomal recessive genes manifest themselves only when homozygous; as a consequence, many carriers of these genes (heterozygous persons) are not identified.

Second only to Down syndrome, **fragile X syndrome** is the most common inherited cause of moderate intellectual disability. Autism spectrum disorder is also prevalent in this condition (Fig. 19-10). Fragile X syndrome has a frequency of 1 in 1500 male births and may account for much of the predominance of males in the mentally challenged population.

Several genetic disorders have been linked to the expansion of **trinucleotides** in specific genes. Examples include myotonic dystrophy, Huntington chorea, spinobulbar atrophy (Kennedy disease), and Friedreich ataxia. X-linked recessive genes are usually manifested in affected (homozygous) males, and occasionally in *carrier (heterozygous) females* (e.g., fragile X syndrome).

The **human genome** comprises an estimated 20,000 to 25,000 genes per haploid set, or 3 billion base pairs. Because of the ***Human Genome Project*** and international research collaboration, many disease-causing and birth

Figure 19–10 Fragile X syndrome. **A,** An 8-year-old, mentally deficient boy with this syndrome exhibiting a relatively normal appearance, with a long face and prominent ears. **B,** His 6-year-old sister also has this syndrome. She has a mild learning disability and similar features of long face and prominent ears. Note the strabismus (crossed right eye).

defect–causing mutations in genes have been and will continue to be identified. Most genes will be sequenced and their specific function determined. Understanding the cause of birth defects will require an improvement in our understanding of gene expression during early development.

Most genes that are expressed in a cell are expressed in a wide variety of cells. These *housekeeping genes* are involved in basic cellular metabolic functions, such as nucleic acid and protein synthesis, cytoskeleton and organelle biogenesis, and nutrient transport and mechanisms. The *specialty genes* are expressed at specific times in specific cells and define the hundreds of different cell types that make up the human organism. An essential aspect of developmental biology is the regulation of gene expression. Regulation is often achieved by transcription factors, which bind to regulatory or promoter elements of specific genes.

Genomic imprinting is an epigenetic process whereby the female and male germ lines confer a sex-specific mark on a chromosome subregion, so that only the paternal or maternal allele of a gene is active in the offspring. In other words, the sex of the transmitting parent influences the expression or nonexpression of certain genes in the offspring.

BIRTH DEFECTS CAUSED BY ENVIRONMENTAL FACTORS

Although the embryo is well protected in the uterus, certain environmental agents—**teratogens**—may cause developmental disruptions after maternal exposure to them (Table 19-4). A teratogen is *any agent that can produce a birth defect or increase the incidence of a defect in a population.* Environmental factors, such as infections and drugs, may simulate genetic conditions, such as when two or more children of normal parents are affected. *The important principle to remember is that not everything that is familial is genetic.*

The organs and parts of an embryo are most sensitive to teratogenic agents during periods of rapid differentiation (Fig. 19-11). Because molecular signaling and embryonic induction precede morphologic differentiation, the period during which structures are sensitive to interference by teratogens often precedes the stage of their visible development.

Teratogens do not appear to be effective in causing birth defects until cellular differentiation has begun; however, their earlier actions may cause the death of an embryo. The exact mechanisms by which many drugs, chemicals, and other environmental factors disrupt embryonic development and induce abnormalities are unclear.

Rapid progress in molecular biology is providing additional information on the genetic control of differentiation, as well as the cascade of molecular signals and factors controlling gene expression and pattern formation. Researchers are now directing increasing attention to the molecular mechanisms of abnormal development in an attempt to understand better the pathogenesis of birth defects.

Principles of Teratogenesis

When considering the possible teratogenicity of an agent, such as a drug or a chemical, three factors are important to consider:

- Critical periods of development (see Fig. 19-11)
- Dose of the drug or chemical
- Genotype (genetic constitution) of the embryo

Table 19–4 Some Teratogens Known to Cause Human Birth Defects

AGENTS	MOST COMMON CONGENITAL BIRTH DEFECTS
Drugs	
Alcohol	Fetal alcohol syndrome; IUGR; mental deficiency; microcephaly; ocular defects; joint abnormalities; short palpebral fissures; fetal alcohol spectrum disorders; cognitive and neurobehavioral disturbances
Androgens and high doses of progestogens	Varying degree of masculinization of female fetuses; ambiguous external genitalia (labial fusion and clitoral hypertrophy)
Cocaine	IUGR; prematurity; microcephaly; cerebral infarction; urogenital defects; neurobehavioral disturbances
Diethylstilbestrol	Abnormalities of uterus and vagina; cervical erosion and ridges
Isotretinoin (13-*cis*-retinoic acid)	Craniofacial abnormalities; neural tube defects such as spina bifida cystica; cardiovascular defects; cleft palate; thymic aplasia
Lithium carbonate	Various birth defects, usually involving the heart and great vessels
Methotrexate	IUGR; multiple birth defects, especially skeletal (involving the face, cranium, limbs, and vertebral column) and renal
Misoprostol	Abnormal development of the limbs; ocular defects; cranial nerve defects; autism spectrum disorders
Phenytoin (Dilantin)	Fetal hydantoin syndrome; IUGR; microcephaly; mental deficiency; ridged metopic suture; inner epicanthal folds; eyelid ptosis; broad, depressed nasal bridge; phalangeal hypoplasia
Tetracycline	Stained teeth; hypoplasia of enamel
Thalidomide	Abnormal development of the limbs: meromelia (partial absence of limb) and amelia (complete absence of limb); facial defects; systemic defects (e.g., cardiac and kidney defects and ocular anomalies)
Trimethadione	Developmental delay; V-shaped eyebrows; low-set ears; cleft lip and/or palate
Valproic acid	Craniofacial defects; neural tube defects; often hydrocephalus; heart and skeletal defects; poor postnatal cognitive development
Warfarin	Nasal hypoplasia; stippled epiphyses; hypoplastic phalanges; eye defects; mental deficiency
Chemicals	
Methylmercury	Cerebral atrophy; spasticity; seizures; mental deficiency
Polychlorinated biphenyls	IUGR; skin discoloration
Infections	
Cytomegalovirus	Microcephaly; chorioretinitis; sensorineural loss; delayed psychomotor and mental development; hepatosplenomegaly; hydrocephaly; cerebral palsy; brain (periventricular) calcification
Hepatitis B virus	Preterm birth; fetal macrosomia
Herpes simplex virus	Skin vesicles and scarring; chorioretinitis; hepatomegaly; thrombocytopenia; petechiae; hemolytic anemia; hydranencephaly
Human parvovirus B19	Fetal anemia; nonimmune hydrops fetalis; fetal death
Rubella virus	IUGR; postnatal growth retardation; cardiac and great vessel abnormalities; microcephaly; sensorineural deafness; cataract; microphthalmos; glaucoma; pigmented retinopathy; mental deficiency; neonatal bleeding; hepatosplenomegaly; osteopathy; tooth defects
Toxoplasma gondii	Microcephaly; mental deficiency; microphthalmia; hydrocephaly; chorioretinitis; cerebral calcifications; hearing loss; neurologic disturbances
Treponema pallidum	Hydrocephalus; congenital deafness; mental deficiency; abnormal teeth and bones
Varicella virus	Cutaneous scars (dermatome distribution); neurologic defects (e.g., limb paresis, hydrocephaly, seizures); cataracts; microphthalmia; Horner syndrome; optic atrophy; nystagmus; chorioretinitis; microcephaly; mental deficiency; skeletal defects (e.g., hypoplasia of limbs, fingers, and toes); urogenital defects
High Levels of Ionizing Radiation	Microcephaly; mental deficiency; skeletal defects; growth retardation; cataracts

IUGR, Intrauterine growth restriction.

Critical Periods of Human Development

An embryo's susceptibility to a teratogen depends on its stage of development when an agent, such as a drug, is present. The most critical period in development is when cell differentiation and morphogenesis are at their peak. *The most critical period for brain development is from 3 to 16 weeks* (see Fig. 19-11), but its development may be disrupted after this time because the brain is differentiating and growing rapidly at birth.

Teratogens (e.g., drugs) may cause limitation of mental development during the embryonic and fetal periods. *Tooth development continues long after birth*; hence, the development of the permanent teeth may be disrupted by *tetracyclines* from 18 weeks prenatal to 16 years of age.

The skeletal system has a prolonged critical period of development, extending into childhood; hence, the growth of skeletal tissues provides a good gauge of general growth. Environmental disturbances during the first 2 weeks after fertilization may interfere with cleavage of the zygote and implantation of the blastocyst, which may cause early death and spontaneous abortion of the embryo (see Fig. 19-11).

Development of the embryo is most easily disrupted when the tissues and organs are forming (see Fig. 19-11). During this **organogenetic period (fourth to eighth weeks)**, teratogenic agents may induce major birth defects. Physiologic defects—minor morphologic defects of the external ear, for example—and functional disturbances, such

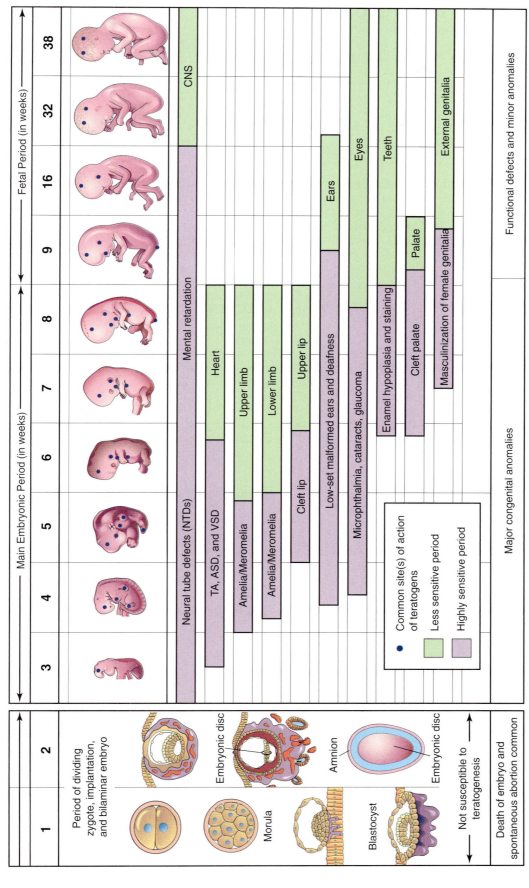

Figure 19–11 Critical periods in human prenatal development. During the first 2 weeks, the embryo is not usually susceptible to teratogens. At this point, a teratogen damages all or most of the cells, resulting in death of the embryo, or damages only a few cells, allowing the conceptus to recover and the embryo to develop without birth defects. The purple areas denote highly sensitive periods, when major defects may be produced (e.g., amelia, absence of limbs). The green sections indicate stages that are less sensitive to teratogens, when minor birth defects may be induced. *ASD*, Atrial septal defect; *CNS*, central nervous system; *TA*, truncus arteriosus; *VSD*, ventricular septal defect.

as limitation of mental development, are likely to result from disruption of development during the fetal period. *Each part, tissue, and organ of an embryo has a critical period during which its development may be disrupted* (see Fig. 19-11). The type of birth defect produced depends on which parts, tissues, and organs are most susceptible at the time the teratogen is active.

Embryologic timetables, such as the one in Fig. 19-11, are helpful when considering the cause of birth defects. However, it is incorrect to assume that defects always result from a single event occurring during the critical period of development, or that it is possible to determine from these timetables the day on which a defect was produced. What is known is that the teratogen would have to disrupt development of the tissue, part, or organ before the end of the critical period. *The critical period of limb development, for example, is 21 to 36 days after fertilization.*

Human Teratogens

Awareness that certain agents can disrupt prenatal development offers the opportunity to prevent some birth defects. For example, if women are made aware of the harmful effects of drugs, alcohol, environmental chemicals, and viruses, most pregnant women will avoid exposure to these teratogenic agents.

Drugs vary considerably in their teratogenicity. Some teratogens, such as thalidomide, cause severe disruption of development if administered during the organogenetic period of certain parts (e.g., the limbs) of the embryo (see Fig. 19-15). Other teratogens cause mental and growth restriction of embryos (see Table 19-4). Drug consumption tends to be higher during the critical periods of development among heavy smokers and drinkers. Despite this, *fewer than 2% of birth defects are caused by drugs and chemicals.* Only a few drugs have been positively implicated as human teratogenic agents, but new agents continue to be identified. It is best for women to avoid using all medications during the first trimester unless a strong medical reason exists for their use.

Cigarette Smoking

Maternal smoking during pregnancy is a well-established cause of **IUGR.** Despite warnings that cigarette smoking is harmful to the embryo/fetus, more than 25% of women continue to smoke during pregnancy. In heavy cigarette smokers (20 per day), premature delivery is twice as frequent as in mothers who do not smoke. In addition, the infants of smokers weigh less than normal.

A population-based case-control study revealed that conotruncal and atrioventricular septal defects occur more frequently in infants of mothers who smoke during the first trimester of pregnancy.

Nicotine constricts the uterine blood vessels, thereby causing a decrease in uterine blood flow and reducing the supply of oxygen and nutrients available to the embryo or fetus from the maternal blood in the intervillous space of the placenta. High levels of *carboxyhemoglobin,* resulting from cigarette smoking, appear in the maternal and fetal blood, and may alter the capacity of the blood to transport oxygen. As a result, chronic fetal hypoxia (decrease in the oxygen level to below normal) may occur, affecting fetal growth and development.

Alcohol

Alcoholism is a drug abuse problem that affects 1% to 2% of women of childbearing age. Both moderate and high levels of alcohol intake during early pregnancy may result in alterations in the growth and morphogenesis of the fetus; the greater the intake, the more severe the signs. Infants born to mothers with chronic alcoholism exhibit a specific pattern of defects, including prenatal and postnatal growth and mental deficiency and other defects (Fig. 19-12). This pattern of defects, **fetal alcohol syndrome,** is detected in 1 to 2 infants per 1000 live births. *Maternal alcohol abuse is now believed to be the most common cause of mental deficiency.*

Even moderate maternal alcohol consumption (e.g., 1–2 oz daily) may produce **fetal alcohol effects**—children with behavioral and learning difficulties, for example—especially if the drinking is associated with malnutrition. **Binge drinking** (heavy consumption of alcohol for 1–3 days) during pregnancy is very likely to produce fetal alcohol effects. The susceptible period of brain development spans the major part of gestation; therefore, **the safest advice is total abstinence from alcohol during pregnancy.**

Androgens and Progestogens

Androgens and progestogens may affect the female fetus, producing masculinization of the external genitalia (Fig. 19-13). The preparations that should be avoided contain

Figure 19–12 Infant with fetal alcohol syndrome. Note the thin upper lip, short palpebral fissures, flat nasal bridge, short nose, and elongated and poorly formed philtrum (vertical groove in the median part of the upper lip). Severe maternal alcohol abuse is believed to be the most common environmental cause of mental deficiency.

Figure 19–13 Masculinized external genitalia of a female infant with a 46,XX chromosome constitution. Observe the enlarged clitoris and fused labia majora. The *arrow* indicates the single orifice of a urogenital sinus. The virilization (mature masculine characteristics in a female) was caused by excessive androgens produced by the suprarenal glands during the fetal period (congenital adrenal hyperplasia).

progestins, ethisterone, or *norethisterone.* From a practical standpoint, the teratogenic risk of these hormones is low. However, progestin exposure during the critical period of development is also associated with an increased prevalence of *cardiovascular defects,* and exposure of male fetuses during this period may double the incidence of *hypospadias* in the offspring (see Chapter 13, Fig. 13-26).

Oral contraceptive (birth control) pills containing progestogens and estrogens, when taken during the early stages of an unrecognized pregnancy, are believed to be teratogenic agents. Many infants of mothers who took *progestogen-estrogen birth control pills* during the critical period of development have been found to exhibit the VACTERL syndrome—*v*ertebral, *a*nal, *c*ardiac, *t*racheal, *e*sophageal, *r*enal, and *l*imb anomalies.

Antibiotics

Tetracyclines cross the placental membrane and are deposited in the embryo's bones and teeth at sites of active calcification. As little as 1 g daily of **tetracycline** during the third trimester of pregnancy can produce yellow staining of the deciduous teeth. Tetracycline therapy during the fourth to ninth months of pregnancy may also cause tooth defects (e.g., enamel hypoplasia—yellow to brown **discoloration of the teeth**) and diminished growth of the long bones (see Chapter 18, Fig. 18-10). Moreover, more than 30 cases of hearing deficit and CN VIII damage have been reported in infants exposed to **streptomycin** derivatives in utero. By contrast, *penicillin* has been used extensively during pregnancy and appears to be harmless to the embryo/fetus.

Anticoagulants

All anticoagulants except heparin cross the placental membrane and may cause hemorrhage in the embryo/fetus. **Warfarin**, an anticoagulant, is definitely a teratogen. The period of greatest sensitivity is 6 to 12 weeks after fertilization, or 8 to 14 weeks after the last normal menstrual period. Second- and third-trimester exposure may result in mental deficiency, optic nerve atrophy, and microcephaly. Heparin does not cross the placental membrane, and so is the drug of choice for pregnant women requiring anticoagulant therapy.

Anticonvulsants

Epilepsy affects approximately 1 in 200 pregnant women, and these women require treatment with an anticonvulsant. Of the anticonvulsant drugs available, **phenytoin** has been definitively identified as a teratogen. **Fetal hydantoin syndrome** occurs in 5% to 10% of children born to mothers treated with phenytoins or hydantoin anticonvulsants (Fig. 19-14).

Valproic acid has been the drug of choice for the management of different types of epilepsy; however, its use by pregnant women has led to a pattern of birth defects consisting of poorer postnatal cognitive development and craniofacial, heart, and limb defects. There is also an increased risk of **neural tube defects**. Phenobarbital is considered to be a safe antiepileptic drug for use during pregnancy.

Antineoplastic Agents

Tumor-inhibiting chemicals are highly teratogenic. This is not surprising because these agents inhibit mitosis in rapidly dividing cells. It is recommended that they be avoided, especially during the first trimester of pregnancy. **Methotrexate**, *a folic acid antagonist* and a derivative of *aminopterin,* is a known potent teratogen that produces major congenital defects.

Angiotensin-Converting Enzyme Inhibitors

Exposure of the fetus to angiotensin-converting enzyme inhibitors, used as antihypertensive agents, causes oligohydramnios, fetal death, long-lasting hypoplasia of the bones of the calvaria, IUGR, and renal dysfunction.

Retinoic Acid (Vitamin A)

Isotretinoin (13-*cis*-retinoic acid), used for the oral treatment of severe cystic acne, is teratogenic in humans, even at very low doses. The critical period for exposure appears to be from the third to the fifth week (5–7 weeks after the last normal menstrual period). The risk of **spontaneous abortion** and birth defects after exposure to **retinoic acid** is high. Postnatal follow-up studies of children exposed to **isotretinoin** in utero showed significant **neuropsychological impairment**. Vitamin A is a valuable and necessary nutrient during pregnancy, but long-term exposure to large doses of vitamin A is unwise because of insufficient evidence to rule out a teratogenic risk.

Salicylates

Acetylsalicylic acid, or **aspirin**, is the most commonly ingested drug during pregnancy. Large doses are

Figure 19–14 Fetal hydantoin syndrome. **A,** This young girl has a learning disability. Note the unusual ears, the wide spacing of the eyes, the epicanthal folds, the short nose, and the long philtrum. Her mother has epilepsy and took phenytoin (Dilantin) throughout her pregnancy. **B,** Right hand of an infant with severe digital hypoplasia (short fingers), born to a mother who took phenytoin (Dilantin) throughout her pregnancy. (**B,** From Chodirker BN, Chudley AE, Persaud TVN: Possible prenatal hydantoin effect in child born to a nonepileptic mother. Am J Med Genet 27:373, 1987.)

potentially harmful to the embryo/fetus. Studies indicate that low doses appear not to be teratogenic.

Acetaminophen

Acetaminophen (paracetamol), a common, over-the-counter medication, is widely used for the treatment of headache, fever, pain, and symptoms of the common cold. A large survey of women who consumed this drug during early pregnancy showed that their offspring had an increased incidence of behavioral problems, including attention-deficit/hyperactivity disorder.

Thyroid Drugs

Iodides readily cross the placental membrane and interfere with thyroxin production. They may also cause thyroid enlargement and **cretinism** (arrested physical and mental development and dystrophy of bones and soft tissue). *Maternal iodine deficiency* may cause *congenital cretinism*. The administration of antithyroid drugs for the treatment of maternal thyroid disorders may cause *congenital goiter* if the dose administered exceeds that required to control the disease.

Tranquilizers

Thalidomide is a potent teratogen. Nearly 12,000 neonates had birth defects caused by this drug. The characteristic feature of *thalidomide syndrome* is **meromelia**—*phocomelia*, or "seal limbs" (Fig. 19-15). It has been well established clinically that the period when thalidomide causes congenital defects is from 20 to 36 days after fertilization (34–50 days after the last normal menstrual period). *Thalidomide is absolutely contraindicated in women of childbearing age.*

Psychotropic Drugs

Lithium is the drug of choice for long-term maintenance therapy in patients with mental illness—*bipolar disorder*; however, it has been known to cause birth defects, mainly of the heart and great vessels, in neonates born to mothers given the drug early in pregnancy. Although **lithium carbonate** is a human teratogen, the U.S. Food and Drug Administration has stated that the agent may be used during pregnancy if "in the opinion of the physician the potential benefits outweigh the possible hazards."

Benzodiazepines are psychoactive drugs that are frequently prescribed for pregnant women. These drugs include *diazepam* and *oxazepam*, which readily cross the placental membrane (see Chapter 8, Fig. 8-7). The use of these drugs during the first trimester of pregnancy is associated with transient withdrawal symptoms and craniofacial defects in neonates. **Selective serotonin reuptake inhibitors** are used to treat depression during pregnancy. Use of these drugs by the mother may lead to transient neurobehavioral disturbances, autism spectrum disorder, and persistent pulmonary hypertension in infants.

Illicit Drugs

Cocaine is one of the most commonly abused illicit drugs in North America, and its increasing use by women of

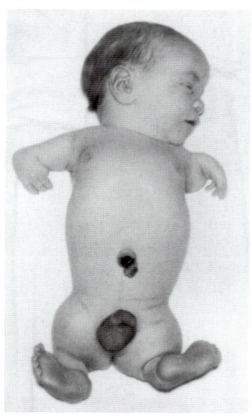

Figure 19–15 Male neonate with malformed limbs (meromelia—congenital absence of parts of the limbs) caused by maternal ingestion of thalidomide during the critical period of limb development. *(From Moore KL: The vulnerable embryo: causes of malformation in man. Manitoba Med Rev 43:306, 1963.)*

childbearing age is of major concern. Many reports deal with the prenatal effects of cocaine; these include spontaneous abortion, prematurity, and diverse birth defects in their infants.

Methadone, used for the treatment of heroin addiction, is considered a "behavioral teratogen," as is heroin. Infants of narcotic-dependent women have lower birth weights, and infants of women receiving maintenance methadone therapy have been found to have *central nervous system dysfunction* and smaller head circumferences than nonexposed infants. There is also concern about the long-term postnatal developmental effects of methadone.

Environmental Chemicals as Teratogens

There has been increasing concern about the possible teratogenicity of environmental, industrial, and agricultural chemicals, pollutants, and food additives. Most of these chemicals have not been positively implicated as teratogens in humans.

Organic Mercury

Infants of mothers whose main diet during pregnancy consists of fish containing abnormally high levels of organic mercury acquire fetal **Minamata disease**—neurologic and behavioral disturbances resembling those associated with cerebral palsy. **Methylmercury** *is a teratogen* that causes cerebral atrophy, spasticity, seizures, and mental retardation.

Lead

Lead is abundantly present in the workplace and the environment. The lead passes the placental membrane and accumulates in fetal tissues. Prenatal exposure to lead is associated with an increased incidence of abortions, fetal defects, IUGR, and functional deficits.

Polychlorinated Biphenyls

Polychlorinated biphenyls (PCBs) are teratogenic chemicals that produce IUGR and skin discoloration in fetuses exposed to these agents. The main dietary source of PCBs in North America is probably sport fish caught in contaminated waters.

Infectious Agents as Teratogens

Rubella (German Measles)

The **rubella virus** crosses the placental membrane and infects the embryo/fetus. In cases of primary maternal infection during the first trimester of pregnancy, the overall risk of embryonic or fetal infection is approximately 20%. The clinical features of **congenital rubella syndrome** are *cataracts, congenital glaucoma, cardiac defects, and deafness* (Fig. 19-16). The earlier in pregnancy that maternal rubella infection occurs, the greater is the danger that the embryo will be malformed.

Cytomegalovirus

This virus is the most common viral infection of the fetus. Because the disease seems to be fatal when it affects the embryo, most pregnancies likely end in spontaneous abortion when the infection occurs during the first trimester. Later in pregnancy, *cytomegalovirus infection may result in IUGR and severe birth defects*. Of particular concern are cases of asymptomatic cytomegalovirus infection, which are often associated with audiologic, neurologic, and neurobehavioral disturbances in infancy.

Herpes Simplex Virus

Maternal infection with **herpes simplex virus** in early pregnancy increases the abortion rate threefold, and infection after the 20th week is associated with an increased rate of prematurity as well as birth defects (e.g., microcephaly and mental deficiency). Infection of the fetus with herpes simplex virus usually occurs very late in pregnancy, probably most often during delivery.

Varicella (Chickenpox)

Varicella and **herpes zoster** (shingles) are caused by the same virus, **varicella-zoster virus, which is highly infectious.** There is convincing evidence that maternal varicella infection during the first 4 months of pregnancy causes several birth defects (muscle atrophy and mental deficiency). There is a 20% incidence of these or other defects when the infection occurs during the critical period of development (see Fig. 19-11).

Figure 19–16   **A,** Typical appearance of a congenital cataract that may have been caused by the rubella virus. Cardiac defects and deafness are other congenital defects common to this infection. **B,** Clouding of the cornea caused by congenital glaucoma. Corneal clouding may also result from infection, trauma, or metabolic disorders. *(From Guercio J, Martyn L: Congenital malformations of the eye and orbit. Otolaryngol Clin North Am 40:113, 2007.)*

Human Immunodeficiency Virus

Human immunodeficiency virus (HIV) is the retrovirus that causes *acquired immunodeficiency syndrome* **(AIDS)**. Infection of pregnant women with HIV is associated with serious health problems in the fetus. These include infection of the fetus, preterm delivery, low birth weight, IUGR, microcephaly, and craniofacial defects. Transmission of the HIV virus to the fetus can occur during pregnancy, labor, or delivery.

Toxoplasmosis

Maternal infection with the intracellular parasite *Toxoplasma gondii* is usually through one of the following routes:

- Eating raw or poorly cooked meat (usually pork or lamb containing *Toxoplasma* cysts)
- Close contact with infected domestic animals (usually cats) or infected soil

The **T. gondii organism** crosses the placental membrane and infects the fetus, causing destructive changes in the brain that result in *mental deficiency* and other birth defects. Mothers of infants with birth defects are often unaware of having had **toxoplasmosis**. Because animals (cats, dogs, rabbits, and other domestic and wild animals) may be infected with this parasite, pregnant women should avoid contact with them. In addition, unpasteurized milk should be avoided.

Congenital Syphilis

Syphilis is increasing in its prevalence in many countries, and pregnant women are consequently often affected. Syphilis infection affects approximately 1 in 10,000 neonates in the United States. *Treponema pallidum*, the small, spiral microorganism that causes syphilis, rapidly crosses the placental membrane as early as 6 to 8 weeks of development. The fetus can become infected at any stage of the disease or at any stage of pregnancy. **Primary maternal infections** (acquired during pregnancy and left untreated) nearly always cause serious fetal infection and birth defects. However, adequate treatment of the mother kills the organism. If the mother remains untreated, only 20% of women will deliver a normal neonate. **Secondary maternal infections** (acquired before pregnancy) seldom result in fetal disease and birth defects.

Radiation as a Teratogen

Exposure to **high levels of ionizing radiation** may injure embryonic cells, resulting in cell death, chromosomal injury, mental deficiency, and deficient physical growth. The severity of the embryonic damage is related to the absorbed dose, the dose rate, and the stage of embryonic or fetal development when the exposure occurs. Accidental exposure of pregnant women to radiation is a common cause for anxiety.

No conclusive proof exists that human congenital defects have been caused by diagnostic levels of radiation (<10 rads). Scattered radiation from a radiographic examination of a part of the body that is not near the uterus (e.g., thorax, sinuses, teeth) produces a dose of only a few millirads, which is not teratogenic to the embryo. The recommended limit of maternal exposure of the whole body to radiation from all sources is 500 mrad (0.005 Gy) for the entire gestational period.

Maternal Factors as Teratogens

Poorly controlled **diabetes mellitus** in the mother with persisting hyperglycemia and ketosis, particularly during embryogenesis, is associated with a two- to threefold higher incidence of birth defects. Neonates of a diabetic mother are usually large (**macrosomia**). The common defects include *holoprosencephaly* (failure of the forebrain to divide into hemispheres), *meroencephaly* (partial absence of the brain), sacral agenesis, vertebral defects, congenital heart defects, and limb defects.

If left untreated, women who are homozygous for phenylalanine hydroxylase deficiency—**phenylketonuria**—and those with **hyperphenylalaninemia** are at increased risk for having offspring with **microcephaly** (abnormal smallness of the head), cardiac defects, mental deficiency, and IUGR. The congenital defects can be prevented if the mother with phenylketonuria follows a phenylalanine-restricted diet before and during pregnancy.

Mechanical Factors as Teratogens

Clubfoot and congenital dislocation of the hip may be caused by mechanical forces, particularly in a malformed uterus. Such birth defects may be caused by any factor that restricts the mobility of the fetus, thereby causing prolonged compression in an abnormal posture. A significantly reduced quantity of amniotic fluid *(oligohydramnios)* may result in mechanically induced deformation of the limbs, such as hyperextension of the knee. **Intrauterine amputations** or other defects caused by local constriction during fetal growth may result from **amniotic bands** (see Chapter 8, Fig. 8-14), rings formed as a result of rupture of the amnion during early pregnancy.

BIRTH DEFECTS CAUSED BY MULTIFACTORIAL INHERITANCE

Many common birth defects (e.g., cleft lip, with or without cleft palate) have familial distributions consistent with multifactorial inheritance (see Fig. 19-1). Multifactorial inheritance may be represented by a model in which one's "liability" for a disorder is a continuous variable determined by a combination of genetic and environmental factors, with a developmental threshold dividing individuals with the defect from those without it. Multifactorial *traits are often single major defects*, such as cleft lip, isolated cleft palate, and neural tube defects. Some of these defects may also occur as part of the phenotype in syndromes determined by single-gene inheritance, chromosomal abnormality, or an environmental teratogen. The recurrence risks used for genetic counseling of families having birth defects that have been determined by multifactorial inheritance are *empirical risks* based on the frequency of the defect in the general population, and in different categories of relatives. In individual families, such estimates may be inaccurate because they are usually averages for the population rather than precise probabilities for the individual family.

CLINICALLY ORIENTED QUESTIONS

1. If a pregnant woman takes aspirin in normal doses, will it cause congenital birth defects?

2. If a woman is a drug addict, will her child show signs of drug addiction?

3. Are all drugs tested for teratogenicity before they are marketed? If the answer is "yes," why are these teratogens still sold?

4. Is cigarette smoking during pregnancy harmful to the embryo or fetus? If the answer is "yes," would refraining from inhaling cigarette smoke be safer?

5. Are any drugs safe to take during pregnancy? If so, what are they?

The answers to these questions are at the back of this book.

The Cellular and Molecular Basis of Development

Jeffrey T. Wigle and David D. Eisenstat

During embryonic development, undifferentiated precursor cells differentiate and organize into the complex structures found in functional adult tissues. This process requires cells to integrate many different cues, both intrinsic and extrinsic, for development to occur properly. These cues control the proliferation, differentiation, and migration of cells to determine the final size and shape of the developing organs. Disruption of these signaling pathways can result in human developmental disorders and birth defects. Interestingly, these key developmental signaling pathways may also be co-opted in the adult by diseases such as cancer.

Although there are diverse changes that occur during embryogenesis, the differentiation of many different cell types is regulated through a relatively restricted set of molecular signaling pathways:

- **Intercellular communication:** Development involves the interaction of a cell with its neighboring cell either directly (gap junctions) or indirectly (cell adhesion molecules).
- **Morphogens:** These are diffusible molecules that specify which cell type will be generated at a specific anatomical location. Morphogens also direct the migration of cells and their processes to their final destination. These include retinoic acid, transforming growth factor-β (TGF-β)/bone morphogenetic proteins (BMPs), and the hedgehog and Wnt protein families (see Table 20-1 for gene and protein nomenclature).

321

Table 20–1		International Nomenclature Standards for Genes and Proteins	
Gene	Human	Italics, all letters capitalized	*PAX6*
	Mouse	Italics, first letter capitalized	*Pax6*
Protein	Human	Roman, all letters capitalized	PAX6
	Mouse	Roman, all letters capitalized	PAX6

- **Receptor tyrosine kinases (RTKs):** Many growth factors signal by binding to and activating membrane-bound RTKs. These kinases are essential for the regulation of cellular proliferation, apoptosis, and migration.
- **Notch-Delta:** This pathway often specifies the fate of precursor cells.
- **Transcription factors:** This set of evolutionarily conserved proteins activates or represses downstream genes that are essential for a number of cellular processes. Many transcription factors are members of the homeobox or helix-loop-helix families. Their activity can be regulated by all of the other pathways described in this chapter.
- **Epigenetics:** Epigenetics relates to the heritable properties of gene function that do not occur as a result of changes to the sequence of the DNA code. This can include variations in DNA packaging and DNA chemical modification.
- **Stem cells:** Stem cells in the embryo can give rise to all cells and tissues in the developing organism. Adult stem cells maintain tissues in the mature organism. These types of stem cells and induced pluripotent stem cells (iPS) are potential sources of cells for regeneration and/or repair of injured or degenerating cells and organs.

INTERCELLULAR COMMUNICATION

Cells communicate with each other in several ways.

Gap Junctions

Gap junctions are channels that permit ions and small molecules (<1 kD) to directly pass from one cell to another, known as gap junctional intercellular communication (GJIC). However, large proteins and nucleic acids cannot transfer through gap junctions. Gap junctions are made from hemi-channels present on the surface of each cell known as *connexons*. Each connexon is made up of six *connexin* molecules that form hexamers. In early development, gap junctions are usually open, permitting exchange of small molecules in relatively large regions. However, as development proceeds, GJIC is more restricted, with establishment of boundaries, such as in the rhombomeres of the developing hindbrain. Gap junctions are particularly important for electrical coupling in the heart and brain. Mutations of specific connexin molecules are associated with human diseases (e.g., mutation of *Cx43* is associated with atherosclerosis).

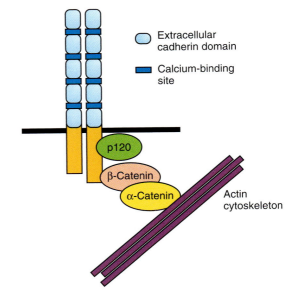

Figure 20–1 Structure of cadherin. The cadherin extracellular domain contains four calcium-binding sites and five repeated domains called extracellular cadherin domains. Each cadherin molecule forms a homodimer. In the intracellular domain, cadherin binds directly to p120-catenin and to β-catenin, which binds to α-catenin. This complex links the cadherin molecules to the actin cytoskeleton.

Cell Adhesion Molecules

Cell adhesion molecules have large extracellular domains that interact with extracellular matrix components or adhesion molecules on neighboring cells. These molecules often contain a transmembrane segment and a short cytoplasmic domain, which regulates intracellular signaling cascades. An example of cell adhesion molecules is the cadherins, which have important roles during embryonic development.

Cadherins are critical for embryonic morphogenesis as they regulate the separation of cell layers (endothelial and epidermal), cell migration, cell sorting, establishment of well-defined boundaries, synaptic connections, and in the growth cones of neurons. These properties result from cadherins mediating the interaction between the cell and its extracellular milieu (both neighboring cells and *extracellular matrix*). Cadherins were originally classified by their site of expression; for example, E-cadherin is highly expressed in epithelial cells, whereas N-cadherin is highly expressed in neural cells.

A typical cadherin molecule has a large extracellular domain, a transmembrane domain, and an intracellular tail (Fig. 20-1). The extracellular domain contains five extracellular repeats and has four Ca^{2+}-binding sites. Cadherins form dimers that interact with cadherin dimers in adjacent cells. These complexes are found clustered in *adherens junctions*, which result in the formation of a tight barrier between epithelial or endothelial cells. Via its intracellular domain, cadherin binds to p120-catenin, β-catenin, and α-catenin. These proteins connect cadherin to the cytoskeleton. E-cadherin expression is lost as epithelial cells transition to mesenchymal cells (this is known as the *epithelial-to-mesenchymal transition*

[EMT]). EMT is required for the formation of neural crest cells during development, and the same process also occurs during tumor development.

MORPHOGENS

Extrinsic signaling by morphogens guides the differentiation and migration of cells during development, determining the morphology and function of developing tissues and organs (see Chapter 6). Many morphogens are found in concentration gradients in the embryo. Different morphogens can be expressed in opposing gradients in the dorsoventral, anteroposterior (AP), and mediolateral axes. The fate of a specific cell can be determined by its location along these different gradients. Cells can also be attracted or repelled by morphogens depending on the set of receptors expressed on the cell surface.

Retinoic Acid

The AP axis of the embryo is crucial for determining the correct location for structures such as limbs and for the patterning of the nervous system. For decades, it has been clinically evident that alterations in the level of vitamin A (retinol) in the diet (excessive or insufficient amounts) can lead to the development of congenital malformations (see Chapter 19). The bioactive form of vitamin A is retinoic acid, which is formed by enzymatic oxidation by retinol aldehyde dehydrogenase and subsequently retinal aldehyde dehydrogenase. Free levels of retinoic acid can be modulated by cellular retinoic acid–binding proteins that sequester retinoic acid. Retinoic acid can also be actively degraded into inactive metabolites by enzymes such as CYP26 (Fig. 20-2).

Normally, retinoic acid acts to "posteriorize" the body plan, and either excessive retinoic acid or inhibition of its degradation leads to a truncated body axis where structures have a more posterior nature. In contrast, insufficient retinoic acid or defects in the enzymes (e.g., retinal aldehyde dehydrogenase) will lead to a more "anteriorized" structure. At the molecular level, retinoic acid binds to its receptors (transcription factors) inside the cell, and their activation will regulate the expression of downstream genes. Hox genes are crucial targets of retinoic acid receptors in development. Because of their profound influence on early development, retinoids are powerful teratogens, especially during the first trimester.

Transforming Growth Factor-β/ Bone Morphogenetic Protein

Members of the TGF-β superfamily include TGF-β, BMPs, and activin. These molecules contribute to the establishment of dorsoventral patterning, cell fate decisions, and formation of specific organs and systems, including the kidneys, nervous system, skeleton, and blood. In humans, there are three different forms of TGF-β (isoforms TGF-β_1, TGF-β_2, and TGF-β_3).

Binding of these ligands to transmembrane kinase receptors results in phosphorylation of intracellular receptor-associated Smad proteins (R-Smads) (Fig. 20-3).

Figure 20–2 Regulation of retinoic acid metabolism and signaling. Dietary retinol (vitamin A) is converted to retinal via the action of retinol dehydrogenases. The concentration of free retinal is controlled by the action of cellular retinal-binding proteins. Similarly, retinal is converted to retinoic acid by retinal dehydrogenases, and its free level is modulated by sequestration by cellular retinoic acid–binding proteins and degradation by CYP26. The bioactive form of retinoic acid is all-*trans* retinoic acid.

The Smad proteins are a large family of intercellular proteins that are divided into three classes: receptor-activated (R-Smads), common-partner Smads (co-Smads [e.g., Smad4]), and inhibitory Smads (I-Smads). R-Smad/Smad4 complexes regulate target gene transcription by interacting with other proteins or as transcription factors by directly binding to DNA. The diversity of TGF-β ligand, receptor, and R-Smad combinations contributes to particular developmental and cell-specific processes, often in combination with other signaling pathways.

Sonic Hedgehog

Sonic hedgehog (Shh) was the first mammalian ortholog of the *Drosophila* gene hedgehog to be identified. Shh and other related proteins, such as desert hedgehog and Indian hedgehog, are secreted morphogens critical for early patterning, cell migration, and differentiation of many cell types and organ systems. Cells have variable thresholds for response to the secreted Shh signal. The primary receptor for Shh is Patched (PTCH in human, PTC family in mouse), a transmembrane domain protein. In the absence of Shh, Patched inhibits transmembrane domain, G-protein–linked protein (Smoothened [Smo]). This results in inhibitions of downstream signaling to the nucleus. However, in the presence of Shh, Ptc inhibition is blocked and downstream events follow, including transcriptional activation of target genes, such as *Ptc-1*, *Engrailed*, and others (Fig. 20-4).

Post-translational modification of Shh protein affects its association with the cell membrane, formation of Shh multimers, and the movement of Shh, which, in turn, alters its tissue distribution and concentration gradients.

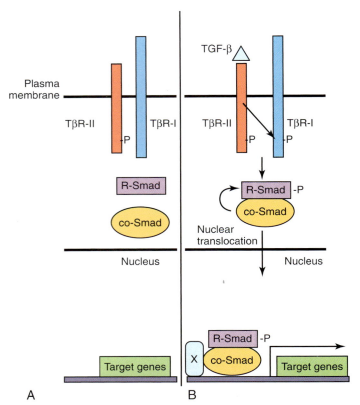

Figure 20–3 Transforming growth factor-β (TGF-β)/Smad signaling pathway. **A,** The type II TGF-β receptor subunit (TβR-II) is constitutively active. **B,** Upon binding of ligand to TβR-II, a type I TGF-β receptor subunit (TβR-I) is recruited to form a heterodimeric receptor complex and the TβR-I kinase domain is transphosphorylated (-P). Signaling from the activated receptor complex phosphorylates R-Smads, which then bind to a co-Smad, translocate from the cytoplasm to the nucleus, and activate gene transcription with cofactor(s) (X).

The role of Shh in patterning of the vertebrate ventral neural tube is one of its best-studied activities. Shh is secreted at high levels by the notochord, and therefore the concentration of Shh is highest in the floor plate of the neural tube and lowest in the roof plate, where members of the TGF-β family are highly expressed. The cell fates of ventral interneuron classes and motor neurons are determined by the relative Shh concentrations in the tissue and other factors.

The understanding of the requirement of Shh pathway signaling for many developmental processes has been enhanced by the discovery of human mutations of members of the Shh pathway. In addition, corresponding phenotypes of genetically modified mice, in which members of the Shh pathway are either inactivated (loss of function/knockout) or overexpressed (gain of function), have also added to this knowledge. Mutations of *SHH* and *PTCH* have been associated with holoprosencephaly in humans, a common congenital brain defect resulting in the fusion of the two cerebral hemispheres, dorsalization of forebrain structures, and anophthalmia or cyclopia (see Chapter 17). In sheep, this same defect

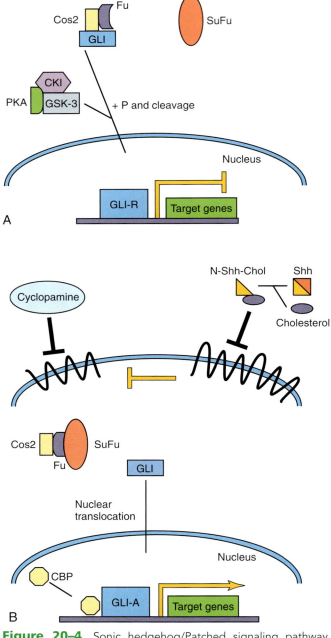

Figure 20–4 Sonic hedgehog/Patched signaling pathway. **A,** The Patched (Ptc) receptor inhibits signaling from the Smoothened (Smo) receptor. In a complex with Costal-2 (Cos2) and Fused (Fu), GLI is modified to become a transcriptional repressor, GLI-R. **B,** Sonic hedgehog (Shh) is cleaved, and cholesterol is added to its N-terminus (N-Shh-Chol). This modified Shh ligand inhibits the Ptc receptor, permitting Smo signaling, and ultimately activated GLI (GLI-A) translocates to the nucleus to activate target genes with CBP. *CBP,* Cyclic AMP–binding protein; *CKI,* casein kinase I; *GSK-3,* glycogen synthase kinase 3; *P,* phosphate group; *PKA,* protein kinase A; *SuFu,* suppressor of Fused.

has been associated with in utero exposure to the teratogen cyclopamine, which disrupts Shh signaling (see Fig. 20-4). Gorlin syndrome, often due to germline *PTCH* mutations, is a constellation of congenital malformations mostly affecting the epidermis, craniofacial structures, and nervous system. Mutations of the *GLI3* gene, encoding a zinc finger that mediates Shh signaling, are associated with autosomal dominant polydactyly syndromes.

Wnt/β-Catenin Pathway

The Wnt-secreted glycoproteins are vertebrate orthologs of the *Drosophila* gene Wingless. Similar to the other morphogens, the 19 Wnt family members control several processes during development, including establishment of cell polarity, proliferation, apoptosis, cell fate specification, and migration. Wnt signaling is a very complex process, and three signaling pathways have been elucidated to date; only the classic or "canonical" β-catenin–dependent pathway is discussed here (Fig. 20-5). Specific Wnts bind to 1 of 10 Frizzled (Fzd) seven-transmembrane domain cell surface receptors, and with low-density, lipoprotein receptor–related proteins 5 and 6 (LRP5/LRP6) coreceptors, thereby activating downstream intracellular signaling events. In the absence of Wnt binding, cytoplasmic β-catenin is phosphorylated by glycogen synthase kinase 3 (GSK-3) and targeted for degradation. In the presence of Wnts, GSK-3 is inactivated, and β-catenin is not phosphorylated and accumulates in the cytoplasm. The β-catenin translocates to the nucleus, where it activates target gene transcription in a complex with T-cell factor (TCF) transcription factors. β-Catenin/TCF target genes include vascular endothelial growth factor *(VEGF)* and matrix metalloproteinases.

Dysregulated Wnt signaling is a prominent feature in many developmental disorders, such as Williams-Beuren syndrome (heart, neurodevelopmental, and facial defects), and in cancer. *LRP5* mutations are found in the osteoporosis-pseudoglioma syndrome (congenital blindness and juvenile osteoporosis). Similar to the Shh pathway, canonical Wnt pathway mutations have been described in children with medulloblastoma, a common malignant brain tumor.

RECEPTOR TYROSINE KINASES

Common Features

Growth factors, such as insulin, epidermal growth factor, nerve growth factor, and other neurotrophins, and members of the platelet-derived growth factor family, bind to cell surface transmembrane receptors found on target cells. These receptors, members of the RTK superfamily, have three domains: (1) an extracellular ligand-binding domain, (2) a transmembrane domain, and (3) an intracellular kinase domain (Fig. 20-6). They are found as monomers in the unbound state but dimerize upon ligand binding. This process of dimerization brings the two intracellular kinase domains into close proximity such that one kinase domain can phosphorylate and activate the other receptor (transphosphorylation), which is required to fully activate the receptors. In turn, this initiates a series of intracellular signaling cascades. An inactivating mutation of one receptor subunit kinase domain results in abolishment of signaling; such a mutation in the kinase domain of the VEGF receptor 3 *(VEGFR-3)* results in the autosomal dominantly inherited lymphatic disorder called Milroy disease.

Figure 20–5 Wnt/β-catenin canonical signaling pathway. **A,** In the absence of Wnt ligand binding to Frizzled (Fzd) receptor, β-catenin is phosphorylated (-P) by a multiprotein complex and targeted for degradation. Target gene expression is repressed by T-cell factor (TCF). **B,** When Wnt binds to the Fzd receptor, LRP coreceptors are recruited, Disheveled (DVL) is phosphorylated, and β-catenin then accumulates in the cytoplasm. Some β-catenin enters the nucleus to activate target gene transcription. *APC,* Adenomatous polyposis coli; *GSK-3,* glycogen synthase kinase 3; *LRP,* lipoprotein receptor–related protein.

Inactive RTKs

Extracellular

Plasma membrane

Cytoplasm

A

Active RTKs in the presence of ligand

P- ⎯ -P

↓

Intracellular signaling pathways

△ Ligand   ▢ Kinase domain

B

Figure 20–6 Receptor tyrosine kinase (RTK) signaling. **A,** In the absence of ligand, the receptors are monomers and are inactive. **B,** Upon binding of ligand, the receptors dimerize and transphosphorylation occurs, which activates downstream signaling cascades. *P,* Phosphorylated.

Regulation of Angiogenesis by Receptor Tyrosine Kinases

Growth factors generally promote cellular proliferation, migration, and survival (i.e., they are antiapoptotic). During embryogenesis, signaling through RTKs is crucial for normal development and affects many different processes, such as the growth of new blood vessels (see Chapter 5), cellular migration, and neuronal axonal guidance.

Endothelial cells are derived from a progenitor cell (the hemangioblast) that can give rise to both the hematopoietic cell lineage and endothelial cells. The early endothelial cells proliferate and eventually coalesce to form the first primitive blood vessels. This process is termed *vasculogenesis*. After the first blood vessels are formed, they undergo intensive remodeling and maturation into the mature blood vessels in a process called angiogenesis. This maturation process involves the recruitment of vascular smooth muscle cells to the vessels to stabilize them. Vasculogenesis and angiogenesis are both dependent on the function of two distinct RTK classes, members of the VEGF and Tie receptor families. VEGF-A was shown to be essential for endothelial and blood cell development; VEGF-A knockout mice fail to develop blood or endothelial cells and die at early embryonic stages. A related molecule, VEGF-C, was shown to be crucial for the

development of lymphatic endothelial cells. VEGF-A signals through three receptors, VEGFR-1, VEGFR-2, and VEGFR-3, which are expressed by endothelial cells.

The process of angiogenic refinement depends on the function of the Angiopoietin/Tie2 signaling pathway. Tie2 is a RTK that is specifically expressed by endothelial cells, and Angiopoietin 1 and Angiopoietin 2 are its ligands that are expressed by the surrounding vascular smooth muscle cells. This represents a paracrine signaling system in which receptor and ligand are expressed in adjacent cells. Both the VEGF/VEGFR-2 and Angiopoietin/Tie2 signaling pathways are co-opted by tumors to stimulate growth of new blood vessels, which in turn stimulate their growth and metastasis. This demonstrates how normal signaling pathways in the embryo can be reused by disease processes, such as cancer.

NOTCH-DELTA PATHWAY

The Notch signaling pathway is integral for cell fate determination, including maintenance of stem cell niches, proliferation, apoptosis, and differentiation. These processes are essential for all aspects of organ development through regulation of lateral and inductive cell-cell signaling. Notch proteins are single transmembrane receptors that interact with membrane-bound Notch ligands (e.g., Delta-like ligands and serrate-like ligands [Jagged]) on adjacent cells (Fig. 20-7). Ligand-receptor binding triggers proteolytic events leading to the release of the Notch intracellular domain (NICD). When the NICD translocates to the nucleus, a series of intranuclear events culminates in the induction of expression of a transcription factor that maintains the progenitor state of the cell.

Lateral inhibition ensures the correct number of two distinct cell types from a population of cells with equivalent developmental potential. In the initial cell-cell interaction, Notch receptor signaling maintains one cell as an uncommitted progenitor. The adjacent cell maintains reduced Notch signaling and undergoes differentiation. Inductive signaling with other surrounding cells expressing morphogens may overcome a cell's commitment to a default fate and lead to an alternative cell fate. Understanding the function of the Notch-Delta signaling pathway in mammalian development has been assisted by loss-of-function studies in the mouse. The findings that mutations in Jagged1 are associated with Alagille syndrome (arteriohepatic dysplasia), with liver, kidney, cardiovascular, ocular, and skeletal malformations, and that *NOTCH-3* gene mutations are found in CADASIL (*ce*rebral *a*utosomal *d*ominant *a*rteriopathy with *s*ubcortical *i*nfarcts and *l*eukoencephalopathy), an adult vascular degenerative disease with a tendency to early-age onset of stroke-like events, support the importance of the Notch signaling pathway in embryonic and postnatal development, respectively.

TRANSCRIPTION FACTORS

Transcription factors belong to a large class of proteins that regulate the expression of many target genes, either

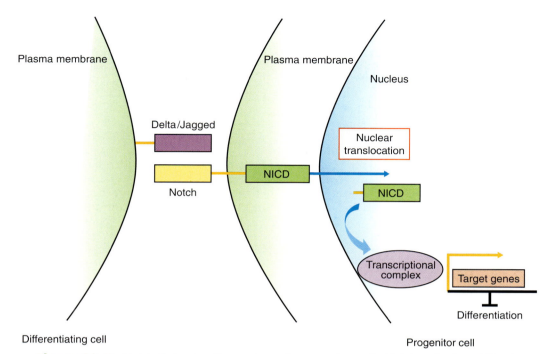

Figure 20–7 Notch-Delta signaling pathway. In progenitor cells *(right)*, activation of Notch signaling leads to cleavage of the Notch intracellular domain (NICD). NICD translocates to the nucleus, binds to a transcriptional complex, and activates target genes, such as the bHLH gene Hes1, that inhibit differentiation. In differentiating cells *(left)*, Notch signaling is not active.

through activation or repression mechanisms. Typically, a transcription factor will bind to specific nucleotide sequences in the promoter/enhancer regions of target genes and regulate the rate of transcription of its target genes via interacting with accessory proteins. Transcription factors can either activate or repress target gene transcription depending on the cell in which they are expressed, the specific promoter, the chromatin context, and the developmental stage. Some transcription factors do not need to bind to DNA to regulate transcription; they may bind to other transcription factors already bound to the promoter DNA, thereby regulating transcription, or bind to and sequester other transcription factors from their target genes, thus repressing their transcription. The transcription factor superfamily is composed of many different classes of proteins. Three examples of this diverse family of proteins are described: Hox/Homeobox, Pax, and basic helix-loop-helix (bHLH) transcription factors.

Hox/Homeobox Proteins

The *Hox* genes were first discovered in the fruit fly, *Drosophila melanogaster*. The order of the Hox genes along the AP axis is faithfully reproduced in their organization at the level of the chromosome. Mutations in these genes of the HOM-C complex lead to dramatic phenotypes (homeotic transformation) such as the Antennapedia gene, in which legs instead of antennae sprout from the head of the fruit fly. In humans, the order of the *Hox* genes along the AP axis and chromosomal location is conserved as well. Defects in *HOXA1* have been shown

to impair human neural development, and mutations in *HOXA13* and *HOXD13* result in limb malformations.

All the *Hox* genes contain a 180-base-pair sequence, the homeobox, which encodes a 60-amino-acid homeodomain composed of three α-helices. The third (recognition) helix binds to DNA sites that contain one or more binding motifs in the promoters of their target genes. The homeodomain is highly conserved across evolution, whereas other regions of the protein are not as well conserved. Mutations in the DNA-binding region of the homeobox gene *NKX2.5* are associated with cardiac atrial septal defects, and mutations in *ARX* are associated with the central nervous system malformation syndrome known as lissencephaly.

Pax Genes

The *Pax* genes all contain conserved bipartite DNA-binding motifs called the Pax (or paired) domain, and most Pax family members also contain a homeodomain. PAX proteins have been shown to both activate and repress transcription of target genes. The *Drosophila melanogaster* ortholog of *Pax6*, eyeless, was shown to be essential for eye development because homozygous mutant flies had no eyes. Eyeless shares a high degree of sequence conservation with its human ortholog *PAX6* and is associated with ocular malformations such as aniridia (absence of the iris) and Peters anomaly. In human eye diseases, the level of *PAX6* expression seems to be crucial because patients with only one functional copy (haploinsufficiency) have ocular defects and patients without *PAX6* function are anophthalmic. This concept of haploinsufficiency is a recurring theme for many different transcription factors and corresponding human malformations.

PAX3 and *PAX7* encode both homeodomain and Pax DNA-binding domains. The human childhood cancer alveolar rhabdomyosarcoma results from a translocation that results in the formation of a chimeric protein wherein PAX3 or PAX7 (including both DNA domains) is fused to the strong activating domains of the Forkhead family transcription factor FOXO1. The autosomal dominant human disease Waardenburg syndrome type I results from mutations in the *PAX3* gene. Patients with this syndrome have hearing deficits, ocular defects (dystopia canthorum), and pigmentation abnormalities best typified by a white forelock.

Basic Helix-Loop-Helix Transcription Factors

The bHLH genes are a class of transcription factors that regulate cell fate determination and differentiation in many different tissues during development. At a molecular level, bHLH proteins contain a basic (positively charged) DNA-binding region that is followed by two α-helices that are separated by a loop. The α-helices have a hydrophilic and a hydrophobic side (amphipathic). The hydrophobic side of the helix is a motif for protein-protein interactions between different members of the bHLH family. This domain is the most conserved region of the bHLH proteins across different species. bHLH proteins often bind other bHLHs (heterodimerize) to regulate transcription. These heterodimers are composed of tissue-specific bHLH proteins bound to ubiquitously expressed bHLH proteins. The powerful prodifferentiation effect of bHLH genes can be repressed by several different mechanisms. For example, inhibitor of differentiation (Id) proteins are HLH proteins that lack the basic DNA-binding motif. When Id proteins heterodimerize with specific bHLH proteins, they prevent binding of these bHLH proteins to their target gene promoter sequences (called E-boxes).

Growth factors, which tend to inhibit differentiation, increase the level of Id proteins that sequester bHLH proteins from their target promoters. In addition, growth factors can stimulate the phosphorylation of the DNA-binding domain of bHLH proteins, which inhibits their ability to bind to DNA. bHLH genes are crucial for the development of tissues such as muscle *(MyoD/Myogenin)* and neurons *(NeuroD/Neurogenin)* in humans. *MyoD* expression was shown to be sufficient to transdifferentiate several different cell lines into muscle cells, demonstrating that it is a master regulator of muscle differentiation. Studies of knockout mice confirmed that *MyoD* and another bHLH, *Myf5*, are crucial for the differentiation of precursor cells into primitive muscle cells (myoblasts). Similarly, *Mash1/Ascl1* and *Neurogenin1* are proneural genes that regulate the formation of neuroblasts from the neuroepithelium. Mouse models have shown that these genes are crucial for the specification of different subpopulations of precursors in the developing central nervous system. For example, *Mash1/Ascl1* knockout mice have defects in forebrain development, whereas *Neurogenin1*

knockout mice have defects in cranial sensory ganglia and ventral spinal cord neurons. Muscle and neuronal differentiation are controlled by a cascade of bHLH genes that function at early and at late stages of cellular differentiation. In addition, both differentiation pathways are inhibited via signaling through the Notch pathway.

EPIGENETICS

Epigenetics refers to inherited modifications that affect gene expression as a result of mechanisms other than changes in the DNA sequence. Examples include DNA methylation and chromatin modifications, such as acetylation, methylation, and phosphorylation of histones. These epigenetic marks (*"epigenetic code"*) are regulated by classes of enzymes that: a) recognize the epigenetic marks (*"readers"*), b) add epigenetic markers to DNA or histone (*"writers"*), or c) remove these epigenetics marks (*"erasers"*). Disorders of chromatin remodeling include Rett, Rubinstein-Taybi, and alpha-thalassemia/X-linked mental retardation syndromes.

DNA Methylation

DNA is methylated at cytosine residues by DNA methyltransferases at CpG sites—where cytosine and guanine nucleotides are directly paired. CpG islands are DNA regions with high concentrations of CpG sites, and are often located in the proximal promoter regions of genes. DNA methylation at CpG sites, in general, leads to reduced gene expression or gene silencing, whereas DNA hypomethylation at CpG sites leads to gene over-expression. Silencing of tumor suppressor genes or over-expression of oncogenes may lead to cancer. Proteins, such as methyl-CpG-binding protein 2 (MECP2), which is mutated in the neurodevelopmental disorder Rett syndrome, function as *"readers"* by binding to methylated DNA and subsequently assembling protein complexes that repress gene expression.

Histone Modifications

Histones are the positively charged nuclear proteins around which genomic DNA is coiled to tightly pack it within the nucleus. Modification of these proteins is a common pathway by which transcription factors regulate the activity of their target promoters. Examples of histone modifications include phosphorylation, ubiquitinylation, sumoylation, acetylation, and methylation. The latter two modifications are discussed here in more depth.

Acetylation

DNA is less tightly bound to acetylated histones, thus allowing for more open access of transcription factors and other proteins to the promoters of their target genes. Histone acetylation status is controlled by genes that add acetyl groups (histone transferase, a *writer*) or remove acetyl groups (histone deacetylase, an *eraser*) (Fig. 20-8). Phosphorylation of histones also leads to an opening of the chromatin structure and activation of gene transcription. These epigenetic marks are recognized (*"read"*)

Transcriptionally inactive chromatin

Transcriptionally active chromatin

Figure 20–8 Histone modifications alter transcriptional properties of chromatin. **A,** In areas of transcriptionally inactive chromatin, the DNA is tightly bound to the histone cores. The histones are not acetylated or phosphorylated. Histone deacetylases (HDACs) are active, whereas histone acetyl transferases (HATs) and histone kinases are inactive. **B,** In areas of transcriptionally active chromatin, the DNA is not as tightly bound to the histone cores. The histone proteins are acetylated (Ac) and phosphorylated (-P). HDACs are inactive, whereas HATs and histone kinases are active.

by both bromodomain proteins and pleckstrin homology domain proteins.

Methylation

Histone methyltransferases, or *"writers,"* catalyze the addition of a methyl group to lysine residues on histone tails. This modification is removed by histone demethylases, or *"erasers."* In contrast to histone acetylation, methylation of histones can result in a) the addition of 1, 2, or 3 methyl groups to an individual lysine residue; and b) either the activation or repression of gene expression depending on the particular lysine residue that is modified. For example, trimethylation of lysine 9 on histone 3 (H3K9me3) is associated with repressed promoters, whereas trimethylation of lysine 4 on histone 3 (H3K4me3) is associated with active promoters. Histone methylation status is *"read"* by a large number of different classes of proteins. Mutations of histone modification *readers, writers, and erasers* can lead to diseases such as neurodevelopmental disorders and cancer.

STEM CELLS: DIFFERENTIATION VERSUS PLURIPOTENCY

Stem cells have the property of self-renewal through symmetric or asymmetric cell divisions, and under specific conditions in the embryo and adult, can give rise to all of the differentiated cell types in the body (totipotent or pluripotent). Several types of stem cell populations have been characterized: **embryonic stem cells** (ESCs), **adult stem cells**, and **cancer stem cells** (CSCs). ESCs, derived from the inner cell mass of the blastula, are **pluripotent** and can give rise to all differentiated cell types from the ectoderm, endoderm, and mesoderm, the primary germ layers (see Chapter 5), but do not contribute to extraembryonic tissues. ESCs express several transcription factors, such as SOX2 and OCT-4, that repress differentiation.

Adult stem cells are found in relative abundance in differentiated tissues and organs that undergo rapid regeneration, such as the bone marrow, hair follicles, and intestinal mucosal epithelium. However, there are "nests" of adult stem cells in many other tissues, including those that have been previously considered nonregenerative, such as the central nervous system and retina; these stem cell populations are small and located in the subventricular zone and ciliary margins, respectively. Hematopoietic stem cells derived from bone marrow, peripheral blood, and umbilical cord sources are now routinely used to treat primary immunodeficiencies and various inherited metabolic disorders, and as a "rescue" strategy following marrow-destroying cancer treatments.

CSCs are under intense study since it has become evident through the study of leukemias and solid tumors (e.g., colorectal cancer, malignant gliomas) that a small population of these cells, identified by various cell surface markers (e.g., CD133 in solid tumors), are often resistant to cancer treatments such as radiation or chemotherapy. Investigators are focusing their efforts on eradicating the CSC population, in addition to standard therapies, in order to increase cure rates.

It is possible to harness the power of stem cells to repair degenerative disorders such as Parkinson disease and tissues severely damaged by ischemia (stroke) and trauma (spinal cord injury). However, researchers have been limited by the available sources of stem cells from the embryo or adult. Hence, there has been tremendous interest in de-differentiating somatic cells such as epithelial cells and fibroblasts from adults into **induced pluripotent stem cells** (iPS cells). Recent studies have identified several key master transcription factors (Fig. 20-9), such as OCT-3/4, SOX2, and KLF4, or Nanog, that can reprogram differentiated cells into pluripotent cells. These iPS cells can be manipulated using nonviral means of gene delivery and have the potential to treat the majority of human diseases in which cell regeneration may restore structure and/or function.

SUMMARY OF COMMON SIGNALING PATHWAYS USED DURING DEVELOPMENT

- There are marked differences among the various signaling pathways, but they share many common features: ligands, membrane-bound receptors and co-receptors, intracellular signaling domains, adapters, and effector molecules.

Figure 20–9 Induced pluripotent stem cells. Stem cells and induced pluripotent stem cells (IPS) have the capacity for self-renewal, for cell death, and/or to become progenitors. Progenitor cells have a more limited capacity for self-renewal, but also can differentiate into various cell types or undergo cell death. Adult, differentiated somatic cells, such as skin fibroblasts, can be reprogrammed into IPS with the introduction of the master transcription factors SOX2, OCT-3/4, or KLF4.

- Signaling pathways are co-opted at various times during development for stem cell renewal, cell proliferation, migration, apoptosis, and differentiation.
- Pathways have "default" settings that result in generation or maintenance of one cell fate rather than another.
- Many genes and signaling pathways are highly conserved throughout evolution.
- Knowledge of gene function has been acquired by reverse genetics using model systems with loss- or gain-of-function transgenic approaches. As well, much insight has been gained by forward genetics that begins with the description of abnormal phenotypes arising spontaneously in mice and humans and then subsequent identification of the mutant gene.
- There is evidence of cross-talk among pathways. This communication among various signaling pathways facilitates our understanding of the far-reaching consequences of single gene mutations that result in malformation syndromes affecting the development of multiple organ systems, or in cancers.

Bibliography and Suggested Reading

CHAPTER 1

Abdelalim EM: Molecular mechanisms controlling the cell cycle in embryonic stem cells. Stem Cell Rev 9:764, 2013.

Abdelalim EM, Bonnefond A, Bennaceur-Griscelli A, et al: Pluripotent stem cells as a potential tool for disease modelling and cell therapy in diabetes. Stem Cell Rev 9:764, 2013.

Gasser R: Atlas of Human Embryos. Hagerstown, MD, Harper & Row, 1975.

Gasser R: Virtual Human Embryo DREM Project. Baltimore, MD, NICHD, 2007.

Hopwood N: A history of normal plates, tables and stages in vertebrate embryology. Int J Dev Biol 51:1, 2007.

Jirásel JE: An Atlas of Human Prenatal Developmental Mechanics: Anatomy and Staging. London, Taylor & Francis, 2004.

O'Rahilly R, Müller F: Developmental Stages in Human Embryos (Publication 637). Washington, DC, Carnegie Institution of Washington, 1987.

Rodrigues AR, Tabin CJ: Deserts and waves in gene expression. Science 340:1181, 2013.

Smith A: Cell biology: potency unchained. Nature 505:622, 2014.

Streeter GL: Developmental horizons in human embryos: description of age group XI, 13 to 20 somites, and age group XII, 21 to 29 somites. Contrib Embryol Carnegie Inst 30:211, 1942.

Yamada S, Samtani RR, Lee ES, et al: Developmental atlas of the early first trimester embryo. Dev Dyn 239:1585, 2010.

Zech NH, Preisegger KH, Hollands P: Stem cell therapeutics—reality versus hype and hope. J Assist Reprod Genet 28:287, 2011.

CHAPTER 2

Buzadzic B, Vucetic M, Jankovic A: New insights into male (in)fertility: the importance of NO. Br J Pharmacol 2014 Mar 7. [Epub ahead of print]

Cameron S: The normal menstrual cycle. In Magowan BA, Owen P, Thomson A (eds): Clinical Obstetrics & Gynaecology, 3rd ed. Philadelphia, Saunders, 2014.

Duggavathi R, Murphy BD: Ovulation signals. Science 324:890, 2009.

Moore KL, Dalley AF, Agur AMR: Clinically Oriented Anatomy, 7th ed. Philadelphia, Lippincott Williams & Wilkins, 2014.

CHAPTER 3

Evans JP: Sperm-egg interaction. Annu Rev Physiol 74:477, 2012.

Gadella BM: Dynamic regulation of sperm interactions with the zona pellucida prior to and after fertilisation. Reprod Fertil Dev 25:26, 2012.

Gleicher N, Kushnir VA, Barad DH: Preimplantation genetic screening (PGS) still in search of a clinical application: a systematic review. Reprod Biol Endocrinol. 12:22, 2014.

Hansen M, Kurinczuk JJ, Milne E, et al: Assisted reproductive technology and birth defects: a systematic review and meta-analysis. Hum Reprod Update 19:330, 2013.

Plaisier M: Decidualisation and angiogenesis. Best Prac Res Clin Obstet Gynaecol 25:259, 2011.

Quenby S, Brosens JJ: Human implantation: a tail of mutual maternal and fetal attraction. Biol Reprod 88:81, 2013.

Rock J, Hertig AT: The human conceptus during the first two weeks of gestation. Am J Obstet Gynecol 55:6, 1948.

Simpson JL: Birth defects and assisted reproductive technology. Semin Fetal Neonatal Med 19:177, 2014.

CHAPTER 4

Hertig AT, Rock J, Adams EC: A description of 34 human ova within the first seventeen days of development. Am J Anat 98:435, 1956.

Kirk E, Bottomley C, Bourne T: Diagnosing ectopic pregnancy and current concepts in the management of pregnancy of unknown location. Hum Reprod Update 20:250, 2014.

Luckett WP: Origin and differentiation of the yolk sac and extraembryonic mesoderm in presomite human and rhesus monkey embryos. Am J Anat 152:59, 1978.

Quenby S, Brosens, JJ: Human implantation: a tail of mutual maternal and fetal attraction. Biol Reprod 88:81, 2013.

Zorn AM, Wells JM: Vertebrate endoderm development and organ formation. Annu Rev Cell Dev Biol 25:221, 2009.

CHAPTER 5

Dias AS, de Almeida I, Belmonte JM: Somites without a clock. Science 343:791, 2014.

Flake AW: The fetus with sacrococcygeal teratoma. In Harrison MR, Evans MI, Adzick NS, Holzgrev W (eds): The Unborn Patient: The Art and Science of Fetal Therapy, 3rd ed. Philadelphia, Saunders, 2001.

Gasser RF: Evidence that some events of mammalian embryogenesis can result from differential growth, making migration unnecessary. Anat Rec New Anat 289B:53, 2006.

Jagannathan-Bogdan M, Zon LI: Hematopoiesis. Development 140:2463, 2013.

Lewis J, Hanisch A, Holder M: Notch signaling, the segmentation clock, and the patterning of vertebrate somites. J Biol 8:44, 2009.

Mayor R, Theveneau E: The neural crest. Development 140:2247, 2013.

Piccolo S: Developmental biology: mechanics in the embryo. Nature 504:223, 2013.

Satoh N, Tagawa K, Takahasi H: How was the notochord born? Evol Dev 14:56, 2012.

Savage P: Gestational trophoblastic disease. In Magowan BA, Owen P, Thomson A (eds): Clinical Obstetrics & Gynaecology, 3rd ed. Philadelphia, Saunders, 2014.

Tovar JA: The neural crest in pediatric surgery. J Pediatr Surg 42:915, 2007.

Van Mieghem T, Al-Ibrahim A, Deprest J, et al: Minimally invasive therapy for fetal sacrococcygeal teratoma: case series and systematic review of the literature. Ultrasound Obstet Gynecol 43:611, 2014.

Wang Y, Steinbeisser H: Molecular basis of morphogenesis during vertebrate gastrulation. Cell Mol Life Sci 66:2263, 2009.

CHAPTER 6

De Bakker BS, de Jong KH, Hagoort J, et al: Towards a 3-dimensional atlas of the developing human embryo: the Amsterdam experience. Reprod Toxicol 34:225, 2012.

FitzPatrick DR: Human embryogenesis. In Magowan BA, Owen P, Thomson A (eds): Clinical Obstetrics & Gynaecology, 3rd ed. Philadelphia, Saunders, 2014.

Gasser R: Virtual Human Embryo DREM Project. New Orleans, Louisiana State University, 2007.

Jirásel JE: An Atlas of Human Prenatal Developmental Mechanics: Anatomy and Staging. London, Taylor & Francis, 2004.

O'Rahilly R, Müller F: Development Stages in Human Embryos (Publication 637). Washington, DC, Carnegie Institution of Washington, 1987.

Persaud TVN, Hay JC: Normal embryonic and fetal development. In Reece EA, Hobbins JC (eds): Clinical Obstetrics: The Fetus and Mother, 3rd ed. Oxford, Blackwell Publishing, 2006.

Pooh RK, Shiota K, Kurjak A: Imaging of the human embryo with magnetic resonance imaging microscopy and high-resolution transvaginal 3-dimensional sonography: human embryology in the 21st century. Am J Obstet Gynecol 204:77.e1, 2011.

Steding G: The Anatomy of the Human Embryo: A Scanning Electron-Microscopic Atlas. Basel, Karger, 2009.

Whitworth M, Bricker L, Neilson JP, et al: Ultrasound for fetal assessment in early pregnancy. Cochrane Database Syst Rev (4): CD007058, 2010.

Yamada S, Samtani RR, Lee ES, et al: Developmental atlas of the early first trimester embryo. Dev Dyn 239:1585, 2010.

CHAPTER 7

FitzPatrick DR: Human embryogenesis. In Magowan BA, Owen P, Thomson A (eds): Clinical Obstetrics & Gynaecology, 3rd ed. Philadelphia, Saunders, 2014.

Jirásel JE: An Atlas of Human Prenatal Developmental Mechanics: Anatomy and Staging. London, Taylor & Francis, 2004.

Khambalia AZ, Roberts CL, Nguyen M, et al: Predicting date of birth and examining the best time to date a pregnancy. Int J Gynaecol Obstet 123:105, 2013.

Kilby M: Prenatal diagnosis. In Magowan BA, Owen P, Thomson A (eds): Clinical Obstetrics & Gynaecology, 3rd ed. Philadelphia, Saunders, 2014.

Korf BR, Rehm HL: New approaches to molecular diagnosis. JAMA 309:1511, 2013.

Moran S, Greene MF, Mello MM: A new era in noninvasive prenatal testing. N Engl J Med 369:2164, 2013.

Owen P: Small babies. In Magowan BA, Owen P, Thomson A (eds): Clinical Obstetrics & Gynaecology, 3rd ed. Philadelphia, Saunders, 2014.

Steding G: The Anatomy of the Human Embryo: A Scanning Electron-Microscopic Atlas. Basel, Karger, 2009.

Whitworth M, Bricker L, Neilson JP, et al: Ultrasound for fetal assessment in early pregnancy. Cochrane Database Syst Rev (4): CD007058, 2010.

CHAPTER 8

Banks CL: Labour. In Magowan BA, Owen P, Thomson A (eds): Clinical Obstetrics & Gynaecology, 3rd ed. Philadelphia, Saunders, 2014.

Collins JH: Umbilical cord accidents: Human studies. Semin Perinatol 26:79, 2002.

Forbes K: IFPA Gabor Than Award lecture: molecular control of placental growth: the emerging role of microRNAs. Placenta 34(Suppl):S27, 2013.

Gibson J: Multiple pregnancy. In Magowan BA, Owen P, Thomson A (eds): Clinical Obstetrics & Gynaecology, 3rd ed.Philadelphia, Saunders, 2014.

Harman CR: Amniotic fluid abnormalities. Semin Perinatol 32:288, 2008.

Jabrane-Ferrat N, Siewiera J: The up side of decidual natural killer cells: new developments in immunology of pregnancy. Immunology 141: 490, 2014.

Knöfler M, Pollheimer J: Human placental trophoblast invasion and differentiation: a particular focus on Wnt signaling. Front Genet 4:190, 2013.

Masselli G, Gualdi G: MRI imaging of the placenta: what a radiologist should know. Abdom Imaging J38:573, 2013.

Redline RW: Placental pathology. In Martin RJ, Fanaroff AA, Walsh MC (eds): Fanaroff and Martin's Neonatal-Perinatal Medicine: Diseases of the Fetus and Infant, 9th ed. Philadelphia, Mosby, 2011.

CHAPTER 9

Badillo A, Gingalewski C: Congenital diaphragmatic hernia: treatment and outcome. Semin Perinatol 38:92, 2014.

Clugston RD, Zhang W, Alvarez S, et al: Understanding abnormal retinoid signaling as a causative mechanism in congenital diaphragmatic hernia. Am J Res Cell Mol Biol 42:276, 2010.

Hedrick HL: Management of prenatally diagnosed congenital diaphragmatic hernia. Semin Pediatr Surg 22:37, 2013.

Kays DW: Congenital diaphragmatic hernia and neonatal lung lesions. Surg Clin North Am 86:329, 2006.

Merrell AJ, Kardon G: Development of the diaphragm—a skeletal muscle essential for mammalian respiration. FEBS J 280:4026, 2013.

Turell DC: Advances with surfactant. Emerg Med Clin North Am 26: 921, 2008.

Wells LJ: Development of the human diaphragm and pleural sacs. Contrib Embryol Carnegie Inst 35:107, 1954.

CHAPTER 10

Bajaj Y, Ifeacho S, Tweedie D, et al: Branchial anomalies in children. Int J Pediatr Otorhinolaryngol 75:1020, 2011.

Berkovitz BKB, Holland GR, Moxham B: Oral Anatomy, Histology, and Embryology, 4th ed. Philadelphia, Mosby, 2009.

Hinrichsen K: The early development of morphology and patterns of the face in the human embryo. Adv Anat Embryol Cell Biol 98:1, 1985.

Jones KL, Jones MC, Campo MD: Smith's Recognizable Patterns of Human Malformation, 7th ed. Philadelphia, Saunders, 2013.

Mueller DT, Callanan VP: Congenital malformations of the oral cavity. Otolaryngol Clin North Am 40:141, 2007.

Nanci A: Ten Cate's Oral Histology: Development, Structure, and Function, 8th ed. Philadelphia, Mosby, 2012.

Parada C, Han D, Chai Y: Molecular and cellular regulatory mechanisms of tongue myogenesis. J Dent Res 91:528, 2012.

Rice DPC: Craniofacial anomalies: from development to molecular pathogenesis. Curr Mol Med 5:699, 2009.

Waldhausen JHT: Branchial cleft and arch anomalies in children. Semin Pediatr Surg 15:70, 2006.

Yatzey KE: DiGeorge syndrome, Tbx1, and retinoic acid signaling come full circle. Circ Res 106:630, 2010.

CHAPTER 11

Brown E, James K: The lung primordium an outpunching from the foregut! Evidence-based dogma or myth. J Pediatr Surg 44:607, 2009.

Gowen CW Jr: Fetal and neonatal medicine (respiratory diseases of the newborn). In Marcdante KJ, Kliegman RM (eds): Nelson Essentials of Pediatrics, 7th ed. Philadelphia, Saunders, 2015.

Herriges M, Morrisey EE: Lung development: orchestrating the generation and regeneration of a complex organ. Development 141:502, 2014.

Jobe AH: Lung development and maturation. In Martin RJ, Fanaroff AA, Walsh MC (eds): Fanaroff and Martin's Neonatal-Perinatal Medicine: Diseases of the Fetus and Infant, 9th ed. Philadelphia, Mosby, 2011.

Morrisey EE, Cardosa WV, Lane RH, et al: Molecular determinants of lung development. Ann Am Thorac Soc 10:S12, 2013.

O'Rahilly R, Boyden E: The timing and sequence of events in the development of the human respiratory system during the embryonic period proper. Z Anat Entwicklungsresch 141:237, 1973.

Rawlins EL: The building blocks of mammalian lung development. Dev Dyn 240:403, 2011.

Warburton D, El-Hashash A, Carraro G, et al: Lung organogenesis. Curr Top Dev Biol 90:73, 2010.

Wells LJ, Boyden EA: The development of the bronchopulmonary segments in human embryos of horizons XVII and XIX. Am J Anat 95:163, 1954.

CHAPTER 12

Baxter KJ, Bhatia AM: Hirschsprung's disease in the preterm infant: implications for diagnosis and outcome. Am Surg 79:734, 2013.

Belo J, Krishnamurthy M, Oakie A, Wang R: The role of SOX9 transcription factor in pancreatic and duodenal development. Stem Cells Dev 22:2935, 2013.

De La Forest A, Duncan SA: Basic science of liver development. In Gumucio DL, Samuelson LC, Spence JR (eds): Translational Research and Discovery in Gastroenterology: Organogenesis to Disease. New York, John Wiley & Sons, 2014.

Keplinger KM, Bloomston M: Anatomy and embryology of the biliary tract. Surg Clin North Am 94:203, 2014.

Klezovitch O, Vasioukhin V: Your gut is right to turn left. Dev Cell 26:553, 2013.

Kluth D, Fiegel HC, Metzger R: Embryology of the hindgut. Semin Pediatr Surg 20:152, 2011.

Ledbetter DJ: Gastroschisis and omphalocele. Surg Clin North Am 86:249, 2006.

Metzger R, Metzger U, Fiegel HC, et al: Embryology of the midgut. Semin Pediatr Surg 20:145, 2011.

Mundt E, Bates MD: Genetics of Hirschsprung disease and anorectal malformations. Semin Pediatr Surg 19:107, 2010.

Naik-Mathuria B, Olutoye OO: Foregut abnormalities. Surg Clin North Am 86:261, 2006.

Vakili K, Pomfret EA: Biliary anatomy and embryology. Surg Clin North Am 88:1159, 2008.

Van den Brink GR: Hedgehog signaling in development and homeostasis of the gastrointestinal tract. Physiol Rev 87:1343, 2007.

Van der Putte SCJ: The development of the human anorectum. Anat Rec 292:952, 2009.

CHAPTER 13

Creighton S: Disorders of sex development. In Magowan BA, Owen P, Thomson A (eds): Clinical Obstetrics & Gynaecology, 3rd ed. Philadelphia, Saunders, 2014.

Haynes JH: Inguinal and scrotal disorders. Surg Clin North Am 86:371, 2006.

Kollin C, Ritzén EM: Cryptorchidism: a clinical perspective. Pediatr Endocrinol Rev 11(Suppl 2):240, 2014.

Lee PA, Houk CP, Ahmed SF, et al: Consensus statement on management of intersex disorders. Pediatrics 118:e4888, 2006.

Mahan JD, Patel HP: Nephrology and urology. In Marcdante KJ, Kliegman KJ (eds): Nelson Essentials of Pediatrics, 7th ed. Philadelphia, Saunders, 2015.

Persaud TVN: Embryology of the female genital tract and gonads. In Copeland LJ, Jarrell J (eds): Textbook of Gynecology, 2nd ed. Philadelphia, Saunders, 2000.

Sisto PAP, Heneghan MK: Endocrinology. In Marcdante KJ, Kliegman KJ (eds): Nelson Essentials of Pediatrics, 7th ed. Philadelphia, Saunders, 2015.

Svingen T, Koopman P: Building the mammalian testis: origins, differentiation, and assembly of the component cell populations. Genes Dev 27:2409, 2013.

Virtanen HE, Toppari J: Embryology and physiology of testicular development and descent. Pediatr Endocrinol Rev 11(Suppl 2):206, 2014.

Woo LL, Thomas JC, Brock JW: Cloacal exstrophy: a comprehensive review of an uncommon problem. J Pediatr Urol 6:102, 2010.

CHAPTER 14

Adams SM, Good MW, DeFranco GM: Sudden infant death syndrome. Am Fam Physician 79:870, 2009.

Dyer LA, Kirby ML: The role of secondary heart field in cardiac development. Dev Dyn 336:137, 2009.

Hildreth V, Anderson RH, Henderson DJH: Autonomic innervations of the developing heart: origins and function. Clin Anat 22:36, 2009.

Horsthuis T, Christoffels VM, Anderson RH, et al: Can recent insights into cardiac development improve our understanding of congenitally malformed heart? Clin Anat 22:4, 2009.

International Society of Ultrasound in Obstetrics and Gynecology (ISUOG): ISUOG Practice Guidelines (updated): sonographic screening examination of the fetal heart. Ultrasound Obstet Gynecol 41:348, 2013.

Kamedia Y: Hoxa3 and signaling molecules involved in aortic arch patterning and remodeling. Cell Tissue Res 336:165, 2010.

Kudo K, Yamagishi H: A decade of advances in the molecular embryology and genetics underlyng congenital heart defects. Circ J 75:2296, 2011.

Loukas M, Bilinsky C, Bilinski E, et al: The normal and abnormal anatomy of the coronary arteries. Clin Anat 22:114, 2009.

Loukas M, Groat C, Khangura R, et al: Cardiac veins: a review of the literature. Clin Anat 22:129, 2009.

Männer J: The anatomy of cardiac looping: a step towards the understanding of the morphogenesis of several forms of congenital cardiac malformations. Clin Anat 22:21, 2009.

Martinsen BJ, Lohr JL: Cardiac development. In Iaizzo PA (ed): Handbook of Cardiac Anatomy, Physiology, and Devices. Totowa, NJ, Humana Press Inc., 2003.

Schneider DS: The cardiovascular system. In Marcdante KJ, Kliegman KJ (eds): Nelson Essentials of Pediatrics, 7th ed. Philadelphia, Saunders, 2015.

Solloway M, Harvey RP: Molecular pathways in myocardial development: a stem cell perspective. Cardiovasc Res 58:264, 2006.

Stoller JZ, Epstein JA: Cardiac neural crest. Semin Cell Dev Biol 16:704, 2005.

Sylva M, van den Hoff MJB, Moorman AFM: Development of the human heart. Am J Med Genet A 164A:1347, 2013.

Watanabe M, Schaefer KS: Cardiac embryology. In Martin RJ, Fanaroff AA, Walsh MC (eds): Fanaroff and Martin's Neonatal-Perinatal Medicine: Diseases of the Fetus and Infant, 9th ed. Philadelphia, Mosby, 2011.

Zaffran S, Kelly RG: New developments in the second heart field. Differentiation 84:17, 2012.

CHAPTER 15

Bentzinger CF, Wang YX, Rudnicki MA: Building muscle: molecular regulation of myogenesis. Cold Spring Harb Perspect Biol 4:a008342, 2012.

Buckingham M, Rigby PWJ: Gene regulatory networks and transcriptional mechanisms that control myogenesis. Dev Cell 28:225, 2014.

Chang KZ, Likes K, Davis K, et al: The significance of cervical ribs in thoracic outlet syndrome. J Vasc Surg 57:771, 2013.

Cole P, Kaufman Y, Hatef DA, et al: Embryology of the hand and upper extremity. J Craniofac Surg 20:992, 2009.

Cohen MM Jr: Perspectives on craniosynostosis: sutural biology, some well-known syndromes and some unusual syndromes. J Craniofac Surg 20:646, 2009.

Cooperman DR, Thompson GH: Musculoskeletal disorders. In Martin RJ, Fanaroff AA, Walsh MC (eds): Fanaroff and Martin's Neonatal-Perinatal Medicine: Diseases of the Fetus and Infant, 9th ed. Philadelphia, Mosby, 2011.

Dallas SL, Bonewald LF: Dynamic of the transition from osteoblast to osteocyte. Ann N Y Acad Sci 1192:437, 2010.

Gillgrass TJ, Welbury RR: Craniofacial growth and development. In Welbury RR, Duggal MS, Hosey MT (eds): Paediatric Dentistry, 4th ed. Oxford, UK, Oxford University Press, 2014.

Hall BK: Bones and Cartilage: Developmental Skeletal Biology. Philadelphia, Elsevier Academic Press, 2005.

Hinrichsen KV, Jacob HJ, Jacob M, et al: Principles of ontogenesis of leg and foot in man. Ann Anat 176:121, 1994.

Jiang Z, Von den Hoff JW, Torensma R, et al: Wnt16 is involved in intramembranous ossification and suppresses osteoblast differentiation through the Wnt/β-catenin pathway. J Cell Physiol 229:384, 2014.

O'Rahilly R, Gardner E: The timing and sequence of events in the development of the limbs of the human embryo. Anat Embryol (Berl) 148:1, 1975.

Towers M, Tickle C: Generation of pattern and form in the developing limb. Int J Dev Biol 53:805, 2009.

CHAPTER 16

Catala M, Kubis N: Gross anatomy and development of the peripheral nervous system. In Said G, Krarup C (eds): Handbook of Clinical Neurology. Amsterdam, Elsevier B.V., 2013.

De Wals P, Tairou F, Van Allen MI, et al: Reduction in neural-tube defects after folic acid fortification in Canada. N Engl J Med 357:135, 2007.

Diaz AL, Gleeson JG: The molecular and genetic mechanisms of neocortex development. Clin Perinatol 36:503, 2009.

Evans OB: Development of the nervous system. In Haines D (ed): Fundamental Neuroscience for Basic and Clinical Applications. Philadelphia, Saunders, 2013.

Haines DE: Fundamental Neuroscience for Basic and Clinical Applications. Philadelphia, Saunders, 2013.

O'Rahilly R, Müller F: Embryonic Human Brain: An Atlas of Developmental Stages, 2nd ed. New York, Wiley-Liss, 1999.

Osterhues A, Ali NS, Michels KB: The role of folic acid fortification in neural tube defects: a review. Crit Rev Food Sci Nutr 53:1180, 2013.

Schiller JH, Shellhaas R: Neurology: congenital anomalies of the central nervous system. In Marcdante KJ, Kliegman KJ (eds): Nelson Essentials of Pediatrics, 7th ed. Philadelphia, Saunders, 2015.

ten Donkelaar HT, Lammens M: Development of the human cerebellum and its disorders. Clin Perinatol 36:513, 2009.

Zhan J, Dinov ID, Li J, et al: Spatial-temporal atlas of human fetal brain development during the early second trimester. Neuroimage 82: 115, 2013.

CHAPTER 17

Barishak YR: Embryology of the Eye and Its Adnexa, 2nd ed. Basel, Karger, 2001.

Bauer PW, MacDonald CB, Melhem ER: Congenital inner ear malformation. Am J Otol 19:669, 1998.

Chung HA, Medina-Ruiz S, Harland RM: Sp8 regulates inner ear development. Proc Natl Acad Sci U S A 111:632, 2014.

FitzPatrick DR, van Heyningen V: Developmental eye disorders. Curr Opin Genet Dev 15:348, 2005.

Jason R, Guercio BS, Martyn LJ: Congenital malformations of the eye and orbit. Otolaryngol Clin North Am 40:113, 2007.

Jones KL, Jones MC, del Campo M: Smith's Recognizable Patterns of Human Malformation, 7th ed. Philadelphia, Saunders, 2013.

Munnamalai V, Fekete DM: Wnt signaling during cochlear development. Semin Cell Dev Biol 24:480, 2013.

O'Rahilly R: The prenatal development of the human eye. Exp Eye Res 21:93, 1975.

Porter CJW, Tan SW: Congenital auricular anomalies: topographic anatomy, embryology, classification, and treatment strategies. Plast Reconstr Surg 115:1701, 2005.

Thompson H, Ohazama A, Sharpe PT, Tucker AS: The origin of the stapes and relationship to the otic capsule and oval window. Dev Dyn 241:1396, 2012.

CHAPTER 18

Caton J, Tucker AS: Current knowledge of tooth development: patterning and mineralization of the murine dentition. J Anat 214:407, 2009.

Chiu YE: Dermatology. In Marcdante KJ, Kliegman KJ (eds): Nelson Essentials of Pediatrics, 7th ed. Philadelphia, Saunders, 2015.

Crawford PJM, Aldred MJ: Anomalies of tooth formation and eruption. In Welbury RR, Duggal MS, Hosey MT (eds): Paediatric Dentistry, 4th ed. Oxford, UK, Oxford University Press, 2014.

Gillgrass TS, Welbery R: Craniofacial growth and development. In Welbury RR, Duggal MS, Hosey MT (eds): Paediatric Dentistry, 4th ed. Oxford, UK, Oxford University Press, 2014.

Harryparsad A, Rahman L, Bunn BK: Amelogenesis imperfecta: a diagnostic and pathological review with case illustration. SADJ 68:404, 2013.

Kawasaki M, Porntaveetus T, Kawasaki K, et al: R-spondins/Lgrs expression in tooth development. Dev Dyn 243:844, 2014.

Nanci A: Ten Cate's Oral Histology: Development, Structure, and Function, 8th ed. Philadelphia, Mosby, 2012.

Paller AS, Mancini AJ: Hurwitz Clinical Pediatric Dermatology: A Textbook of Skin Disorders of Childhood and Adolescence, 3rd ed. Philadelphia, Saunders, 2006.

Papagerakis P, Mitsiadis T: Development and structure of teeth and periodontal tissues. In Rosen CJ (ed): Primer on the Metabolic Bone Diseases and Disorders of Mineral Metabolism, 8th ed. New York, John Wiley & Sons, 2013.

Patil S, Doni B, Kaswan S, Rahman F: Prevalence of dental anomalies in Indian population. J Clin Exp Dent 5:e183, 2013.

Smolinski KN: Hemangiomas of infancy: clinical and biological characteristics. Clin Pediatr 44:747, 2005.

CHAPTER 19

Benedum CM, Yazdy MM, Mitchell AA, et al: Risk of spina bifida and maternal cigarette, alcohol, and coffee use during the first month of pregnancy. Int J Environ Res Public Health 10:3263, 2013.

Briggs GG, Freeman RK, Yaffe SJ: Drugs in Pregnancy and Lactation, 8th ed. Baltimore, Lippincott, Williams & Wilkins, 2011.

Dolk H, Loane M, Garne E: The prevalence of congenital anomalies in Europe. Adv Exp Med Biol 686:349, 2010.

Holbrook BD, Rayburn WF: Teratogenic risks from exposure to illicit drugs. Obstet Gynecol Clin N Am 41:229, 2014.

Holloway AC, Salomon A, Soares MJ, et al: Characterization of the adverse effects of nicotine on placental development: in vivo and in vitro studies. Am J Physiol Endocrinol Metab 306:E443, 2014.

Jia J, Geng L, Zong Y: Birth defects in assisted reproductive technology and spontaneously conceived children: a meta-analysis. J Reprod Contraception 24:237, 2013.

Levine DA: Growth and development. In Marcdante KJ, Kliegman KJ (eds): Nelson Essentials of Pediatrics, 7th ed. Philadelphia, Saunders, 2015.

Levy PA, Marion RW: Human genetics and dysmorphology. In Marcdante KJ, Kliegman KJ (eds): Nelson Essentials of Pediatrics, 7th ed. Philadelphia, Saunders, 2015.

Medicode, Inc: Medicodes' Hospital and Payer: International Classification of Diseases, Clinical Modification, ICD-9-CM 2006, vols. 1-3. Salt Lake City, Medicode, 2006.

Rasmussen SA: Human teratogens update 2011: can we ensure safety during pregnancy? Birth Defects Res A Clin Mol Teratol 94:123, 2012.

Rasmussen SA, Erickson JD, Reef SE, et al: Principles and practice of teratology for the obstetrician. Clin Obstet Gynecol 51:106, 2009.

Simpson JL: Birth defects and assisted reproductive technology. Semin Fetal Neonatal Med 19:177, 2014.

Slaughter SR, Hearns-Stokes R, van der Vlugt T, et al: FDA approval of doxylamine-pyridoxine therapy for use in pregnancy. N Engl J Med 370:1081, 2014.

Turnpenny P, Ellard S: Emery's Elements of Medical Genetics, 14th ed. Philadelphia, Churchill Livingstone, 2012.

Waldorf KMA, McAdams RM: Influence of infection during pregnancy on fetal development. Reproduction 146:R151, 2013.

CHAPTER 20

Alvarez-Buylla A, Ihrie RA: Sonic hedgehog signaling in the postnatal brain. Semin Cell Dev Biol 33:105, 2014.

Amakye D, Jagani Z, Dorsch M: Unraveling the therapeutic potential of the Hedgehog pathway in cancer. Nat Med 19:1410, 2013.

Andersson ER, Lendahl U: Therapeutic modulation of Notch signalling—are we there yet? Nat Rev Drug Discov 13:357, 2014.

Aster JC: In brief: Notch signalling in health and disease. J Pathol 232:1, 2014.

Beets K, Huylebroeck D, Moya IM, et al: Robustness in angiogenesis: Notch and BMP shaping waves. Trends Genet 29:140, 2013.

Benoit YD, Guezguez B, Boyd AL, Bhatia M: Molecular Pathways: epigenetic modulation of Wnt/glycogen synthase kinase-3 signaling to target human cancer stem cells. Clin Cancer Res 20(21):1, 2014.

Berdasco M, Esteller M: Genetic syndromes caused by mutations in epigenetic genes. Hum Genet 132:359, 2013.

Blake JA, Ziman MR: Pax genes: regulators of lineage specification and progenitor cell maintenance. Development 141:737, 2014.

Castro DS, Guillemot F: Old and new functions of proneural factors revealed by the genome-wide characterization of their transcriptional targets. Cell Cycle 10:4026, 2011.

Das BC, Thapa P, Karki R, et al: Retinoic acid signaling pathways in development and diseases. Bioorg Med Chem 22:673, 2014.

De Robertis EM: Spemann's organizer and the self-regulation of embryonic fields. Mech Dev 126:925, 2009.

Dekanty A, Milán M: The interplay between morphogens and tissue growth. EMBO Rep 12:1003, 2011.

Dhanak D, Jackson P: Development and classes of epigenetic drugs for cancer. Biochem Biophys Res Commun 2014 Jul 10. [Epub ahead of print]

Gaarenstroom T, Hill CS: TGF-β signaling to chromatin: how Smads regulate transcription during self-renewal and differentiation. Semin Cell Dev Biol 32C:107, 2014.

Giannotta M, Trani M, Dejana E: VE-cadherin and endothelial adherens junctions: active guardians of vascular integrity. Dev Cell 26:441, 2013.

Goldman D: Regeneration, morphogenesis and self-organization. Development 141:2745, 2014.

Guillot C, Lecuit T: Mechanics of epithelial tissue homeostasis and morphogenesis. Science 340:1185, 2013.

Gutierrez-Mazariegos J, Theodosiou M, Campo-Paysaa F, Schubert M: Vitamin A: a multifunctional tool for development. Semin Cell Dev Biol 22:603, 2011.

Hendriks WJ, Pulido R: Protein tyrosine phosphatase variants in human hereditary disorders and disease susceptibilities. Biochim Biophys Acta 1832:1673, 2013.

Hori K, Sen A, Artavanis-Tsakonas S: Notch signaling at a glance. J Cell Sci 126(Pt 10):2135, 2013.

Imayoshi I, Kageyama R: bHLH factors in self-renewal, multipotency, and fate choice of neural progenitor cells. Neuron 82:9, 2014.

Inoue H, Nagata N, Kurokawa H, Yamanaka S: iPS cells: a game changer for future medicine. EMBO J 33:409, 2014.

Kieran MW: Targeted treatment for sonic hedgehog-dependent medulloblastoma. Neuro Oncol 16:1037, 2014.

Kim W, Kim M, Jho EH: Wnt/β-catenin signalling: from plasma membrane to nucleus. Biochem J 450:9, 2013.

Lamouille S, Xu J, Derynck R: Molecular mechanisms of epithelial-mesenchymal transition. Nat Rev Mol Cell Biol 15:178, 2014.

Le Dréau G, Martí E: The multiple activities of BMPs during spinal cord development. Cell Mol Life Sci 70:4293, 2013.

Li CG, Eccles MR: PAX genes in cancer: friends or foes? Front Genet 3:6, 2012.

Lien WH, Fuchs E: Wnt some lose some: stem cell governance of stem cells by Wnt/β-catenin signaling [review]. Genes Dev 28:1517, 2014.

Lim J, Thiery JP: Epithelial-mesenchymal transitions: insights from development. Development 139:3471, 2012.

MacGrogan D, Luxán G, de la Pompa JL: Genetic and functional genomics approaches targeting the Notch pathway in cardiac development and congenital heart disease. Brief Funct Genomics 13:15, 2014.

Mallo M, Alonso CR: The regulation of Hox gene expression during animal development. Development 140:3951, 2013.

Mallo M, Wellik DM, Deschamps J: Hox genes and regional patterning of the vertebrate body plan. Dev Biol 344:7, 2010.

Manoranjan B, Venugopal C, McFarlane N, et al: Medulloblastoma stem cells: where development and cancer cross pathways. Pediatr Res 71(4 Pt 2):516, 2012.

Maze I, Noh KM, Soshnev AA, Allis CD: Every amino acid matters: essential contributions of histone variants to mammalian development and disease. Nat Rev Genet 15:259, 2014.

Meijer DH, Kane MF, Mehta S, et al: Separated at birth? The functional and molecular divergence of OLIG1 and OLIG2. Nat Rev Neurosci 13:819, 2012.

O'Brien P, Morin P Jr, Ouellette RJ, Robichaud GA: The Pax-5 gene: a pluripotent regulator of B-cell differentiation and cancer disease. Cancer Res 71:7345, 2011.

Park KM, Gerecht S: Harnessing developmental processes for vascular engineering and regeneration. Development 141:2760, 2014.

Pignatti E, Zeller R, Zuniga A: To BMP or not to BMP during vertebrate limb bud development. Semin Cell Dev Biol 32C:119, 2014.

Rhinn M, Dollé P: Retinoic acid signalling during development. Development 139:843, 2012.

Ring A, Kim YM, Kahn M: Wnt/catenin signaling in adult stem cell physiology and disease. Stem Cell Rev 10:512, 2014.

Roussel MF, Robinson GW: Role of MYC in medulloblastoma. Cold Spring Harb Perspect Med 3(11), 2013.

Sánchez Alvarado A, Yamanaka S: Rethinking differentiation: stem cells, regeneration, and plasticity. Cell 157:110, 2014.

Scadden DT: Nice neighborhood: emerging concepts of the stem cell niche. Cell 157:41, 2014.

Schlessinger J: Receptor tyrosine kinases: legacy of the first two decades. Cold Spring Harb Perspect Biol 6(3), 2014.

Shah N, Sukumar S: The Hox genes and their roles in oncogenesis. Nat Rev Cancer 10:361, 2010.

Shearer KD, Stoney PN, Morgan PJ, McCaffery PJ: A vitamin for the brain. Trends Neurosci 35:733, 2012.

Sotomayor M, Gaudet R, Corey DP: Sorting out a promiscuous superfamily: towards cadherin connectomics. Trends Cell Biol 24:524, 2014.

Steffen PA, Ringrose L: What are memories made of? How Polycomb and Trithorax proteins mediate epigenetic memory. Nat Rev Mol Cell Biol 15:340, 2014.

Tee WW, Reinberg D: Chromatin features and the epigenetic regulation of pluripotency states in ESCs. Development 141:2376, 2014.

Thompson JA, Ziman M: Pax genes during neural development and their potential role in neuroregeneration. Prog Neurobiol 95:334, 2011.

Torres-Padilla ME, Chambers I: Transcription factor heterogeneity in pluripotent stem cells: a stochastic advantage. Development 141:2173, 2014.

Verstraete K, Savvides SN: Extracellular assembly and activation principles of oncogenic class III receptor tyrosine kinases. Nat Rev Cancer 12:753, 2012.

Wilkinson G, Dennis D, Schuurmans C: Proneural genes in neocortical development. Neuroscience 253:256, 2013.

Willaredt MA, Tasouri E, Tucker KL: Primary cilia and forebrain development. Mech Dev 130:373, 2013.

Wu MY, Hill CS: Tgf-beta superfamily signaling in embryonic development and homeostasis. Dev Cell 16:329, 2009.

Yang Y, Oliver G: Development of the mammalian lymphatic vasculature. J Clin Invest 124:888, 2014.

Zagozewski JL, Zhang Q, Pinto VI, et al: The role of homeobox genes in retinal development and disease. Dev Biol 393:195, 2014.

Answers to Clinically Oriented Questions

CHAPTER 1

1. Everyone, especially those in the health-care professions, needs to know about conception, contraception, and how embryos and fetuses develop, both normally and abnormally. Health-care professionals are expected to give intelligent answers to the questions people ask, such as, "When does the baby's heart start to beat?" "When does it move its limbs?" "When is the embryo most at risk for effects from alcohol?" For prenatal diagnosis and any medical treatment before birth, physicians—especially family doctors, obstetricians, and pediatricians—need to know how the embryo and fetus develop, and also what might cause developmental defects. Moreover, research in embryology supports the application of stem cells for the treatment of certain chronic diseases.

2. Physicians date pregnancies from the first day of the last normal menstrual period because this date is usually remembered by women. It is not possible to detect the precise time of ovulation (discharge of ovum) or of fertilization (when development begins). Laboratory tests and ultrasound imaging can be performed to detect when ovulation is likely to occur and when pregnancy has occurred.

CHAPTER 2

1. Pregnant women do not menstruate, even though there may be some bleeding at the usual time of menstruation. This blood may be leaking from the intervillous space of the placenta because of partial separation of the placenta from the endometrium of the uterine wall. Because there is no shedding of endometrium, this blood is not menstrual fluid; it is maternal blood that escaped from the intervillous space of the placenta.

2. It depends on when she forgot to take the oral contraceptive. If it was at mid-cycle, ovulation may occur and pregnancy could result. Taking two doses the next day would not prevent ovulation.

3. Coitus interruptus refers to withdrawal of the penis from the vagina before ejaculation occurs. This method is not reliable. Often, a few sperms are expelled from the penis with the secretions of the auxiliary sex glands (e.g., seminal glands) before ejaculation occurs. One of these sperms may fertilize the oocyte.

4. Spermatogenesis refers to the complete process of sperm formation. Spermiogenesis is the transformation of a spermatid into a sperm. Therefore, spermiogenesis is the final stage of spermatogenesis.

5. A copper-releasing intrauterine device (IUD) may inhibit the capacitation of sperms and their transport through the uterus to the fertilization site in the uterine tube; in this case, it would be a contraceptive device. A hormone-releasing IUD (e.g., levonorgestrel) may cause changes that alter the morphologic features of the endometrium; as a result, the blastocyst does not implant. In this case, the intrauterine device could be called a "contra-implantation" device.

CHAPTER 3

1. The ovarian and menstrual cycles typically cease between 48 and 55 years of age, with the average age being 51 years. Menopause results from the gradual cessation of gonadotropin production by the pituitary gland; however, it does not mean that the ovaries have exhausted their supply of oocytes. The risk of Down syndrome and other trisomies is increased in the children of women who are 39 years or older (see Chapter 19, Table 19-2). Spermatogenesis also decreases after the age of 45 years, and the number of nonviable and abnormal sperms increases. Nevertheless, sperm production continues until old age. The risk of producing abnormal gametes is much less common in men than in women; however, older men may accumulate mutations that the child might inherit. Mutations may produce birth defects (see Chapter 19).

2. Considerable research on new contraceptive methods is being conducted, including the development of oral contraceptives for men. This research includes experimental work on hormonal and nonhormonal prevention of spermatogenesis and stimulation of immune responses to sperms. Arresting the development of millions of sperms on a continuous basis has proven much more difficult than arresting the monthly development of a single oocyte. The results of molecular approaches, such as pharmacologic antagonism of the P2X1-purinoceptor and α_1A-adrenoceptor, may eventually provide a safe and reversible male contraceptive.

3. It is not known whether polar bodies are ever fertilized; however, it has been suggested that dispermic chimeras result from the fusion of a fertilized oocyte

with a fertilized polar body. Chimeras are rare individuals who are composed of a mixture of cells from two zygotes. More likely, dispermic chimeras result from the fusion of dizygotic twin zygotes early in development. Dizygotic twins are derived from two zygotes. If a polar body were fertilized and remained separate from the normal zygote, it could form an embryo.

4. The most common cause of spontaneous abortion during the first week is chromosomal abnormality, such as the abnormalities resulting from nondisjunction (see Chapter 2). Failure of the syncytiotrophoblast to produce an adequate amount of human chorionic gonadotropin to maintain the corpus luteum in the ovary could also result in early spontaneous abortion.

5. Yes, it is possible for women to have dissimilar twins; however, this phenomenon is extremely rare. The term *superfecundation* indicates fertilization (during separate acts of coitus) of two or more oocytes that are ovulated at approximately the same time.

6. Mitosis is the usual process of cell reproduction that results in the formation of daughter cells of the zygote. Cleavage is the series of mitotic cell divisions of the zygote. This process results in the formation of daughter cells—blastomeres. The expressions *cleavage division* and *mitotic division* have the same meaning when referring to the dividing zygote.

7. The nutritional requirements of the dividing zygote are not great. The nutrients are derived mainly from the secretions of the uterine tubes.

8. Yes. One of the blastomeres could be removed, and a Y chromosome could be identified by fluorescence staining with quinacrine mustard, or by molecular techniques (see Chapter 7). This technique could be made available to couples with a family history of sex-linked genetic diseases (e.g., hemophilia, muscular dystrophy), and to women who have already given birth to a child with such a disease and are reluctant to have more children. In these cases, only female embryos developing in vitro would be transferred to the uterus.

CHAPTER 4

1. Implantation bleeding refers to the loss of small amounts of blood from the implantation site of a blastocyst that occurs a few days after the expected time of menstruation. Women unfamiliar with this possible occurrence may interpret the bleeding as a light menstrual flow. In such cases, they may give the physician the wrong date for their last normal menstrual period. This blood is not menstrual fluid; it is blood from the intervillous space of the developing placenta. Blood loss could also result from the rupture of chorionic arteries, veins, or both (see Chapter 8).

2. Drugs or other agents may cause early abortion of an embryo, but they do not cause birth defects if taken during the first 2 weeks. A drug or other agent either damages all the embryonic cells, killing the embryo, or injures only a few cells, in which case the embryo recovers to develop normally.

3. Intrauterine devices are typically very effective at preventing pregnancy by altering sperm capacitation or motility, or by altering the morphologic features of the endometrium. However, an intrauterine device does not physically block a sperm from entering the uterine tube and fertilizing an oocyte, if one is present. Although the endometrium could be hostile to implantation, a blastocyst could develop and implant in the uterine tube (i.e., ectopic tubal pregnancy). If fertilization occurs in a woman who is using an intrauterine device, the risk of ectopic pregnancy is approximately 5%.

4. Abdominal pregnancies are very uncommon, but such a pregnancy may result from primary implantation of a blastocyst in the abdomen. In most cases, it is believed to result from ectopic implantation of a blastocyst that spontaneously aborts from the uterine tube and enters the peritoneal cavity. The risk of severe maternal bleeding and fetal mortality is high in cases of abdominal pregnancy. However, if the diagnosis is made late in pregnancy and the patient (mother) is free of symptoms, the pregnancy may be allowed to continue until the viability of the fetus is ensured, at which time it would be delivered by cesarean section.

CHAPTER 5

1. Yes, certain drugs can produce birth defects if administered during the third week after the last normal menstrual period (see Chapter 19). For instance, antineoplastic agents (chemotherapy or antitumor drugs) can produce severe skeletal and neural tube defects in the embryo, such as acrania and meroencephaly (partial absence of brain), if administered during the third week.

2. Yes, risks to the mother 40 years or older and the embryo are increased. Advanced maternal age is a predisposing factor to certain medical conditions. For example, preeclampsia, a hypertensive disorder of pregnancy characterized by increased blood pressure and edema, occurs more frequently in older pregnant women than in younger ones. Advanced maternal age is also associated with a significantly increased risk to the embryo or fetus. The most common risks are birth defects associated with chromosomal abnormalities, such as Down syndrome and trisomy 13 (see Chapter 19); however, women older than 40 years may have normal children.

CHAPTER 6

1. Early in the eighth week, embryos have webbed toes and stubby, tail-like caudal eminences and look different from 9-week fetuses; however, by the end of the eighth week, embryos and early fetuses appear similar. The name change is arbitrarily made to indicate that a new phase of development (rapid growth

and differentiation) has begun and that the most critical period of development has been completed.

2. There are different opinions of when an embryo becomes a human being because opinions are often affected by religious and personal views. The scientific answer is that the embryo is a human being from the time of fertilization because of its human chromosomal constitution. The zygote is the beginning of a developing human. Some people consider that the embryo becomes human only after birth.

3. No, it cannot. During the embryonic period, more similarities than differences exist in the external genitalia (see Chapter 13). It is impossible to tell by ultrasound examination whether the primordial sexual organ (genital tubercle at 5 weeks and phallus at 7 weeks) will become a penis or a clitoris. Sex differences are not clear until the early fetal period (10th–12th week). Sex chromatin patterns and chromosomal analysis (fluorescence in situ hybridization) of embryonic cells obtained during amniocentesis can show the chromosomal sex of the embryo (see Chapter 7).

■ CHAPTER **7**

1. Ultrasound examinations have shown that mature embryos (8 weeks) and young fetuses (9 weeks) show spontaneous movements, such as twitching (sudden jerking movements) of the trunk and limbs. Although the fetus begins to move its back and limbs during the 12th week, the mother cannot feel the fetus move until the 16th to 20th week. Women who have had several children usually detect this movement, called quickening, sooner than women who are pregnant for the first time because they know what fetal movements feel like. Quickening is often perceived as a faint flutter or a quivering motion.

2. Folic acid supplementation before conception and during early pregnancy is effective in reducing the incidence of neural tube defects (e.g., spina bifida). It has been shown that the risk of having a child with neural tube defect is significantly lower when a vitamin supplement containing 400 mg of folic acid is consumed daily. However, no consensus exists that vitamins are helpful in preventing these defects in most at-risk pregnancies.

3. Direct injury to the fetus from the needle during amniocentesis is very uncommon when ultrasound guidance is used to locate the position of the fetus and monitor needle insertion. The risk of inducing an abortion is slight (approximately 0.5%) in second-trimester pregnancies. Maternal or fetal infection is also an uncommon complication.

■ CHAPTER **8**

1. A stillbirth is the birth of a fetus that was dead before delivery, weighs at least 500 g, and is at least 20 weeks old. The incidence of having a stillborn infant is approximately three times greater among mothers older than 40 years than among women 20 to 30 years. More male fetuses than female fetuses are stillborn. The reason for this is unknown.

2. Sometimes the umbilical cord is abnormally long and wraps around part of the fetus, such as the neck or a limb. This cord accident may obstruct the flow of high-oxygen blood in the umbilical vein to the fetus and in the umbilical arteries from the fetus to the placenta. If this obstruction causes the fetus to receive insufficient oxygen and nutrients, then the fetus is likely to die. A true knot in the umbilical cord, formed when the fetus passes through a loop in the cord, also obstructs blood flow through the cord. Prolapse of the umbilical cord into the cervix at the level of a presenting part (often the head) may also be considered a cord accident. This creates pressure on the cord and prevents the fetus from receiving adequate oxygen. Entanglement of the cord around the fetus can also cause birth defects (e.g., absence of a forearm).

3. Most over-the-counter pregnancy tests are based on the detection of relatively large amounts of human chorionic gonadotropin in the woman's urine. The results of such tests are positive for a short time (approximately 1 week) after the first missed menstrual period (after embryo implantation). Human chorionic gonadotropin is produced by the syncytiotrophoblast of the chorion. These tests usually give an accurate diagnosis of pregnancy; however, a physician should be consulted as soon as possible to confirm pregnancy because some tumors (choriocarcinomas) also produce this hormone.

4. The "bag of water" is a colloquial term for the amniotic sac, which contains amniotic fluid (largely composed of water). Sometimes the amniochorionic sac ruptures before labor begins, allowing fluid to escape. Premature rupture of the membranes is the most common event leading to premature labor and birth. Premature rupture of the membranes may complicate the birth process, or it may allow a vaginal infection to spread to the fetus. Sometimes sterile saline is infused into the uterus by way of a catheter—*amnioinfusion*—to alleviate fetal distress. The term *dry birth* is used to describe a low volume of amniotic fluid.

5. Fetal distress is synonymous with fetal hypoxia, indicating decreased oxygenation to the fetus as a result of a general decrease of maternal oxygen content in the blood, decreased oxygen-carrying capacity, or diminished blood flow. Fetal distress exists when the fetal heart rate is less than 100 beats/min. Pressure on the umbilical cord may also cause fetal distress secondary to impairment of the blood supply to the fetus in approximately 1 in 200 deliveries. In these cases, the fetal body compresses the umbilical cord as it passes through the cervix and vagina.

6. The incidence of dizygotic twins increases with maternal age. This twinning is an autosomal recessive trait that is carried by the daughters of mothers of twins; hence, dizygotic twinning is hereditary. Monozygotic

twinning, on the other hand, is a random occurrence that is not genetically controlled.

CHAPTER 9

1. Yes, it is. When a neonate is born with a congenital diaphragmatic hernia, part of its stomach and liver may enter the thorax (chest); however, this is uncommon. Usually, the abnormally placed viscera are the intestines. The viscera enter the thorax through a posterolateral defect in the diaphragm, usually on the left side.

2. Congenital diaphragmatic hernia (CDH) occurs in 1 in 3000 neonates. A neonate with a CDH may survive; however, the mortality rate is relatively high (approximately 76%). Treatment must be given immediately. A feeding tube is inserted into the stomach, and the air and the gastric contents are aspirated with continuous suction. Intubation of the airway, mechanical ventilation, and stabilization of the neonate are critical until surgery can be performed. The displaced viscera are replaced into the abdominal cavity, and the defect in the diaphragm is surgically repaired. Infants with large diaphragmatic hernias who are operated on within 24 hours after birth have survival rates of 40% to 70%. Intrauterine surgical repair of a CDH has been attempted; however, this intervention carries considerable risk to the fetus and mother. The developing use of minimally invasive surgical techniques may reduce this risk.

3. It depends on the degree of herniation of the abdominal viscera. With a moderate hernia, the lungs may be mature, but small. With a severe degree of herniation, lung development is impaired. Most infants with a congenital diaphragmatic hernia die, but not because of the defect in the diaphragm or viscera in the thorax; they die because the lung on the affected side is hypoplastic (underdeveloped).

4. Yes, it is possible to have a small congenital diaphragmatic hernia and not be aware of it. Some small hernias may remain asymptomatic into adulthood and may be discovered only during routine radiographic or ultrasound examination of the thorax. The lung on the affected side would probably develop normally because there would be little or no pressure on it during prenatal development.

CHAPTER 10

1. No, both statements are inaccurate. All embryos have grooves in their upper lips where the maxillary prominences meet the merged medial nasal prominences; however, normal embryos do not have cleft lips. When lip development is abnormal, the tissue in the floor of the labial groove breaks down, forming a cleft lip.

2. The risk in this case is the same as in the general population, approximately 1 in 1000.

3. Although environmental factors may be involved, it is reasonable to assume that the son's cleft lip and

cleft palate were hereditary and recessive in their expression. This would mean that the father also carried a concealed gene for cleft lip and that his family genetics were equally responsible for the son's anomalies.

4. Minor anomalies of the auricle of the external ear are common and usually they are of no serious medical or cosmetic consequence. Approximately 14% of neonates have minor birth defects; less than 1% of them have other defects. The child's abnormal ears could be considered pharyngeal (branchial) arches anomalies because the six small auricular hillocks (swellings) of the first two pairs of pharyngeal arches contribute to the auricles; however, such minor abnormalities of ear shape would not normally be classified in this way.

CHAPTER 11

1. Multiple stimuli initiate breathing at birth. Slapping the buttocks used to be a common physical stimulus; however, this action is usually unnecessary. Under normal circumstances, the neonate's breathing begins promptly, which suggests that it is a reflex response to the sensory stimuli of exposure to air and touching. The changes in blood gases after interruption of the placental circulation, such as the decrease in oxygen tension and pH and the increase in partial pressure of carbon dioxide, are also important in stimulating breathing.

2. Hyaline membrane disease, another name for respiratory distress syndrome, occurs after the onset of breathing in infants with immature lungs and a deficiency of pulmonary surfactant. The incidence of respiratory distress syndrome is approximately 1% of all live births, and it is the leading cause of death in newborn infants. It occurs mainly in infants who are born prematurely. Hyaline membrane disease is caused mainly by surfactant deficiency.

3. A 22-week fetus is viable and, if born prematurely and given special care in a neonatal intensive care unit, may survive. The chances of survival, however, are poor for infants who weigh less than 600 g because the lungs are immature and incapable of adequate alveolar-capillary gas exchange. Furthermore, the fetus's brain is not usually differentiated sufficiently to permit regular respiration. Administration of exogenous surfactant (surfactant replacement therapy) reduces the severity of respiratory distress syndrome and neonatal mortality.

CHAPTER 12

1. Undoubtedly, the infant has congenital hypertrophic pyloric stenosis, a diffuse hypertrophy (enlargement) and hyperplasia of smooth muscle in the pyloric part of the stomach. This condition produces a hard palpable mass; however, it is a benign enlargement and is definitely not a malignant tumor. The muscular enlargement causes narrowing of the exit canal (pyloric canal). In response to the outflow obstruction

and vigorous peristalsis, the vomiting is projectile, as in the case of the infant described. Surgical relief of the pyloric obstruction is the usual treatment. The cause of pyloric stenosis is not known; however, it is believed to have a multifactorial pattern of inheritance (i.e., genetic and environmental factors are probably involved).

2. It is true that infants with Down syndrome have an increased incidence of duodenal atresia. They are also more likely to have imperforate anus and other birth defects (e.g., atrial septal defects). These birth defects are likely caused by their abnormal chromosomal constitution (i.e., three instead of two copies of chromosome 21). Duodenal atresia can be corrected surgically by bypassing the pyloric obstruction (duodenoduodenostomy).

3. In very uncommon cases, when the intestines return to the abdomen after physiologic umbilical herniation, they may rotate in a clockwise direction rather than in the usual counterclockwise manner. As a result, the cecum and appendix are located on the left side, a condition called situs inversus abdominis. A left-sided cecum and appendix can also result from a mobile cecum. If the cecum is not fixed to the posterior abdominal wall during the fetal period, the cecum and appendix are freely movable and could migrate to the left side.

4. Undoubtedly, the individual described had an ileal (Meckel) diverticulum, a finger-like outpouching of the ileum. This common anomaly is sometimes referred to as a second appendix, which is a misnomer. An ileal diverticulum produces symptoms that are similar to those of appendicitis. It is also possible, although rare, that the person had a duplication of the cecum, which would result in two appendices.

5. Hirschsprung disease, or congenital megacolon, is the most common cause of obstruction of the descending colon in newborn infants. The cause of the condition is failure of migration of neural crest cells into the wall of the intestine. The neural crest cells normally form neurons, so there is a deficiency of the nerve cells that innervate the muscular wall of the bowel—congenital aganglionosis. When the bowel wall collapses, obstruction occurs and constipation results. Bowel over distention and perforation may also occur.

6. If the infant had an umbilico-ileal fistula, the abnormal canal connecting the ileum and the umbilicus could permit the passage of the contents of the ileum to the umbilicus. This occurrence would be an important diagnostic clue to the presence of this canal. The fistula results from the persistence of the intra-abdominal part of the omphaloenteric duct.

CHAPTER **13**

1. Most people with a horseshoe kidney have no urinary problems. The abnormal position of the fused kidneys is usually discovered postmortem or during diagnostic imaging procedures. Nothing needs to be done with the abnormal kidney unless the person has an uncontrolled infection of the urinary tract. In some cases, the urologist may divide the kidney into two parts and fix them in positions that do not result in urinary stagnation.

2. His developing kidneys probably fused during the sixth to eighth weeks as they "migrated" from the pelvis. The fused kidneys then ascended toward the normal position on one side or the other. Usually, no problems are associated with fused kidneys; however, surgeons must be conscious of the possibility of this condition and recognize it for what it is. This abnormality is called crossed renal ectopia.

3. Affected individuals have both ovarian and testicular tissue. Although spermatogenesis is uncommon, ovulation is not. Pregnancy and childbirth have been observed in a few patients; however, this is very unusual.

4. By 48 hours after birth, a definite sex assignment can be made in most cases. The parents are told that their infant's genital development is incomplete and that tests are needed to determine whether the infant is a boy or a girl. They are usually advised against announcing their infant's birth to their friends until the appropriate sex has been assigned. Karyotyping (chromosomal staining, visualization, and counting) from whole blood lymphocytes is conducted, as well as identification of the *SRY* gene (sex-determining region of the Y chromosome) by either fluorescence in situ hybridization or polymerase chain reaction amplification. Hormone studies may also be required.

5. Virilization (masculinization) of a female fetus as a result of congenital adrenal hyperplasia is the most common cause of ambiguous external genitalia. In other cases, androgens enter the fetal circulation after maternal ingestion of androgenic hormones. In unusual cases, these hormones are produced by a tumor on one of the mother's suprarenal glands. Partial or complete fusion of the urogenital folds or labioscrotal swellings is the result of exposure to androgens before the 12th week of development. Clitoral enlargement occurs after this point; however, androgens do not cause sexual ambiguity because the other external genitalia are fully formed by this time.

CHAPTER **14**

1. Heart murmurs are sounds transmitted to the thoracic wall from turbulence of blood in the heart or great arteries. Loud murmurs often represent stenosis of one of the semilunar valves (aortic or pulmonary valve). A ventricular septal defect or a patent oval foramen (foramen ovale) may also produce a murmur.

2. Congenital heart defects are common. They occur in 6 to 8 in 1000 newborn infants and represent approximately 10% of all congenital anomalies. Ventricular septal defects are the most common type of heart anomaly. They occur more frequently in males than in females, but the reason for this is unknown.

3. The cause of most congenital anomalies of the cardiovascular system is unknown. In approximately 8% of children with heart disease, a genetic basis is clear. Most of these anomalies are associated with obvious chromosomal abnormalities (e.g., trisomy 21) and deletion of parts of chromosomes. Down syndrome is associated with congenital heart disease in 50% of cases. Maternal ingestion of drugs, such as antimetabolites and warfarin (an anticoagulant), has been shown to be associated with a high incidence of cardiac defects. Heavy consumption of alcohol during pregnancy may cause heart defects.

4. Several viral infections are associated with congenital cardiac defects; however, only rubella virus (German measles) is known to cause cardiovascular disease (e.g., patent ductus arteriosus). Rubeola (common measles) does not cause cardiovascular defects. Rubella virus vaccine is available and is effective in preventing the development of rubella infection in a woman who has not had the disease and is planning to have a baby. It will subsequently prevent rubella syndrome from developing in her infant as well. Because of the potential hazard of the vaccine to the embryo, the vaccine is given only if there is assurance that there is no likelihood of pregnancy for the next 2 months.

5. This anomaly is called transposition of the great arteries because the positions of the great vessels (aorta and pulmonary trunk) are reversed. Survival after birth depends on mixing between the pulmonary and systemic circulations (e.g., through an atrial septal defect—patent oval foramen). Transposition of the great arteries occurs in slightly more than 1 in 5000 live births and is more common in male infants than in female infants (by almost 2 to 1). Most infants with this severe cardiac anomaly die during the first months of life; however, corrective surgery can be performed in those who survive for several months. Initially, an atrial septal defect may be created to increase mixing between the systemic and pulmonary circulations. Later, an arterial switch operation (reversing the aorta and the pulmonary trunk) can be performed. However, more commonly, a baffle (a device used to restrain the flow of blood) is inserted into the atrium to divert systemic venous blood through the mitral valve, left ventricle, and pulmonary artery to the lungs, and to divert pulmonary venous blood through the tricuspid valve, right ventricle, and aorta. This physiologically corrects the circulation.

6. Very likely, one twin has dextrocardia, which usually is of no clinical significance. The heart is simply displaced to the right. In the individual described, the heart presents a mirror image of the normal cardiac structure. This occurs during the fourth week of development, when the heart tube rotates to the left rather than to the right. Dextrocardia is a relatively common anomaly in monozygotic twins.

CHAPTER **15**

1. An accessory rib associated with the seventh cervical vertebra is of clinical importance because it may compress the subclavian artery, the brachial plexus, or both, producing symptoms of artery and nerve compression. The most common type of accessory rib is a lumbar rib, but it usually causes no problems.

2. A hemivertebra can produce lateral curvature of the vertebral column (scoliosis). A hemivertebra is composed of one half of a body, a pedicle, and a lamina. This anomaly occurs when mesenchymal cells from the sclerotomes on one side do not form the primordium of half of a vertebra. As a result, more growth centers are found on one side of the vertebral column; this imbalance causes the vertebral column to bend laterally.

3. Craniosynostosis indicates premature closure of one or more of the cranial sutures. This developmental abnormality results in cranial malformations. Scaphocephaly or dolichocephaly—a long, narrow cranium—results from premature closure of the sagittal suture. This type of craniosynostosis accounts for approximately 50% of cases of premature closure of cranial sutures and is more commonly seen in males.

4. The features of Klippel-Feil syndrome are a short neck, a low hairline, and restricted neck movements. In most cases, fewer than normal cervical vertebrae are present.

5. Prune-belly syndrome results from partial or complete absence of the abdominal musculature. Usually the abdominal wall is thin. This syndrome is usually associated with malformations of the urinary tract, especially the urinary bladder (e.g., exstrophy). In males, almost all patients have cryptorchidism (failure of one or both testes to descend into the scrotum).

6. Absence of the sternocostal part of the left pectoralis major muscle is usually the cause of an abnormally low nipple and areola. Despite its numerous and important actions, absence of all or part of the pectoralis major muscle usually causes no disability. The actions of other muscles associated with the shoulder joint compensate for the partial absence of this muscle.

7. The girl has a prominent sternocleidomastoid muscle. This muscle attaches the mastoid process to the clavicle and sternum; hence, continued growth of the side of the neck results in tilting and rotation of the head. This relatively common condition—congenital torticollis (wry neck)—may occur because of injury to the muscle during birth. Stretching and tearing of some muscle fibers may have occurred during delivery, resulting in bleeding into the muscle. Over several weeks, necrosis of some fibers occurs and the

blood is replaced by fibrous tissue. This results in shortening of the muscle and pulling of the child's head to one side. If the condition is not corrected, the shortened muscle also could distort the shape of the face on the affected side.

8. The young athlete probably had an accessory soleus muscle. It is present in approximately 6% of people. This anomaly probably results from splitting of the primordium of the soleus muscle into two parts.

9. The ingestion of drugs did not cause the child's short limbs. The infant has a skeletal disorder known as achondroplasia. This type of short-limbed dwarfism has an incidence of 1 in 10,000 and shows an autosomal dominant inheritance. Approximately 80% of affected infants are born to normal parents and, presumably, the condition results from fresh mutations (changes in the genetic material) in the parents' germ cells. Most people with achondroplasia have normal intelligence and lead normal lives within their physical capabilities. If the parents of an achondroplastic child have more children, the risk of having another child with this condition is slightly higher than the risk in the general population; however, the risk for the achondroplastic person's own children is 50%.

10. Brachydactyly is an autosomal dominant trait. If the woman (likely bb) marries the brachydactylous man (likely Bb), the risk is 50% for a brachydactylous child and 50% for a normal child. It would be best for them to discuss their obvious concern with a medical geneticist.

11. Bendectin, an antinauseant mixture of doxylamine, dicyclomine, and pyridoxine, does not produce limb defects in human embryos. Several epidemiologic studies have not shown an increased risk of birth defects after exposure to Bendectin or its separate ingredients during early pregnancy. In the case described, the mother took the drug more than 3 weeks after the end of the critical period of limb development (24–36 days after fertilization). Most limb reduction defects have a genetic basis.

12. Cutaneous syndactyly is the most common type of limb anomaly. It varies from cutaneous webbing between the digits to synostosis (union of the phalanges, the bones of the digits). This anomaly occurs when separate digital rays do not form in the fifth week or when the tissue between the developing digits does not undergo apoptosis. Simple cutaneous syndactyly is easy to correct surgically.

13. The most common type of clubfoot is talipes equinovarus, occurring in approximately 1 in 1000 newborn infants. In this deformity, the soles of the feet are turned medially and the feet are plantar flexed. The feet are fixed in the tiptoe position, resembling the foot of a horse (Latin *equinus*, horse).

CHAPTER 16

1. Neural tube defects (NTDs) have a multifactorial inheritance pattern. Although only a few environmental factors have been shown to be directly related (such as folic acid), studies indicate that there are also genetic components. After the birth of one child with an NTD, the risk of a subsequent child having an NTD is much higher. The recurrence risk in the United Kingdom, where NTDs are common (7.6 per 1000 in South Wales and 8.6 per 1000 in Northern Ireland), is approximately 1 in 25. NTDs can be detected prenatally by a combination of ultrasound scanning and measurement of levels of alpha fetoprotein in the amniotic fluid and maternal serum.

2. Mental deficiency and growth restriction are the most serious aspects of fetal alcohol syndrome. Average IQ scores in affected children are 60 to 70. It has been estimated that the incidence of mental deficiency resulting from heavy drinking during pregnancy may be as high as 1 in 400 live births. Heavy drinkers are those who consume five or more drinks on one occasion, with a consistent daily average of 45 mL of absolute alcohol. Currently, no safe threshold for alcohol consumption during pregnancy is known. Physicians recommend complete abstinence from alcohol during pregnancy.

3. No conclusive evidence indicates that maternal smoking affects the mental development of a fetus; however, cigarette smoking compromises the oxygen supply to the fetus because blood flow to the placenta is decreased during smoking. Because it is well established that heavy maternal smoking seriously affects the physical growth of the fetus and is a major cause of intrauterine growth restriction, it is not wise for mothers to smoke during pregnancy. The reduced oxygen supply to the brain could affect fetal intellectual development, even though the effect may be undetectable. Abstinence gives the fetus the best chance for normal development.

4. Most laypeople use the term *spina bifida* in a general way. They are unaware that the common type, spina bifida occulta, is usually clinically insignificant. It is an isolated finding in up to 20% of radiographically examined vertebral columns. Most people are unaware that they have this vertebral defect because it produces no symptoms unless it is associated with a neural tube defect or abnormality of the spinal nerve roots. The various types of spina bifida cystica are of clinical significance. Meningomyelocele is a more severe defect than meningocele because neural tissue is included in the lesion. Because of this, the function of the abdominal and limb muscles may be affected. Meningoceles are usually covered with skin, and motor function in the limbs is usually normal unless associated developmental defects of the spinal cord or brain are present. Management of infants with spina bifida cystica is complex and involves

several medical and surgical specialties. Spinal meningocele is easier to correct surgically than spinal meningomyelocele, and the prognosis is also better.

CHAPTER 17

1. The chance of significant damage to an embryo or fetus after rubella infection depends primarily on the timing of the viral infection. In cases of primary maternal infection during the first trimester of pregnancy, the overall risk of embryonic or fetal infection is approximately 20%. It is estimated that approximately 50% of such pregnancies end in spontaneous abortion, stillbirth, or birth defects (deafness, cataract, glaucoma, and mental retardation). When infection occurs at the end of the first trimester, the probability of birth defects is only slightly higher than that for an uncomplicated pregnancy. Certain infections occurring late in the first trimester, however, may result in severe eye infections (e.g., chorioretinitis), which may affect visual development. Deafness is the most common manifestation of late fetal rubella infection (i.e., during the second and third trimesters). If a pregnant woman is exposed to rubella, an antibody test can be performed. If she is determined to be immune, she can be reassured that her embryo or fetus will not be affected by the virus. Preventive measures are essential for the protection of the embryo. It is especially important for girls to obtain immunity to rubella (e.g., by active immunization) before they reach childbearing age.

2. The purposeful exposure of young girls to rubella (German measles) is not recommended. Although complications resulting from such infections are uncommon, neuritis and arthritis (inflammation of the nerves and joints, respectively) occasionally occur. Encephalitis (inflammation of the brain) occurs in approximately 1 in 6000 cases. Rubella infection is often subclinical (difficult to detect), yet children with such infections represent an exposure risk to pregnant women. There is a chance of injury to embryos because the danger period is greatest when the eyes and ears are developing. This occurs early enough in pregnancy that some women might be unaware that they are pregnant. A much better way of providing immunization against rubella is the administration of live virus vaccine to children older than 15 months and to nonpregnant postpubertal females who can be reasonably relied on not to become pregnant within 3 months of immunization.

3. Congenital syphilis (fetal syphilis) results from transplacental transmission of the microorganism *Treponema pallidum*. Transfer of this microorganism from untreated pregnant women may occur throughout pregnancy; however, it usually takes place during the last trimester. Deafness and tooth deformities commonly develop in these children. These birth defects can be prevented by treating the mother early in pregnancy. The microorganism that causes syphilis is very sensitive to penicillin, an antibiotic that does not harm the fetus.

4. Several viruses in the herpesvirus family can cause fetal blindness and deafness during infancy. Cytomegalovirus can cross the placenta, be transmitted to the infant during birth, and be passed to the infant in breast milk. Herpes simplex viruses (usually type 2, or genital herpes) are usually transmitted just before or during birth. The chances of normal development in infected infants are not good. Some infants have microcephaly, seizures, deafness, and blindness.

5. Methyl mercury is teratogenic (causing birth defects) in human embryos, especially to the developing brain. Because the eyes and internal ears develop as outgrowths from the brain, it is understandable that their development is also affected. Besides the methyl mercury that passes from the mother to the embryo or fetus through the placenta, the neonate may receive additional methyl mercury from breast milk. Sources of methyl mercury include fish from contaminated water, flour made from methyl mercury–treated seed grain, and meat from animals raised on contaminated food.

CHAPTER 18

1. Congenital absence of the skin is very uncommon. Patches of skin may be absent, most often from the scalp, or sometimes from the trunk and limbs. Affected infants usually survive because healing of the lesions is uneventful and takes 1 to 2 months. A hairless scar persists. The cause of congenital absence of hair, termed *aplasia cutis congenita*, is usually unknown. Most cases are sporadic; however, several well-documented pedigrees show autosomal dominant transmission of this skin defect.

2. The white patches of skin on a dark-skinned person result from partial albinism (piebaldism). This defect, which also affects light-skinned persons, is a heritable disorder transmitted by an autosomal dominant gene. Ultrastructural studies show an absence of melanocytes in the depigmented areas of skin. Presumably, the cause is a genetic defect in the differentiation of melanoblasts. These skin and hair defects are not amenable to treatment; however, they can be covered with cosmetics and hair dyes.

3. The breasts, including the mammary glands within them, of males and females are similar at birth. Slight breast enlargement in a neonate is common and results from stimulation by maternal hormones that enter the infant's blood through the placenta. Therefore, enlarged breasts are a normal occurrence in young male infants and do not indicate abnormal sex development.

4. An extra breast (polymastia) or nipple (polythelia) is common. The axillary breast may enlarge during puberty, or it may not be noticed until pregnancy occurs. The embryologic basis of extra breasts and nipples is the presence of mammary crests (ridges) that extend from the axillary to the inguinal regions. Usually, only one pair of breasts develops; however, breasts can develop anywhere along the mammary

crests. The extra breast or nipple is usually just superior or inferior to the normal breast. An axillary breast or nipple is very uncommon.

5. Teeth that are present at birth are termed *natal teeth* and are observed in approximately 1 in 2000 newborn infants. Usually, two mandibular medial (central) incisors are present. The presence of natal teeth usually suggests that early eruption of other teeth may occur. Often, they fall out on their own. Because there is a danger that they may be aspirated, natal teeth are sometimes extracted.

CHAPTER **19**

1. No evidence indicates that the occasional use of aspirin in recommended therapeutic dosages is harmful during pregnancy; however, large doses at subtoxic levels (e.g., for rheumatoid arthritis) have not been proven to be harmless to the embryo and fetus. Pregnant women should discuss the use of over-the-counter medications with their physicians.

2. A woman who is addicted to habit-forming drugs (e.g., heroin) and takes them during pregnancy is almost certain to give birth to a child who shows signs of drug addiction. The fetus's chances of survival until birth, however, are not good; mortality and premature birth rates are high among fetuses of drug-addicted mothers.

3. All drugs prescribed in North America are tested for teratogenicity before they are marketed. The thalidomide tragedy clearly showed the need for improved methods for detecting potential human teratogens. Thalidomide was not found to be teratogenic in pregnant mice and rats—yet it is a potent teratogen in humans during the fourth to sixth weeks of pregnancy. Because it is unethical to test the effects of drugs on human embryos, no way exists to guarantee that some drugs that may be human teratogens will not be marketed. Human teratologic evaluation depends on retrospective epidemiologic studies and reports of astute physicians. This is the way that the teratogenicity of thalidomide was detected. Most new drugs contain a disclaimer in the accompanying package insert, such as, "This drug has not been proven safe for pregnant women." Some drugs may be used if, in the opinion of the physician, the potential benefits outweigh the possible hazards. All known teratogenic drugs that may be taken by a pregnant woman are available only through prescription by a physician.

4. Cigarette smoking during pregnancy is harmful to embryos and fetuses. Its most adverse effect is intrauterine growth restriction. Women who stop smoking during the first half of pregnancy have infants with birth weights closer to the birth weights of infants of nonsmokers. Decreased placental blood flow, believed to be a nicotine-mediated effect, is believed to cause decreased intrauterine blood flow. No conclusive evidence exists that maternal smoking causes birth defects. The growth of the fetus of a woman who smokes but does not inhale is still endangered because nicotine, carbon monoxide, and other harmful substances are also absorbed into the maternal bloodstream through the mucous membranes of the mouth and throat. These substances are then transferred to the embryos or fetuses through the placenta. Smoking in any manner during pregnancy is not advisable.

5. Ample evidence indicates that most drugs do not cause birth defects in human embryos and fetuses; however, a pregnant woman should take only drugs that are essential and are recommended by her physician. A pregnant woman with a severe lower respiratory infection, for example, would be unwise to refuse drugs recommended by her physician to cure her illness; her health and that of her embryo or fetus could be endangered by the infection. Most drugs, including sulfonamides, meclizine, penicillin, and antihistamines, are considered safe drugs. Similarly, local anesthetic agents, killed vaccines, and salicylates (e.g., aspirin) in low doses are not known to cause birth defects.

Index

Page numbers followed by f indicate figures; b, boxes; t, tables.

Arteriocapillary venous system, in chorionic
 villi, 74–75, 77f
Artery (arteries)
 aorta. *see* Aorta; Aortic arches
 axial, primary, 246f
 brachial, 244, 246f
 carotid
  common, 213f, 214, 215f, 217f
  external, 215f–216f
  internal, 214, 215f
 celiac trunk, 92, 138
 chorionic, 74–75
 deep
  of arm, 246f
  of thigh, 244, 246f
 endometrial, 72, 76f
 foregut, 94f
 great, transposition of, 208, 211b, 211f
 hyaloid, 277–279, 278f, 281f
 iliac
  common, 166, 167f, 193
  internal, 193, 219f–220f
 intercostal, 193
 intersegmental, 190f, 193
 lumbar, 193
 maxillary, 213f, 214
 mesenteric
  inferior, 92
  superior, 92
 midgut, 94f
 radial, 244, 246f
 renal, 166, 167f–168f
  accessory, 166b
 retinal, central, 277–279, 279b
 sacral, 193
 spiral, 72–74, 76f
 stapedial, 214
 subclavian, 218f
  right, anomalous, 216b
 ulnar, 244, 246f
 umbilical, 74–75, 76f, 78f, 221
  absence of, 82b, 82f
  at birth, 221
  fate of, 190f, 193
 vertebral, 193
 vitelline, fate of, 190f, 193
Arthrogryposis, 247b
Arytenoid swellings, 129
Asphyxia, intrauterine, surfactant deficiency,
 135b
Aspirin, fetal effects of, 315–316
Astroblasts, 255
Atrial septal defects (ASDs), 206b, 210f,
 313f
Atrioventricular canal, partitioning of, 197,
 197f
Atrioventricular node and bundle, 203–204,
 206f
Atrioventricular septum, primordial, 199,
 200f–201f
Atrioventricular valves, 203
Atrium, 203–204
 common, 206
 left, formation of, 199, 203f
 primordial, 197, 197f, 202f
  partitioning of, 198f, 199, 200f–201f
Auditory ossicles, 285
Auditory (pharyngotympanic) tube, 106

Auricle (ear), 286
 development of, 288f
Auricular abnormalities, 287b
Auricular appendages, 287b
Auricular hillocks, 58, 116, 286
Autonomic ganglia, 272
Autonomic nervous system, 158, 251
 development of, 275
Autosomal recessive inheritance, 310
Autosomes, 304
Axial artery, primary, 244, 246f
Axial skeleton
 congenital anomalies of, 232b, 235b–
  236b, 235f–236f
 development of, 229–235, 230f–231f, 233f
Axons
 ganglion cell, 280f
 motor, 244
 olfactory, 120
 sensory, 244
Azygos vein, 192f, 193

B
Balanced translocation carriers, 309
Bartholin glands, 163t
Basal layer
 of endometrium, 9f, 10
 in skin development, 291–292, 292f
Basal plates, 255–256, 262f–264f, 273
Basic helix-loop-helix transcription factors,
 328
"Behavioral teratogen," 317
Bell stage, of tooth development, 297–298,
 298f–299f
Benzodiazepines, as teratogens, 316
Bifid ureter, 168, 169f
Bilaminar embryonic disc, 29, 30f
Bile duct, 143
Bile formation, 141
Biliary apparatus, development of, 141–143
Biliary atresia, extrahepatic, 142b
Binge drinking, during pregnancy, 314
Biparental inheritance, 23
Birth(s)
 multiple, 88
 placenta and fetal membranes after, 80–82
Birth defects, 303–319
 anorectal, 158b, 159f
  high, 160b
 chromosomal abnormalities and
  numerical, 304–307, 305f
  structural, 308–310, 309f
 environmental factors in, 304f, 311–319
 genetic factors in, 304–311, 304f
 infant deaths and, 304
 multifactorial inheritance and, 304, 304f,
  319
 rectal, low, 159b
 teratology in, 303–304
Birth-weight, low, 66
Blastocyst
 attachment of, to endometrial epithelium,
  23, 25f
 extrauterine, 32b
 formation of, 23–24, 24f
 implantation of, 29, 30f
 inhibition of, 33b
 sites of, 33, 33f–34f

Blastocystic cavity, 23, 24f
Blastomeres, 23, 24f
Blink-startle responses, 65–66
Blood-air barrier, 134
Blood islands, 43, 44f
Blood vessels
 development of, 190–193
 formation of, 43, 44f
Body cavities. *see also specific body cavities*
 embryonic, 91–93, 92f, 94f
  division of, 92–93
Bone marrow, development of, 227
Bone matrix, 227
Bone morphogenetic protein (BMP), 323
Bone(s)
 age of, 236b
 development of, 227–229
  endochondral ossification and, 227–229,
   228f
  membranous ossification and, 227, 227f
 histogenesis of, 227–229
 lengthening of, 227–228
Bony labyrinth, of internal ear, 285, 286f
Brachial artery, 244, 246f
Brachiocephalic vein, left, 191f, 193
Brachycephaly, 236, 236f, 307t
Brain
 congenital anomalies of, 268
 development of, 259–268, 262f–265f
 fetal, lateral and medial surfaces of, 270f
 herniation of, 271f
 primordium of, 51
 protective case of (neurocranium),
  232–233
 vesicles, 262f
Brain flexures, 259, 262f
Branch chorionic villi, 45, 74, 76f–77f
Breasts
 development of, 295, 296f
 excessive development in males, 295b, 308f
 supernumerary, 295b
Breathing movements, fetal, 66, 134
Brevicollis, 232b
Broad ligament, 179–180
Bronchi
 development of, 130–134
 main, 132
 secondary, 132
 segmental, 132
Bronchial buds, 92, 132f
Bronchioles, respiratory, 132
Bronchopulmonary segment, 132
Brown fat, fetal, 65
Bud stage, of tooth development, 296,
 297f–298f
Bulbar ridges, 199, 201–203, 205f, 207f
Bulbourethral glands, 178f, 179
Bulboventricular groove, 197f, 199
Bulboventricular loop, 194, 195f
Bulbus cordis
 partitioning of, 201–203
 in ventricle walls, 203, 205f
Bundle branches, 203–204, 206f

C
Cadherins, 322, 322f
Calcitonin, C cell production, 108
Calcium phosphate, 227

05609639